LIVING WITH POLIO

Living with Polio

THE EPIDEMIC AND ITS SURVIVORS

Daniel J. Wilson

The University of Chicago Press | Chicago and London

DANIEL J. WILSON is professor of history at Muhlenberg College. His previous books include *Science, Community, and the Transformation of American Philosophy* (University of Chicago Press, 1990).

All photographs are reproduced by permission of the March of Dimes Birth Defects Foundation, White Plains, New York.

The University of Chicago Press, Chicago 60637
The University of Chicago Press, Ltd., London
© 2005 by The University of Chicago
All rights reserved. Published 2005
Printed in the United States of America
14 13 12 11 10 09 08 07 06 05   2 3 4 5
ISBN: 0-226-90103-3 (cloth)

Library of Congress Cataloging-in-Publication Data

Wilson, Daniel J., 1949-
    Living with polio : the epidemic and its survivors / Daniel J. Wilson.
       p. cm.
    Includes bibliographical references and index.
    ISBN 0-226-90103-3 (cloth : alk. paper)
    1. Poliomyelitis—Popular works.   2. Postpoliomyelitis syndrome—Popular works.
I. Title.
RC180.2.W47 2005
616.8'35—dc22   2004024170

For Carol

Contents

Acknowledgments

I began this study in the late 1980s when two developments reminded me forcefully of the polio epidemics. First, the fears associated with the early years of the AIDS epidemic seemed eerily reminiscent of fears from the polio era. Second, I began to develop the symptoms of post-polio syndrome some thirty years after I had polio in 1955. I began to look into the historical literature on the polio epidemics and discovered that much had been written from the medical and scientific perspective of understanding the virus and the disease and about the dramatic story of the development of the polio vaccines by Jonas Salk and Albert Sabin. Little, however, had been written about the experience of having polio, of living with a polio-related disability, and of developing new impairments decades after the initial disease. I decided that I would focus on the experiences of the men and women who had had polio as children, adolescents, or young adults. The book you hold is the result of that decision.

First, I want to thank all the polio survivors who wrote their narratives, recorded their oral histories, or shared memories on the Internet. Without their desire to record their memories, this book could not have been written.

Many individuals and institutions have helped me during the researching and writing of Living with Polio and I would like to acknowledge and thank them. I particularly want to thank those who provided the financial assistance that allowed me to take time away from teaching to focus on research and writing. Without the opportunities provided by this funding the book would still be unwritten. I want especially to thank the National Endowment for the Humanities (NEH). Early in the research an NEH Travel to Collections Grant (FE-26992–92) funded a research trip to the Franklin D. Roosevelt Library in Hyde Park, New York. In the summer of 2000 I attended an NEH Summer Institute on Disability Studies at San Francisco State University. Then, in 2002–2003, the NEH and the Agency for Healthcare Research and Quality (AHRQ) awarded me a fellowship (FB-37553–02) that allowed me to complete the writing of the manuscript. I am grateful to both the NEH and the AHRQ for their continued support. My research at the Roosevelt Library was also aided by a Beeke-Levy Research Fellowship from the Franklin and Eleanor Roosevelt Institute, for which I am also grateful. Muhlenberg College has also been very supportive of the project. During the project's long gestation I have had a year and a half of sabbatical leave and the College granted me a leave of absence to take up the NEH/AHRQ Fellowship. In addition, I have been the beneficiary of several Faculty Summer Research Grants that supported both research and writing. I very much appreciate the willingness of the College to support the project with funding and time released from teaching.

I also owe heartfelt thanks to a number of people at Muhlenberg College who helped make this volume possible. I have had the strong support of four presidents, Jonathan Messerli, Arthur Taylor, James Steffy, and Randy Helm, for which I am grateful. Several deans have also lent their support in many ways, especially Nelvin Vos, Richard Hatch, Curtis Dretsch, and Marjorie Hass. I also appreciate the assistance of several heads of the History Department who helped make it possible for me to leave the classroom. These include Edwin Baldrige, who preceded me as department head; William Tighe, who served as interim head during my leave of absence; and John Malsberger, who followed me into the position. I appreciate the fact that my other History Department colleagues took up some of my responsibilities while I was away. Others at the College who helped include Kelly Cannon, a reference librarian in Trexler Library; three interlibrary loan librarians, Scherelene Schatz, Douglas Moore, and Kristin Harakal, who tracked down and obtained sometimes obscure sources; and Anne Hochella and Kent Dyer, who facilitated arrangements for the NEH/AHRQ Fellowship. Colleagues at the College who have been particularly supportive include disability specialists Wendy Cole and Priscilla Howard, as well as faculty colleagues Charles Richter and Kathy Wixon. I also want to thank the students in my Disease and Medicine in American History classes, whose curiosity about the polio epidemics always reminds me why it is important to remember those decades. I especially want to acknowledge Lauren Dobrowalski, Alyssa Picard, and Jennifer Baldwin.

I have been grateful for the support I have received from other scholars working on the history of polio, disability history, and the history of medicine. Naomi Rogers, Amy Fairchild, Walton O. Schalick III, and Christopher Rutty have all offered good advice and support. Paul Longmore and Rosemarie Garland Thomson were superb directors of the NEH Summer Institute on Disability Studies, and I have appreciated their advice and support since. The other members of the Institute helped usher me into disability studies, and I am particularly grateful to the historians Catherine Kudlick, Sandy Sufian, Jerold Hirsh, and Rebecca Edwards. In addition, the many conversations I had with Jim Ferris, Stephen Fox, Martha Stoddard Holmes, Lori Kelly, Carrie Sandahl, and Susan Schweik helped me think through the issues of disability in connection with polio. I am also grateful to Edmund J. Sass, whose collection of polio oral histories proved particularly useful, and to Joan Headley at GINI/Post Polio Health International. I also want to thank Dr. Jean Maurice Poitras, who made available to me his extensive clipping file on the polio epidemics. I also want to thank David Rose, archivist of the March of Dimes, for his assistance in choosing the images used, and the March of Dimes Birth Defects Foundation for permission to print them. Finally, Dr. Julie Silver has graciously shared with me her insights on post-polio syndrome and her work on polio oral history. I appreciate the willingness of Alyssa Picard, Julie Silver, Beverly Solomon, and Carol Wilson to read the entire manuscript and to offer useful suggestions. The readers for the University of Chicago Press also made a number of very helpful recommendations. Any problems that remain are no fault of theirs. Working with Douglas Mitchell at the University of Chicago Press has been a pleasure whether we are discussing philosophy or polio. Finally, I appreciate Carol Saller's fine work editing the manuscript.

Many friends outside the world of scholarship have also supported and encouraged me during this long process. I want to thank my friends and colleagues at the Post Polio Support Group of the Lehigh Valley, especially Beverly Solomon, and at the Lehigh Valley Center for Independent Living, especially its director, Amy Beck. Friends and family, especially Arthur and Phoebe Altman, Melissa Barker, Kathleen Dalton, Lynne Dunphy, Roger Ekirch, David and Sally Keehn, Louise and Carl Kempka, Richard and Kay Klausmeier, Dotty and George Kriebel, Alan and Judy Morrison, Paul and June Schlueter, Bart and Diane Shaw, Mare Shell, Larry Shiner, Robert Streich, Joseph and Emily Vincent, and Carolyn Ditte Wagner have all patiently listened to me talk about polio and have asked intelligent and provocative questions. I appreciated Richard Selzer's early encouragement that there was a book to be written and that I was the one to write it. Paul and Beth Paskoff have been good friends since graduate school, and I value their continuing support and friendship.

Finally, I want to thank my family. First, I am grateful to my deceased parents, Russell S. and Mary P. Wilson, who sustained me through polio and subsequent surgeries and who always encouraged me to use the abilities left unimpaired by the poliovirus. My sister Marjorie and brother Stewart have likewise been especially supportive and encouraging. Finally, I particularly want to thank my wife, Carol, who has helped in so many ways to make this book possible.

Introduction

D URING THE MIDDLE DECADES of the twentieth century, polio, or infantile paralysis, was the most feared disease of childhood and adolescence. Every summer, when the poliovirus circulated most freely, parents warned their children not to drink from public water fountains, to avoid swimming pools and swimming holes in ponds and rivers, and to stay away from movie theaters and other crowded public places. Although polio was sometimes fatal, parents more typically feared the crippling paralysis that was so characteristic of the disease. At a time when American society made few accommodations for the disabled, parents dreaded the potential of polio to cripple young lives full of promise. But, until the development of the Salk and Sabin vaccines, there was little parents could do to protect their children from exposure to the poliovirus.[1]

Polio begins innocently enough with the symptoms of an intestinal virus, fatigue, nausea, and a fever. In more than 90 percent of the infections, the virus remains in the alimentary and intestinal tract, does no permanent damage, and conveys lifelong immunity to that type of poliovirus. However, in less than 2 percent of the cases, the virus invades the nervous system, where it damages or destroys the anterior horn cells of the spinal cord.[2] These spinal cord cells are part of the motor neuron system, and their damage or destruction produces the paralysis associated with polio. Because polio is highly contagious, children, adolescents, and adults diagnosed with polio were usually quickly whisked away to the isolation wards of the nearest hospital accepting polio patients. Here, separated from the support of parents and family, these patients endured creeping paralysis as doctors and nurses stood by unable to do more than make them comfortable while the disease ran its course. Only when the acute infection waned could patients and doctors begin to assess how much paralysis had resulted from the damage done by the virus. Polio patients whose muscles were paralyzed faced months, perhaps years, of arduous physical therapy to strengthen weakened muscles and to compensate for those atrophied because their motor neurons had been destroyed. In addition, many polio survivors would undergo repeated surgeries to fuse bones or to transplant ligaments and muscles in an effort to improve function.

In spite of the best efforts of the patients, their therapists and surgeons, many survivors ended rehabilitation still significantly disabled by their paralyzed muscles. At that point, polio survivors confronted the challenge of reconstructing lives so abruptly altered by the disease and of finding ways to live, to succeed in school and work, and to have a family in spite of their disabilities. And then, after having lived with their familiar impairments for decades, polio survivors discovered to their dismay that their bodies were failing them once again. After pushing their bodies for two to three decades, many began to experience new pain, fatigue, and muscle weakness with what came to be called post-polio syndrome. Many survivors came to view post-polio syndrome as a second disability. Paralytic polio was thus a disease whose physical and emotional consequences shadowed the entire lives of those who had contracted it.

Although polio is associated in the public mind with the period from 1930 to 1960, when epidemics occurred every summer somewhere in the United States, poliomyelitis is actually a very old disease. There is some visual evidence of the crippling typical of polio in ancient Egypt and other evidence suggestive of the disease in the classical world. Until the advent of modern sanitation in Europe and North America in the late nineteenth century, polio was apparently endemic, and most individuals were exposed to the virus as young children when they possessed some protection through maternal antibodies. The poliovirus is an intestinal virus that is spread largely through contaminated fecal material. The mouth is the normal entry portal for the virus, which in the vast majority of infections causes only a minor case of stomach flu. Ninety to ninety-five percent of infections are "completely inapparent." Four to eight percent produce "abortive" cases of "minor illness" and only one to two percent produce a major illness and paralysis.[3] Poliomyelitis became epidemic in Northern Europe and in the United States in the late nineteen and early twentieth centuries when modern sanitation practices increasingly kept children from coming into contact with the poliovirus. This meant the development of a population of older children, no longer protected by maternal antibodies, who were vulnerable to the virus. When the virus appeared in a community where it had been absent for some time, the result was an epidemic among those born since the previous epidemic and thus susceptible to the disease.[4]

In addition to becoming epidemic, poliomyelitis was changing in other significant ways in the twentieth century. The age distribution of those who contracted the disease was shifting and becoming older. Whereas the vast majority of cases in the great 1916 epidemic had been under the age of four, by the 1940s and 1950s a significant number of cases were between five and nine or older than ten. This was significant because there was good evidence that the older one contracted the disease, the more likely it was to be paralytic. The rate of polio also increased in the 1940s and 1950s. While the 1916 epidemic remained the most severe in American history, the years from 1944 to 1955 recorded ten of the worst epidemic years in the United States between 1912 and 1970, and the 1952 epidemic was second only to 1916 in severity.[5] From 1937 to 1955 there were 415,624 reported cases and 361,555 (87 percent) of these occurred from 1944 to 1955.[6] Thus, although the rates of poliomyelitis remained well below those of such diseases as tuberculosis, scarlet fever, whooping cough, and measles, the increase in the number and severity of cases was real in the 1940s and 1950s and gave Americans considerable reason to fear the disease.

I focus on the polio epidemics that occurred between 1930 and 1960 because I have found few narratives from the earlier epidemics and because the polio experience changed in the middle decades of the twentieth century.[7] Two things, in particular, altered the experience after about 1930. First, Franklin D. Roosevelt, whose legs had been paralyzed by polio in 1921 when he was thirty-nine, entered the national political stage first as governor of New York in 1929 and after 1933 as president of the United States. Roosevelt, who always portrayed himself as having recovered from polio, gave the disease new prominence and served as a role model for the many thousands who contracted the disease every year.[8] In addition, by establishing a polio rehabilitation facility at a run-down resort in Warm Springs, Georgia, Roosevelt helped initiate a new approach in which restoring the confidence and determination of the survivors was as important as rehabilitating their bodies.[9]

The second development that changed the polio experience was the establishment of the National Foundation for Infantile Paralysis (NFIP) under Roosevelt's sponsorship in 1938. Through the fund-raising efforts of the March of Dimes, the NFIP under the leadership of Basil O'Connor sponsored and funded scientific and medical research to understand the virus and its actions in the body and to develop a vaccine to prevent the disease. In addition, the NFIP spent substantial sums every year to pay for the care of the children, adolescents, and adults who developed paralytic polio.[10] The publicity machine of the NFIP—with its March of Dimes posters, newsreels, and magazine and newspaper articles describing the latest scientific discoveries and offering advice on how to protect children against polio and what to do if the disease struck—soon made infantile paralysis both widely known and widely feared. Although polio treatment and rehabilitation were never fully standardized, the national and local efforts of the NFIP clearly shaped the way polio was experienced from the early 1940s to the end of the epidemics. Mothers learned the warning signs of polio, children learned to avoid water fountains and swimming pools, and adolescents with a summer flu feared the worst. Beginning in the early 1940s, the NFIP tried to ensure that the medical community was informed of the best methods of treating polio. In addition, by paying much of the cost of treatment the NFIP tried to guarantee that polio patients received proper care and appropriate rehabilitation. While the amount and quality of care during both the acute and rehabilitative phases of the disease still varied widely from place to place, the efforts of the NFIP nonetheless established a kind of template for the polio experience, even though every patient's experience had its unique aspects. The implications of the Roosevelt model for what was expected of polio patients and the work of the NFIP to fight polio and care for its victims meant that the polio experience from 1930 to 1960 was different from that in the earlier epidemics.

This book is an exploration of lives altered by their encounter with the poliovirus. It tells the story of polio from the perspective of the polio patient and polio survivor.[11] The book is organized around the experience of having polio, recovering from the disease, and living with a disability in the second half of the twentieth century. The separate chapters deal with the phases of the polio experience from the diagnosis and acute illness through recovery and rehabilitation; reentry into the worlds of home, school, and work; life with a permanent disability; and the physical and emotional consequences of the late effects of polio. I have sought to portray the range of experiences of polio patients and polio survivors as they have moved through the stages of the disease and its consequences. I have not tried to construct a typical polio experience because I don't think there was one. Some cases were quickly diagnosed and sent to isolation hospitals. For others, there was a considerable delay in diagnosing the disease. And some polio patients were treated at home and never hospitalized. Many polio patients experienced recovery and rehabilitation in large wards segregated by age and gender, but others had private or semi-private rooms or recovered at home using a mixture of orthodox and unorthodox treatments. Some polio survivors were welcomed back to schools or jobs, while others experienced prejudice in school and discrimination seeking work. Many polio survivors, but not all, succeeded in finishing their educations, having careers, marrying, and raising families. And while many survivors have experienced the distressing symptoms of post-polio syndrome, others have thus far escaped. Each polio experience was, to some extent, unique, but elements of the experience were shared, and I have tried to bring out the central characteristics of each phase of living with this disease and its crippling aftermath.

Living with Polio is based on over 150 polio narratives. The narratives are almost evenly divided between men and women. These narratives take many forms. Some are full-scale autobiographies that treat the life before and after polio. Most book-length narratives, however, begin with polio and take the story forward to cover the disease, recovery, and rehabilitation.[12] Many of the longer narratives written during and immediately after the period of the epidemics, which ended in the early 1960s, concluded with rehabilitation and the return to home, school, and work. However, narratives written in the 1980s and after usually continue the account through the writer's development of post-polio syndrome. These book-length polio narratives vary widely in literary quality, tone, and openness to discussing difficult and often painful issues involving treatment and mistreatment and feelings of shame, anger, fear, and resentment. The earlier narratives tend to be narratives of triumph with an uplifting account of how the author overcame polio through hard work, a strong will, and determination. The later narratives are more likely to be forthcoming about the powerful emotions engendered by polio, the pain and difficulty of polio rehabilitation, anger at treatment and mistreatment by medical personnel, and the shame of living with a disabled body caused by a highly feared disease.[13] I have also relied on shorter narratives and articles published in popular magazines such as the *Saturday Evening Post, Life,* and *Reader's Digest,* and in newspapers such as the *Los Angeles Times* and the *Philadelphia Inquirer.* Other sources include short essays reflecting on the author's experience and the recollections of polio survivors published in the newsletters of post-polio support groups. Oral histories of polio survivors constitute an additional source as do two documentary films. And, finally, I have used the Internet, where polio survivors on discussion lists carry on threads reminiscing about the hospitals, pranks on the rehabilitation wards, the smell of hot, wet wool, and nurses to hate or love. While some of these narratives are carefully crafted autobiographies or reflective essays by professional writers, the oral histories, support group newsletters, and Internet sources give voice to the experiences of men and women who would have been unlikely to write a formal autobiography. I have also drawn on my own experience of having polio in 1955 when I was five, undergoing a spinal fusion in 1960, and developing post-polio symptoms in the mid-1980s.

By relying on these varied narrative sources I have sought to give voice to the polio patients and the polio survivors. Scholars of illness narratives have argued that such narratives allow us to get inside the experience of illness and the rigorous rehabilitation that followed. As Anne Hunsaker Hawkins has observed about what she calls "pathographies," illness narratives "show us the drastic interruption of a life of meaning and purpose by an illness that often seems arbitrary, cruel, and senseless; and by treatment procedures that too often can appear as likewise arbitrary, cruel, and senseless—especially to the person undergoing them." Hawkins argues, however, that the task of the pathographer is not simply to describe but also "to restore to reality its lost coherence and to discover, or create, a meaning that can bind it together again." Illness narrative restores "the person ignored or canceled out in the medical enterprise and it places that person at the very center." In a very real way, pathography "gives that ill person a voice." Likewise, Arthur Frank, in *The Wounded Storyteller,* suggests that "the ill person who turns illness into story transforms fate into experience." Stories, he writes, "have to *repair* the damage that illness has done to the ill person's sense of where she is in life, and where she may be going. Stories are a way of redrawing maps and finding new destinations." And, finally, G. Thomas Couser has noted that "one of the most fundamental functions of the illness narrative . . . is to validate the experience of illness—to put it on record, to exemplify living with bodily dysfunction, to offer lasting testimony."[14] Relying on polio narratives, then, provides a way to understand what it was like to contract a greatly feared disease in mid-twentieth-century America, to undergo polio recovery and rehabilitation largely isolated from friends, family, and all that was familiar, and to live with a significant disability in the decades before and after the Americans with Disabilities Act of 1990.

Although these narratives allow us to see and understand the lived experience of polio in the mid-twentieth century, as sources they also have some limitations. The vast majority of narratives that I have found and used are by polio survivors who are white. There are a handful of brief accounts from African Americans, but none from Hispanics. Most of the writers were at least middle class in terms of their economic and social positions at the time of writing. Their middle-class standing is consistent with what other scholars who have used illness narratives have discovered. Both Anne Hawkins and Thomas Couser have noted the predominance of middle-class writers among the authors of illness narratives because they are more likely to have the education and opportunity to write and publish. This is less true of some of the narratives, the oral histories, and the Internet sources. Many of these reveal a background that was distinctly limited in its pre-polio economic status and social aspiration. In fact, the disabilities of polio, by forcing young men and women to focus their energies on their educations, enabled some polio survivors to improve their social and economic status.[15]

The narratives also slight the experience of polio patients who died during the acute phase of the illness or who failed to work hard to recreate life after polio. There are suggestive comments in these narratives about fellow patients or survivors who died early or simply gave up and withdrew into their own private worlds. Although not all the narratives I have used are explicitly "overcoming narratives," they at the very least reflect the experiences of men and women who in some sense came through their polio experience and gained sufficient critical distance to be able to be able to write about it. As Harlan Hahn has observed about the autobiographies of physically disabled individuals, "Few autobiographies are written by persons who consider themselves a failure in life, and the disabled men and women portrayed in these works seemed to be especially assertive, determined, and capable of getting what they wanted in life."[16] Nonetheless, a few sources discuss fellow patients who died early in the illness or who were unable or unwilling to strive to fight and overcome their illness and disability, and I have tried to encompass this aspect of the polio experience as well.

One of the challenges to relying on published polio narratives is that in some measure the earliest narratives shape those that follow. Published narratives, whether book length or article length, can help those who had polio understand their experience, but they can also influence the way in which readers of these narratives begin to mold the memories of their own experience. As Arthur Frank observes, "Published stories also have a particular influence; they affect how others tell their stories, creating a social rhetoric of illness." He notes that "a published narrative of an illness is not the illness itself, but it can become the experience of an illness." Accordingly, certain aspects of the polio experience become almost set pieces in the narratives—getting sick, finding out you had polio, being separated from parents and family, enduring the hot wool treatments—and most writers of polio narratives incorporate their own experience into the expected elements of a polio story. These narrative patterns make it possible to generalize about the experience of having polio, but there are also enough variations in the experiences and published memories to keep a reader's interest. For all their similarities, no polio experiences were ever the same. In addition, as Amy Fairchild has pointed out, the narrative patterns of polio memoirs changed over time because of the aging of the polio cohorts, changing social and cultural attitudes about medicine, and evolving social expectations regarding revealing in print powerful emotions such as anger, fear, and shame. She argues that early polio narratives, those written in the 1940s and 1950s shortly after the disease struck, were often accounts of the "acute, painful stages of the disease," with some going on "to tell stories of either full or substantial recovery." The narratives written after the mid-1950s more often "reflect a lifetime of coping with chronic disability." The perspective of these later writers was often influenced by social and political developments such as the civil rights movement or the struggles for women's rights, patients' rights, and disability rights. In addition, "polio's second wave of narrators were part of a culture in which it became increasingly acceptable to express sadness, discontent, and even resentment."[17] These later narratives are less triumphal and more complexly nuanced regarding the lifelong struggle of living with a permanent disability. Thus, literary, social, and cultural influences have helped create the distinct style and tone of the polio narratives and, in turn, the published memoirs have helped fashion both individual and collective memories of polio.

There is also the question of the truth of these stories and the reliability of these narratives. In one sense, these narratives cannot be literally true. Almost all of them include significant quoted dialogue recalled several years or even several decades after the conversations took place. Polio patients and survivors did not have tape recorders available to record conversations with parents, spouses, doctors, and nurses. Clearly the dialogue is a reconstruction based on their memories of the incidents being described. However, if the words quoted in the narratives are not precisely the same as the ones uttered at a polio bedside, I am convinced that they generally reflect the tenor and meaning of those remembered conversations. Scholars of illness narratives have acknowledged the impossibility of literal truthfulness in these stories, but they have also argued that in an important sense we can regard them as true nonetheless. Anne Hawkins, for example, has argued that "pathographies may indeed be read as 'true stories,' but the emphasis must be as much on the word 'stories' as the word 'true.' For these books cannot be taken as accurate records of experience: they are too highly charged, as the ambivalence and prosaic quality of everyday living is resolved into sharp contrasts and clear-cut issues." She also notes that "the narrative description of illness is both less and more than the actual experience: less, in that remembering and writing are selective processes—certain facts are dropped because they are forgotten or because they do not fit the author's narrative design; and more, in that the act of committing experience to narrative form inevitably confers upon it a particular sequence of events and endows it with a significance that was probably only latent in the original experience." She acknowledges that "writing about an experience—any experience—inevitably changes it." Arthur Frank also acknowledges that the truth of illness narratives does not lie in a literal fidelity to the actual experience. "The truth of stories," he writes, "is not only what *was* experienced, but equally what *becomes* experience in the telling and its reception. The stories we tell about our lives are not necessarily those lives as they were lived, but these stories become our experience of those lives."[18] I have tried to be sensitive to the reconstructed nature of these accounts of polio and have sought to emphasize patterns, themes, and shared or similar experiences remembered by the authors of these narratives. While the details described and the conversations recounted may not fully or completely accurately replicate the actual lived experience of polio, these narratives nonetheless offer reliable testimony about what it was like to be a polio patient and polio survivor in the last two-thirds of the twentieth century.

Let me note several subjects *Living with Polio* addresses only tangentially. First, I don't take up the case of the most famous American polio survivor, Franklin D. Roosevelt. Roosevelt's case differed so significantly from the experience of the vast majority of polio patients that it is not an appropriate model of the polio experience in America. Roosevelt's wealth and later his position as governor of New York and president of the United States provided him with a level of support and care impossible for ordinary citizens with the disease to emulate. There are in addition, a number of good accounts of Roosevelt's illness and recovery.[19] I have tried to focus, instead, on the range of experiences of individuals lacking Roosevelt's advantages of wealth and power. Second, the polio rehabilitation facility Roosevelt established at Warm Springs, Georgia, is treated only as another facility where polio patients might seek rehabilitation. There is no doubt that Warm Springs was unusual for the time in its approach to rehabilitation, and that it served as a model for what polio rehabilitation could achieve. However, the capacity of Warm Springs was very limited, and only a small portion of polio survivors were ever treated at the facility.[20] Most polio survivors underwent rehabilitation in facilities less well endowed, furnished, and staffed than Warm Springs. Third, I address the work of the National Foundation for Infantile Paralysis (NFIP) and the March of Dimes only through the perceptions of polio patients and their families. A history of NFIP, the March of Dimes, and the work of Basil O'Connor is needed, but that is another book entirely.[21] Finally, the long effort of scientists and physicians to understand the workings of the poliovirus and to develop the ultimately successful Salk and Sabin vaccines plays little role in *Living with Polio*. John R. Paul's *A History of Poliomyelitis* remains the standard source on the scientific and medical aspects of polio, and several other recent books have also traced the work of Jonas Salk and Albert Sabin in developing their vaccines.[22] The vaccines, after all, came too late for the men and women who wrote the polio narratives.

In *Living with Polio,* then, the focus is squarely on the experiences of the men and women who remembered and recorded memories of being diagnosed with the most feared childhood disease, of their hospitalization and long, painful rehabilitation, of their struggle to rebuild lives painfully interrupted by disease, and, in some cases, of their dismay at acquiring a second polio-related disability late in life. Paralytic polio is not a disease that one recovered from easily. Its physical and emotional consequences were long-lasting and profound, even when polio survivors appeared to have overcome their disability, reconstructed their lives, and entered the American cultural and social mainstream. Accepting the cultural value of individual willpower, hard work, and determination, many polio survivors appeared to have triumphed over the disease that had weakened and paralyzed their muscles. And by the conventional markers of education, careers, marriage, and children, polio survivors were remarkably successful considering the severity of many of their disabilities and the social impediments they faced. That March of Dimes image of the little girl rising out of her wheelchair to walk once again was only part of the story, but it is the part that has dominated the history of polio patients and survivors to date. The public story has emphasized the drama of Franklin Roosevelt's political success in spite of his paralyzed legs, the miracles of rehabilitation wrought at Warm Springs, the fund-raising efforts of the March of Dimes, the NFIP's support for research and polio care, and the excitement of Jonas Salk and Albert Sabin developing and proving the success of their vaccines. In *Living with Polio* those undeniably dramatic events fade and the attention shifts to the children, adolescents, and adults whose bodies were paralyzed by the virus and who slowly, painfully, and determinedly rebuilt lives shattered by polio. It is their story, the story of ordinary Americans in their encounter with a feared disease, that is the subject of this book.

"I'm Afraid It's Polio"

IT BEGAN ALMOST WITHOUT NOTICE, perhaps on a fine day in late summer. The initial symptoms were like so many of the common illnesses of children and adults that it was easy to ignore them, confident in the belief that the headache, fatigue, or nausea would go away in a few hours, or at most a day or two, as it always had before. There didn't appear to be any immediate need to leave work early, stay home from school, or cancel the date for Friday night. It was just a touch of the flu, nothing to worry about. Except, this time, as the hours passed, the headache got worse, the fatigue became overwhelming, a high fever developed, and weakness began to appear, especially in legs and arms. Aspirin didn't really help, and it was hard to find a comfortable place in bed. Then, in the middle of the night, getting up to go to the bathroom, your legs no longer supported you and you fell. Now a sliver of fear lodged in the recesses of consciousness: could it be polio? But no, of course not; you hadn't been swimming in weeks. Concerned parents quickly called the family doctor, who made a house call in the morning. After checking reflexes, taking your temperature, and asking you to touch your chin to your chest, the doctor had a whispered conversation with your parents. Soon you were bundled into the family car for a quick ride to the hospital. Still, no one had said what was wrong, but the sense of fear was omnipresent, from parents, doctor, and the nurses who wheeled you down long corridors, past closed doors to the isolation ward. The pervasive fear of polio in postwar America had once again become a terrifying reality for another family.

The widespread fear of polio and its attendant crippling made any summer illness in these decades a cause for concern. Because the onset of polio could be so gradual and innocuous, it was easy for infected children and young adults to continue their daily activities in the hope that it was only a minor flu. Children, who may have heard the repeated injunctions to avoid swimming, water fountains, and crowded movie theaters, did not necessarily connect

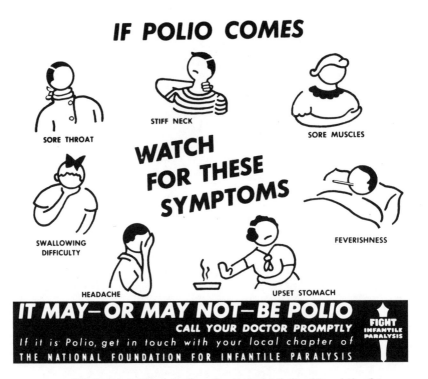

FIG. 1. "If Polio Comes, Watch for These Symptoms." A National Foundation for Infantile Paralysis poster of the warning signs of polio, ca. early 1950s. Many polio narratives mention one or more of these symptoms.

these flu-like symptoms with polio. Parents were more likely to fear a connection, but their children had so often been sick with minor intestinal viruses that it was easier to wait and to hope for the best. Even doctors, knowing how a diagnosis of polio was dreaded, were often inclined to wait until the illness more clearly revealed itself before offering a definitive diagnosis. Fear often created an implicit conspiracy among patient, parents, and physician to hold the disease at bay as long as possible by withholding a diagnosis until paralysis meant that polio could no longer be denied. When the diagnosis came it not only shattered the often-comfortable world of the family and child, it also set them on a long journey through acute and rehabilitation hospitals and the often-difficult readjustment to home, school, and work. How patients, parents, and physicians negotiated that fearful diagnosis is the subject of this chapter.

The fear of polio was widespread in midcentury America, and during epidemic years it could approach hysteria. While the fear of crippling and death was well founded, the overwhelming dread of polio was driven by more than the medical reality. Cultural and social factors including the absence of accommodations for the handicapped, the successful fund-raising and educational campaigns of the NFIP, the cold war mentality in which stealthy enemies threatened the American way of life, and the successes of modern medicine in preventing and curing disease, all contributed to making polio the most feared childhood disease. Certain epidemiological features of polio only heightened fears. In any epidemic, most of the cases were inapparent. The individual was infected, perhaps suffered a mild case of summer flu, and recovered without any evidence of paralysis. However, these inapparent or abortive cases were carriers and could infect others. One study has suggested that in the United States at midcentury only 1 to 3 percent of infections produced paralysis.[1] Thus the polio epidemics at midcentury bore a striking similarity to the concurrent cold war fears of Communist subversion in which convicted spies were seen as only the visible tip of a vast hidden conspiracy. Ironically, the information campaigns of the NFIP contributed to these anxieties in the same way that exposés of supposed Communists contributed to the fear of communism. By making the disease more prominent through its fund-raising and information campaigns, the NFIP both successfully raised large sums of money to support care and research and fanned the widespread dread of this crippling disease.

Even before the establishment of the NFIP, polio epidemics had received considerable attention from newspapers and magazines. Papers and journals closely tracked the spread of epidemics, depicted the efforts of doctors to care for their patients, portrayed the anguish of parents whose children had been diagnosed and isolated in hospitals, and cited experts who described what was known about the disease. Careful readers from the late 1930s on would have known that polio was an exclusively human disease, that inapparent cases far outnumbered obvious paralytic cases, and that polio was primarily an intestinal disease that caused paralysis only in the small percentage of cases where the virus entered the central nervous system. By the early 1940s they could have learned that the polio patients shed the virus in their feces, thus raising the specter of contaminated water supplies. This discovery gave force to the familiar injunction of so many doctors and parents to avoid swimming holes and pools during the summer polio season.[2]

The establishment of the NFIP provided a new source for the dissemination of information about polio. From its very beginning, the organization published a widely distributed series of pamphlets providing both physicians and the general public with the latest information on preventing the disease, on caring for polio patients, and on the progress being made to find an effective preventive. Journalists often used these publications as the basis for articles that further spread knowledge of the disease. For example, in the August 1941 edition of *Good Housekeeping* Maxine Davis used NFIP material to review the causes of polio, the ways to contract the disease and to reduce the chances of contracting it, and the symptoms, treatment, and methods of paying for care.[3]

The anxiety about polio was not entirely misplaced. Following a major outbreak in 1931, when the rate was 12.8 per 100,000, the rate of polio dropped to 8.5 by 1935 and to a low of 1.3 by 1938. But the figures climbed from there, reaching 9.3 in 1943 and increasing to a peak of 37.2 in 1952, the second worst epidemic year after 1916, when the rate was 41.1. Between 1943 and 1956, when the Salk vaccine began to make inroads against the disease, the polio rate dropped below 10 per 100,000 only once (1947) and saw four years when the rate was in the twenties (1949, 1950, 1953, 1954). There were 415,624 reported cases of polio between 1937 and 1955. In the worst postwar year, 1952, there were 57,879 reported cases nationwide. By comparison, other serious diseases that could kill and sometimes cripple had much higher rates of incidence. Tuberculosis, whooping cough, and measles all had significantly higher rates of incidence in these years.[4]

There were other epidemiological features of polio that set it apart from diseases with higher incidence rates. Because of the large number of inapparent polio cases, the characteristic crippling paralysis was a relatively rare complication (1–3 percent) of a fairly common disease. In addition, polio was fatal in only a small percentage of the paralytic cases. A study from the late 1940s reveals that in most years there were between eleven and thirteen paralytic cases for every death.[5] More worrisome, the increased incidence of polio at midcentury was accompanied by significant change in the age distribution. For example, in Massachusetts in the period from 1912 to 1916, about 70 percent of the cases occurred in children four or younger and only about 10 percent in children ten and older. By contrast, in the period from 1948 to 1952, about 20 percent of the cases were four and younger and approximately 55 percent were ten and older. This is significant, for "the older a susceptible individual is when infection is acquired, the more likely is the illness to be serious."[6] What made a diagnosis of polio so frightening was that no physician at the time of diagnosis, and for some time afterward, could predict with any certainty how severe the outcome of the disease would be. Only time and the course of the infection would tell.

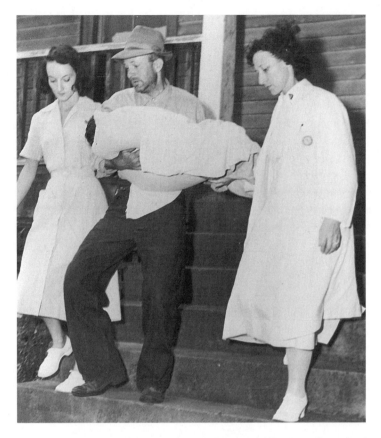

FIG. 2. Leslie Arnold carrying his son Zan to the hospital following a diagnosis of polio in Wytheville, Virginia, 1950. Father and son are accompanied by nurse Peggy Williams and physical therapist Hilda Traina.

Another feature of polio epidemiology that fostered fear of the disease was the unpredictability of its occurrence. As suggested by the figures cited above, "the annual incidence of poliomyelitis in the United States was irregular, with years of high incidence mingled amongst average or low years." Scientists and physicians were never able to develop a good explanation for this irregularity, in spite of its being one of the greatest reasons for fear of the disease. Even within a single polio season, the rate of polio could vary tremendously from state to state and city to city. In 1948, for example, when the national case rate was 19 per 100,000 population, the case rate in the different states ranged from a high of 142.8 per 100,000 in South Dakota to a low of 1.1 in Rhode Island.[7] The variability and unpredictability of the polio epidemic meant that neither doctors and health officials nor parents could prepare or relax their vigilance. It also meant that at midcentury virtually every year saw serious polio epidemics somewhere in the country that were featured in the national news media, reminding everyone of the ever present danger.[8]

Parents, especially, feared polio's ability to permanently cripple its victims. Many Americans in this period knew someone who was crippled by polio and who struggled with braces or a wheelchair. The use of poster children by the NFIP to raise funds kept the image of the crippled polio survivor before the public, even though many of those initially paralyzed were left with relatively minor or nearly invisible deformities. As David Sills points out, the "high visibility of polio's crippling aftereffects" meant that polio victims were relatively easy to identify, which contributed to the fear of the disease and its crippling.[9] The increased incidence of polio at midcentury, and the determination of survivors to rebuild their lives and enter the mainstream of school and work, meant that more and more people were likely to encounter someone crippled by polio and be reminded of the disease.

The activities of the NFIP following its establishment in 1938 also contributed to keeping polio before the public, even as they sought to allay fears and support research and care. Especially in its early years, in the estimation of polio researcher Dr. John Paul, the foundation "seemed to have placed more emphasis on promoting the specter of paralytic poliomyelitis and on fundraising activities than on anything else." In his study of the foundation, David Sills found that one of the reasons that polio evoked such high levels of anxiety was that it received so much media attention. In the four cities Sills studied, "a majority (64 percent) of the public reported having heard more about polio in the past year than any other disease." The foundation was sensitive to the charge that its fund-raising and educational efforts heightened fears unnecessarily. Addressing this allegation, Sills discovered that "polio information, in effect, serves to mitigate against the influence of scare headlines or back-fence gossip." Still, impressions derived from the headlines, newsreels, and the foundation's crippled poster children often overrode rational considerations. In his classic study of fourteen Baltimore families in which a son or daughter had polio, Fred Davis concluded that for parents, "the popular polio imagery of iron lung, crippling, and death proved too potent to afford them much consolation once they realized that their child had contracted the disease."[10]

Many American families feared that polio, along with two other postwar specters, communism and nuclear war, threatened their chance to achieve the American dream. Elaine Tyler May observed that in the postwar culture of the baby boom era, children "provided tangible results of a successful marriage and family life; they gave evidence of responsibility, patriotism, and achievement." Because the American dream envisioned only healthy children, not ones wearing braces and using wheelchairs, Steven Mintz and Susan Kellogg discovered that child care manuals of the period expressed "much anxiety and fear about children's health, safety, and happiness."[11] Several features of the midcentury polio epidemics heightened parental and communal anxiety. As Fred Davis wrote, "It was primarily a disease of children, persons least meriting ill fortune and upon whom altruism could be showered unstintingly. Moreover, by midcentury polio had come to strike disproportionately large numbers of children from middle-class families, that is, families whose life-style most vividly displayed core American values." Thus, polio's epidemiological characteristics meant that it often struck hardest at those families most favorably situated to take advantage of the postwar American dreams of peace, progress, and prosperity. As one father put it, "Polio kills that. It stops the dream."[12]

By keeping their children out of harm's way, parents tried their best to prevent polio from striking their families. Dr. Hart Van Riper, medical director of the NFIP tried to calm fears while at the same time urging caution. He advised that "mixing with crowds or close contact with strangers increases the risk of infection," but he also cautioned parents that "to overshelter your child is unfair." Still, if polio was in the vicinity, "be cautious." Regardless of the advice issued by the NFIP, many parents had their own strong convictions concerning the dangers of summer and what they would or would not allow their children to do. Annie Dillard's mother made her and her sister go to bed early and wash their hands frequently during the polio season. When the girls asked why, Dillard remembers, "Mother would kneel to look us in the eyes and answer in a low, urgent voice, So you do not get polio." Gerald Shepherd's parents kept him out of movie theaters and away from a yo-yo tournament he had a chance of winning. When he cut his hand on glass, his father grounded him for a week out of fear that "polio germs might filter in through the sutures." Noreen Linduska's mother boiled the family's drinking water after reading polio stories in the newspaper.[13] Other parents kept their children away from drinking fountains, amusement parks, county fairs, baseball games, libraries, downtown stores, churches, and even the beginning of the school year. Teachers warned their students to avoid dangers such as swimming and becoming badly sun-burned. But life could not cease entirely, and children, and sometimes their parents, were willing to take chances, especially as the polio season wound down in late summer or early fall. Charlene Pugleasa's mother, for example, allowed her thirteen-year-old daughter to have a slumber party in September. Pugleasa remembers that it was "really kind of a scary thing to have because it was polio season. But it was the end of polio season so parents were more relaxed and more willing to let girls get together."[14] A week later Pugleasa was diagnosed with polio. Parental warnings and precautions undoubtedly prevented many cases of polio, but when the virus was present in a community, it was virtually impossible to prevent all exposure.

In spite of its potential severity, polio could be a difficult disease to diagnose, especially in its early stages, when the typical symptoms of headache, sore throat, nausea, and muscle pains could be indicative of a wide range of diseases, many of them minor. Arriving at a definite diagnosis of polio was often a matter of negotiation between the patient, his or her parents, spouse, other family members, or friends, and the physician or physicians eventually consulted. Because the initial symptoms were so commonplace, the first "negotiation" often took place entirely within the mind of the patient. How serious is this headache that won't quit? Do I need to stay home from school or work? Do I need to tell Mom or call a doctor? Others, especially parents or spouses, were brought into the conversation when the symptoms persisted or increased in severity, or when more disturbing symptoms began to develop, such as the inability to stand or to hold a glass. Depending upon the severity of the symptoms, the parental attitude toward doctors, the family's reliance on traditional and common home remedies, and their knowledge of the early signs of polio, there might be a delay of several days before a physician was called. Older individuals often resisted suggestions to call in a doctor, believing that the illness was minor and that the symptoms would soon begin to diminish. Adolescents and young adults often resisted seeking medical help out of a desire not to miss out on school, sports, social engagements, and work. Unless clear evidence of paralysis had set in when the doctor was consulted, and sometimes even then, the process of arriving at a diagnosis of polio often entailed some negotiation between patients, family, and doctor. Families, of course, did not want to hear a diagnosis of polio, and doctors did not like having to make such a diagnosis.[15] The result was that doctors and families sometimes discussed for days the meaning and significance of the symptoms before polio was finally diagnosed and the patient was rushed to the hospital. This process took a substantial emotional toll on the patient and family. They did not know precisely what was happening or why; they were still hoping for the best and increasingly fearing the worst. A diagnosis of polio ended the agony of not knowing and ushered in a very uncertain future.

In spite of its potential to cripple and to kill, polio usually began innocuously. Many polio victims did not immediately suspect that their headaches or nausea were the initial signs of a life-threatening disease. Although many polio victims experienced the entire gamut of initial symptoms, a severe headache was often the first sign that one was getting ill. John Lindell's polio began as a headache on a Tuesday while he was working as a soil conservationist in Nebraska. His headache persisted through the week, although Lindell dragged himself to work every day until Friday. Eventually, the thought of polio crossed Lindell's mind because it was an epidemic year in Nebraska, but he dismissed it, believing only children got it.[16] Most expected these terrible headaches to go away with aspirin and rest. It was only when the headache persisted and began to be accompanied by other disturbing symptoms that concern about polio began to emerge.

Like a headache, a sore throat or nausea did not ordinarily cause undue concern. When John Lindell developed a sore throat in addition to his headache, he began to worry a bit more about his symptoms, although he went ahead with his weekend naval reserve training after having felt ill since the previous Tuesday. Other polio survivors recalled that nausea and a flu-like feeling were their first symptoms. Mark Sauer's parents had taken him and his sister to a nearby park were they could picnic and play in the water. As they left, six-year-old Mark was so "dizzy and disoriented" that he walked into a sign. Nonetheless, that evening, the family went to a drive-in movie. It was during the movie that Mark "got violently ill and began vomiting and had sweats and a fever."[17] Doctors were seldom called at this stage. It was only when these symptoms persisted, a high fever developed, or pain and muscle weakness became apparent that anxiety increased and the family doctor was called.

Excruciating pain was one of the indications that the virus had begun to invade the central nervous system and that the developing illness might be more than a mild summer flu. For some children, the pain from the developing polio took the form of muscle cramps or a "charley horse," only more persistent and intense. The narratives of both Regina Woods and Hugh Gallagher illuminate how painful the onset of polio could be as well as the kind of negotiation that could occur among patient, family, and health professionals. For Regina Woods, polio began with a sudden pain in her lower back. The next day the pain was worse and she developed a severe headache. In spite of fears that "something was radically wrong," Regina's mother allowed her daughter to go to school. Because she was bused fifteen miles to school, Woods remained at school all day in spite of the increasing pain and the nausea. Hugh Gallagher was in his first semester at Haverford College in spring of 1952 when he acquired an "annoying and painful" backache accompanied by a stiff neck. The pain continued for two days of increasing intensity. Following two sleepless nights, Gallagher finally saw the college physician, who wanted to place him in the infirmary immediately. Gallagher, however, made a deal with the doctor to return to the infirmary later that evening after greeting his parents who were coming for the weekend.[18] In both these cases, the better judgment of mother or physician was overridden in favor of a bargain that allowed Woods and Gallagher to carry on normally, at least for the short run.

Younger patients as well as older ones experienced the severe pains of developing polio. But these younger patients could not describe their pain. The parents' first sign of illness often came when they picked up their child and she screamed. Kay Brutger's mother remembered that when she changed her daughter's diaper she started to scream. She then noticed that her daughter's leg "dropped down" and she couldn't raise it.[19]

Given the pervasive fear of polio and its crippling paralysis, it is not at all odd that parents and patients alike would allow the hope that these symptoms derived from a minor illness to override the terrible possibility that they were the initial stages of polio. In addition, home and folk remedies were often the first recourse in the effort to reduce the symptoms. Sarah Hunt's mother tried to bring down her fever by covering her daughter with "dew-laden peach leaves" and by tying cloth-wrapped sliced onions to the soles of her feet. Only when these home remedies failed to work did her mother call in the county nurse, who diagnosed the illness as polio. Charlene Pugleasa's parents were Finnish and believed in the power of saunas. When their daughter developed a severe headache, sore throat, and muscle pains in September 1953 they took her to their nearby cabin in the woods for a sauna. Only after the sauna provided no relief did they call the doctor. Arvid Schwartz probably summed up the feelings of many, especially of those in rural areas or with limited incomes, when he observed that "in 1952 in rural Minnesota you didn't go to the doctor the minute you ran a fever. You waited until you were sure something was wrong."[20]

Some parents and physicians used the ability of the patient to touch her chin to her chest as a definitive test. A stiff neck was often symptomatic of polio, and if the patient could not touch her chin to her chest, polio was a likely cause. Every day throughout the summer Linda Atkins's mother, like many others, had her touch her chin to her chest as "constant proof that her children were still healthy—safe from the death moving all around us," until, of course, she could no longer pass the test. Soon the ten-year-old was in an ambulance rushing to a hospital in Boston. However, even this fairly reliable sign of developing polio could be a matter of negotiation between patient and doctor. Seven-year-old Carol Meyer had heard her parents mention that a stiff neck was a symptom of polio, so when the doctor who examined her asked if her neck was stiff she lied and said no. Her mother, however, was convinced her daughter had polio, and, once her legs collapsed, insisted that the doctor meet them at the hospital, where a spinal tap soon confirmed polio.[21]

If headaches, sore throats, and painful muscles were commonplace, falling down without warning or reason was not. The inability to stand or walk was often the first sign that the illness was serious. Richard Owen recalled that he had stayed home from school and gone back to bed with what he "thought was a cold with a fever." When he awoke later in the morning and tried to get out of bed he "fell to the floor and . . . couldn't get up." He felt "rather limp" and worried that "something was awfully wrong." Arms as well as legs could give out in disconcerting fashion. Paul Longmore went to bed with symptoms of the flu, but when he awoke the next morning and tried to dress himself he discovered that his left arm was paralyzed. He went into his mother's bedroom and told her, " 'Mommy, my arm doesn't work. Could you put on my sock for me?' Instead of putting on the sock, she called the doctor."[22] Once arms or legs failed, the doctor was almost always called.

Due to the confusing character of the early symptoms of polio, the patient's resistance to confronting the severity of his or her developing illness, and the lack of a definitive early test for polio, the negotiations that led to a final diagnosis and the confirmatory spinal tap could be quite protracted. The cases of Regina Woods and Hugh Gallagher, discussed briefly above, are good examples of how patient, family, and physician all conspired to delay a diagnosis of polio. After Woods made her way home from school after a very long day of increasing pain, her mother called a "typical country doctor." The physician diagnosed the illness as polio and prescribed castor oil. When the symptoms persisted for another day, a different doctor was called. This second physician diagnosed the problem as just a "virus." After a difficult night, Regina could no longer walk without assistance, and she was beginning to develop problems breathing and urinating. Only when she was unable to get out of bed by herself did the family take her to the hospital. Like Woods, Hugh Gallagher refused to surrender to his terrible pains and growing weakness. After meeting his parents, Gallagher checked into the infirmary. His father feared polio and wanted the doctor called. Gallagher gave the doctor a full account of his increasingly painful and frightening symptoms and pleaded for some relief from the pain. The doctor gave him morphine to sleep. In the night Gallagher took his last steps when he managed to make it to the bathroom and back. Only in the morning as paralysis began to spread across his body was he taken to the hospital, where polio was finally confirmed.[23]

Clearly the process of negotiating a diagnosis was more elaborate and protracted for Woods and Gallagher than was the case with most individuals who contracted polio. However, many of the other narratives also reveal considerable delay between the onset of symptoms and the ultimate diagnosis of polio. In most cases, it seems to have been a matter of waiting until the symptoms increased in severity or until they more clearly pointed to a diagnosis of polio rather than any of the other possible illnesses. Arvid Schwartz remembers that his family "debated" for several days the significance of his flu-like symptoms and called the doctor only when the twelve-year-old did not improve. On his first visit, the doctor decided the youngster had "some kind of flu," and his parents continued their usual home flu remedies. Finally, when Arvid fell down trying to get out of bed, they called the doctor again. This time, the doctor "brought up the possibility of polio" and recommended that they take their son to the Sister Kenny Institute in St. Paul, several hours away. John Lindell, as we have already seen, had endured a work week with a headache, sore throat, and muscle pain, and then did two days of naval reserve duty. On Monday morning when his ten-year-old son woke up with similar symptoms Lindell's wife took both father and son to the doctor. The physicians immediately diagnosed the son's polio, but doubted that Lindell's ailment was polio, because "polio was a childhood disease." They sent him home and prescribed antibiotics and rest. Overnight his pains increased, and he began to see double. The next day when he again went to the doctors, they finally agreed that Lindell might have polio and recommended hospitalization.[24]

Even once the physician was called and had conducted an examination, a diagnosis of polio was by no means a certainty. Perhaps he was not looking for polio, and other diagnoses seemed equally plausible. Perhaps he was reluctant to pronounce such a fearful diagnosis until he was absolutely certain, but in either case it is clear that some physicians' reluctance to diagnose polio delayed the possibility of early treatment and the possible mitigation of permanent paralysis.

Even when physicians ventured a diagnosis of the increasingly debilitating symptoms, their initial diagnosis was not always polio. The narratives reveal a wide range of maladies initially proposed by doctors as the cause of the patient's distress. Appendicitis with spinal meningitis, strep throat, rheumatic fever, meningitis, the flu, some unspecified virus, kidney infection, pleurisy, throat abscess, tonsillitis, and pneumonia were among the diagnoses offered by doctors to explain the symptoms.[25] In most of these cases, the doctors eventually settled on a diagnosis of polio, often after the symptoms had progressed or had continued without abatement, and often with the aid of a spinal tap. Nine-year-old Millie Teders, for example, was misdiagnosed before her polio was correctly identified. When, after two days of headaches, Millie awoke with a stiff neck her parents took her to the doctor. The doctor found a spot on her lung, so he treated her with sulfa drugs for pneumonia. He suspected polio, but since her reflexes were still good, was unwilling to make the diagnosis. He did put her in the local hospital, where he checked her reflexes and had her walk each day. Finally, on the third day in the hospital, her reflexes disappeared and she collapsed on the floor when she tried to walk. Because the polio hospitals in Minneapolis were not accepting any new patients due to an epidemic, the doctor suggested that her parents drive her to the university hospital "in the middle of the night, feeling that they would not turn a sick child away." She was admitted, and a spinal tap confirmed the polio diagnosis.[26] Teders came from a small community in rural Minnesota where the local doctor no doubt saw relatively few cases of polio. Other illnesses and conditions could easily come to mind first, at least until paralysis developed, or the patient could not touch chin to chest, or stand unaided. For these families and their physicians, getting to a diagnosis of polio was a matter of painful waiting until the picture had come into focus and the doctor could be more confident of his diagnosis. Because of the fear of polio, no doctor wanted to give a false diagnosis of polio.

Early and prompt diagnosis was important for both the patient and the community. By midcentury, many specialists believed that rest and a cessation of physical activity helped reduce the severity of paralysis. Conversely, continuing to exercise, or even continuing one's normal daily routines increased the risk of more severe paralysis.[27] Second, since polio was contagious, a correct diagnosis, followed by the immediate isolation of the patient in the home or hospital, limited the spread of the disease. In the late forties and in the early fifties, numerous articles in medical journals, as well as publications of the NFIP, stressed both the necessity and the difficulty of early diagnosis.

The key to prompt and correct diagnosis of poliomyelitis was recognizing the early symptoms and then differentiating a case of polio from the other illnesses that began with the same or similar symptoms. Nearly every physician who addressed the subject conceded that polio was "one of the most difficult of all diseases to recognize accurately." Even as the polio epidemics were nearing their end in the mid-1950s, physicians still had "no infallible method . . . for making a definite diagnosis of poliomyelitis during the earlier phases of the infection. The physician must rely on clinical judgment for interpretation and evaluation of the findings in each individual case."[28]

Several characteristics of a polio infection made the diagnosis more complicated and difficult. Many patients experienced the infection in the two phases first identified by George Draper in 1917.[29] First, there was an early phase characterized by slight fever, respiratory and intestinal distress, and slightly stiff neck. This was often followed by an abatement of the symptoms for one to three days. For most patients infected with the poliovirus, the illness ended here in either the abortive or nonparalytic stage. However, for a minority of patients the lessening of symptoms was followed by a more serious phase that involved the central nervous system and often resulted in temporary or permanent paralysis. In this second phase, the usual symptoms of headache, vomiting, high fever, muscle aches, and stiffness were often present, along with muscle weakness and paralysis. Abortive poliomyelitis was almost impossible to diagnose except during an epidemic and in individuals known to have been exposed. It was a brief flu-like illness with fever, nausea, headache, sore throat, and fatigue among the common symptoms. Nonparalytic polio had similar symptoms, "except that headache, nausea or vomiting becomes more intense, together with soreness and stiffness of the posterior muscles of the neck, trunk, and limbs." Rigidity of the neck and spine were key markers for a diagnosis of nonparalytic polio. In making a diagnosis of nonparalytic poliomyelitis, the physician had to differentiate the illness from a variety of other possibilities, including various forms of meningitis, Coxsackie viruses, infectious mononucleosis, viral encephalitis, rheumatic fever, pneumonia, and acute tonsillitis. The only way to definitively eliminate these other possibilities, even during a polio epidemic, was through a spinal tap and examination of the cerebrospinal fluid.[30]

A spinal tap was the only reliable laboratory test to diagnose polio and was usually done shortly after a patient arrived at the hospital. The patient lay on her side in a fetal position and the physician inserted a long needle into the spinal column to draw off some of the fluid for analysis. The laboratory looked for certain changes in the composition of the fluid characteristic of polio. The spinal tap was most effective when done early in the disease before paralysis set in, and it was especially useful in diagnosing nonparalytic forms of the disease. Although doctors believed that "a carefully performed spinal puncture is harmless" and may be "beneficial," patients feared the long needle when they were already in considerable pain and discomfort from the advancing disease. All too often, the spinal puncture was very painful and the procedure was etched in the memories of many polio survivors.[31]

In theory, paralytic polio was easier to diagnose, especially during epidemics, because of the distinguishing paralysis. However, here the conscientious physician needed to consider whether the illness was taking the spinal form, which involved the nerves of the spinal cord; the bulbar form, which affected the cranial nerves; the bulbospinal form, which involved both cranial and spinal nerves; or the rare encephalitic form, which affected the brain. In addition, certain other diseases also produced muscle weakness and/or paralysis and had to be eliminated. These included Guillain-Barré syndrome, viral encephalitis, spinal cord tumors, unrecognized trauma, acute rheumatic fever, scurvy, and osteomyelitis.[32] Here again, the testing of the cerebrospinal fluid as the result of a spinal tap was the most certain tool in the diagnosis of polio. However, because the spinal tap was often quite painful, some experts argued that if a careful differential diagnosis was conducted, especially during a polio epidemic, the lumbar puncture was not necessary.

Given the commonplace symptoms, it is not surprising that many of the narratives reveal an initial misdiagnosis or uncertainty on the part of the physician. Since other childhood diseases could also cause paralysis, even doctors who initially diagnosed paralytic polio as some other illness may have had good reasons. Two studies done during the early fifties suggest that physicians had an error rate of between 15 and 22 percent in diagnosing poliomyelitis. Doctors in these studies misdiagnosed poliomyelitis as pneumonia, rheumatoid arthritis, hysteria, encephalitis, bacterial meningitis, meningococcic meningitis, brain tumor, Guillain-Barré syndrome, osteomyelitis, and scurvy.[33] The misdiagnoses uncovered in these two hospital studies are consistent with those recalled by the authors of the polio narratives.

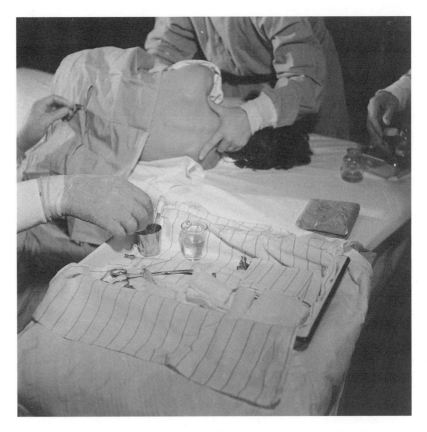

FIG. 3. Preparations for a spinal tap in Alexandria, Louisiana, 1956. Spinal taps
were often used to provide a definitive diagnosis of polio. Many narratives mention
the painful procedure.

Because of the fear polio created, delivering a diagnosis of polio was difficult for many physicians. Part of the difficulty, as we have seen, lay in clearly
identifying a case of poliomyelitis in its early stages. However, the difficulty
was compounded by the public's concern to limit the spread of the disease. A
missed diagnosis meant that the individual remained in the family and community and had the very real potential to infect others. The difficulties did not
end when the physician was sure of his diagnosis; the individual and his or her
family still had to be told. Dr. Richard Aldrich recalled that "then the worst
part of the whole thing came, and that's when you had to talk to the parents.
Those were some of the most awful experiences I ever had in my life . . . sitting

down with a mother and father whose child you just diagnosed as having polio." In the view of Fred Davis, there were three reasons why doctors, especially
family doctors, sometimes withheld a definitive diagnosis of polio. First, "it afforded the doctors some protection in the event that their tentative diagnosis
was proved wrong," which, as several studies demonstrated, was always possible. Second, "it relieved the doctor to some extent of the unpleasant task of
'breaking the bad news,' to the parents." That "bit of 'dirty work'" was left to
the physicians at the hospital where the spinal tap was performed. And third,
some doctors felt that the family could better deal with the diagnosis if it came
to them gradually.[34] The family doctor raised the possibility of polio when he
sent the patient to the hospital. Thus, the physician gave those involved some
time to get used to the possibility before the hospital staff confirmed the diagnosis following the spinal tap.

In some cases, polio was suspected before the physician was called or before a definite judgment was rendered. Families and individuals had different
levels of awareness regarding polio, in spite of the widespread educational
campaigns of the NFIP. Some were aware of the early potential signs of polio,
or of the existence of an epidemic in their community, while others seemed
largely unaware of either. Of the fourteen families in Fred Davis's study, only
one knew very much about polio. Both parents in that family were college educated and the father had worked in military hospitals during World War II
and had come in contact with polio patients. Most people knew someone who
had had polio and were thus aware of its potential to cripple, but otherwise
their knowledge of the disease was "relatively meager." [35] But even if families
lacked substantial knowledge about polio, their very real fear of the disease
led many families, and some patients, to suspect polio as the symptoms persisted and increased in severity.

Although family members might suspect and fear that an ill child or
spouse had polio, their concern was not always voiced either to the patient or
to the physician. It was almost as if the illness would turn out to be something
relatively benign as long as it were not named. Robert Hall had consulted a specialist for what he thought was a sinus infection. When the specialist sent him
to his family doctor, Hall began to worry about polio. Sent to a hospital for
observation, his worries only increased. He remembered that at the time he
"didn't know a thing about it except that if you got it some awful things could
happen. It killed quite a few people, and it disabled a lot more in some awful
ways. Arms and legs shriveled up. I didn't want to dwell on it too much."
Shortly after a spinal tap was taken, "a nurse came to the door of my room and

closed it. She did so without saying a word. That is how I learned I had polio." After the doctor examined Dorothea Nudelman he went into the kitchen to talk to her parents. She caught only a few words of the hushed conversation. No one mentioned polio, but she remembers "*thinking* it. And I was sure everyone else was too. I was *afraid* to ask." [36]

If for some families polio was too dreadful even to be spoken, in others parents were more willing than doctors to raise the possibility that their child might have polio. Although their fear of polio was no doubt as great, these parents, by mentioning the possibility of polio and by pushing the physician for a decision, were hoping that early diagnosis and treatment would alleviate the pain and lessen the severity of the disease. Twenty-three-year-old June Radosovich contracted polio in 1952. When her family called the doctor after several days of increasing symptoms and growing weakness, her sister, aware of the symptoms because of the news reports of the serious epidemic, told the physician, "I think she has polio." The doctor was less certain, but he did admit Radosovich to the hospital where the spinal tap confirmed the sister's suspicion.[37] Parents had little to lose and much to gain from pushing the physicians for a diagnosis, even if the diagnosis was for something as feared as polio. Knowing what their children had was in some measure easier to deal with than the awful uncertainty of watching them get increasingly ill and not knowing what caused it or what could be done about it. Little could be done to stop the spread of the virus, and palliative measures such as hot packs only partially relieved the pain of muscle spasms, but there was some comfort in knowing that doctors and nurses were doing all they could.

Whether or not families and patients articulated suspicions that the illness might be polio depended on such things as the level of knowledge of polio, family roles and dynamics, and pivotal clues such as a stiff neck or the beginning of paralysis. News reports during epidemic years were a major source of information about the symptoms of polio. Many parents and some patients suspected polio because the developing illness matched descriptions in the newspapers. Conversely, when there was no local epidemic and the papers were not filled with warnings about what to watch for in their children's behavior, parents could miss the warning signs and assume that their child's illness was merely a "summer virus." [38] Knowledge of polio's symptoms was sometimes acquired in unusual ways. Mary-Lou Whitaker's mother had seen a movie in which a child was diagnosed with polio: when Mary-Lou exhibited the same symptoms as the actress, her mother, certain her daughter had polio, called the doctor. In other cases, members of the family had medical training as nurses or physicians and thus recognized the early symptoms as likely signs of polio. For example, Ray Gullickson's sister recognized his symptoms because she had worked in a Shrine Hospital where she had cared for polio patients. Others had equally direct knowledge of polio. Marlene Krumrie's mother immediately recognized her daughter's nausea, stiff neck, and back pains as polio because her husband had had the disease. She remembers her mother "weeping and crying, saying 'Oh no! It can't be polio again!'" But it was.[39]

If some patients knew or suspected from the very beginning that polio was the cause of their distress, others did not learn the diagnosis of their illness until somewhat later. By the early fifties, at least, experts recommended that physicians tell patients of the diagnosis immediately rather than deferring an explanation. Because patients were already quite aware that they were seriously ill, not telling them the cause of the problem only increased their anxiety. When physicians withheld a diagnosis, patients tended to assume the worst, which exacted an unnecessary psychological toll.[40]

Doctors usually told an adult patient the diagnosis at the time that it was made. Other doctors preferred to wait until a spinal tap had provided a definitive diagnosis. With children and adolescents, doctors were not the only ones to decide when and how to tell the patient the diagnosis. Parents, who were almost always told immediately, played a key role in telling their children. Some parents, like Luther Robinson and his wife, asked the doctor to tell their daughter immediately. In other families, the child overheard the doctor tell the parents that their son or daughter had infantile paralysis. In some cases, when the child or adolescent was told, the significance of the diagnosis was not immediately apparent. For example, Richard Owen, who was twelve at the time, recalls being told that he had "poliomyelitis," but he did not connect that term with "infantile paralysis," the disease of President Roosevelt. Only later did he learn that he and Roosevelt shared illnesses. Leonard Kriegel saw the fear in his mother's face when she told him that the doctor had diagnosed polio, but not until he had been sent to the rehabilitation hospital did Kriegel connect polio with infantile paralysis, a term his "eleven-year-old mind heard with dread."[41]

When adolescent patients were not told what caused their illness they sometimes found other ways to learn the diagnosis. Hugh Gallagher's physicians, in spite of his significant paralysis, deflected his inquiries. Since the doctors would not answer him directly, Gallagher "decided to probe indirectly." When a new resident examined him, Gallagher asked him how severe his polio was. When the resident replied that they did not yet know, Gallagher had his suspicions confirmed. Nine-year-old Dorothea Nudelman learned that she had polio only after the acute illness had abated. When she began to feel somewhat better, she asked her mother if she had polio. Her mother replied yes and assured her daughter that she was going to be fine. Dorothea's response captured the feelings of many for whom the anxiety of not knowing was worse than knowing: "I thought so. But no one would say it to me. I feel better being able to name it. Now I don't have to worry about what's wrong with me anymore."[42]

Because they knew how devastating a diagnosis of polio could be, doctors and parents often tried to soften the blow when telling a patient or child. The mothers of both Dorothea Nudelman and Leonard Kriegel tried to comfort their children, assuring them that the doctor thought they would soon be "fine." Polio left both of them needing braces permanently. Louis Sternburg's physician initially told the thirty-year-old father of two that his was a "mild case. Nonparalytic." His "mild case" left him permanently dependent on an iron lung or rocking bed. However much comfort these reassuring words offered, assessments offered at the time of diagnosis were not always accurate predictions of the course of the disease. Until the virus had run its course, and sometimes for months afterward, physicians had no sure way of knowing how much damage was done and what kind of permanent weakness or paralysis, if any, would remain.[43]

In spite of the efforts of some physicians and parents to minimize the seriousness of the illness, children were sensitive to other clues that revealed parental concern and fear. Mark Sauer recalled that "when the physician used the word polio, my mother looked over to my father and I immediately saw tears welling in his eyes." When Grace Audet's father sped through the Iowa countryside at 80 miles an hour, far beyond his usual sedate speed, she sensed the seriousness of her illness.[44] Some parents tried to hide their own anxieties as they comforted their children in the brief time between diagnosis and admission to the hospital. However, directly or indirectly, many children knew from the words and behavior of their physicians and their parents that this disease was more serious than any they had previously experienced.

Several contemporary studies confirm that most patients and families experienced significant emotional distress when polio was diagnosed. The pervasive fear of the disease and the uncertainty of prognosis regarding the outcome in any particular case contributed substantially to the psychological impact. One small study of patients between fourteen and thirty-seven years of age revealed that almost all recalled "a conscious feeling of shock and fear for their lives when they first learned their illness was poliomyelitis." Most of the sixteen patients in the study reacted to the diagnosis with "varying degrees of affective depression and tearfulness or a desire to cry." Parents, like their sons and daughters, had powerful emotional reactions on learning their children had polio. Men and women alike wept. Fred Davis found that "the imagery of crippling, iron lungs, and death" underlay the parents' emotional responses.[45] A diagnosis of polio meant uncertainty had been replaced by awful reality.

One of the common responses to a diagnosis of polio was a sense of guilt. Many children, and some older patients, felt guilty for having done something forbidden—playing in the stream, sneaking off to a movie, drinking from a water fountain. Others felt that they were being punished for some unrelated transgression. Parents often felt guilt for failing to protect their children from the virus. These guilt feelings emerge both in the narratives and in the psychological studies conducted on polio survivors. For example, Dorothea Nudelman's parents had told her not to carry a doll carriage upstairs. A few days before polio struck she had done so, and when she became ill she was certain that her aching back was God's punishment for disobeying her parents. When Leonard Kriegel saw his mother for the first time in the hospital, and watched her "make her frightened way across the room," he felt responsible for what had happened, for what he had done: "I yelled, 'Momma, I'm sorry.' She had the unconscious grace to cry. And I cried with her, relieved that I had won forgiveness." Parents often replayed the events of preceding days to see what they might have done differently to have protected their sons and daughters from exposure to the virus. They wanted desperately to find "the answer to that plaguing question—how did it happen."[46]

Studies of polio patients and their families in the forties and fifties also demonstrated that guilt was a significant component of the psychological response to a diagnosis of polio. Several studies revealed that children often interpreted sickness as "punishment for their misdeeds." William Langford argued that children develop this guilt from repeated parental admonitions that doing certain things, for example, getting wet, will produce illnesses such as colds. He argues that it is not surprising that children interpret more serious illnesses to be the result of their own actions and misdeeds. Similarly, the patients in Fred Davis's study tended to view their paralysis "as a kind of punishment for a behavioral transgression." A parental sense of guilt usually derived from their sense of responsibility to protect their children from harm. Davis suggested that parents were often trapped in "the American value scheme: namely, that misfortune rarely touches those who take the proper precautionary measures."[47] Such a devastating disease should not happen in modern America, and when it did, children and parents often reverted to an older religious paradigm of understanding disease which interpreted illness as divine punishment for sin. This tendency to connect sin, illness, and guilt was fostered in the case of polio by the difficulty of determining precisely where the individual acquired the virus. That uncertainty, combined with the dread of the disease, allowed the older religious paradigm to flourish.

A diagnosis of polio, though it most directly affected the sick individual, also had a significant and immediate impact on the family. Families, especially parents, had to deal with the many emotional, psychological, and logistical implications of the diagnosis. They needed and wanted to comfort their son or daughter, but they were frightened about the immediate prospects for recovery and the long-term possibilities for the future. Their fears were often accompanied by feelings of helplessness and even rage at the unfairness of it all.[48] More practical problems also loomed large in those early hours and days following a diagnosis. Was anybody else in the family infected? What about neighbors and friends? Were they at risk? Who would take care of the children at home if the parents stayed in the hospital? If it was the father or mother who was stricken, how would the family survive without an income or with a mother permanently paralyzed? In addition, families had to confront this serious, sometimes life-threatening illness largely by themselves, as they were often stigmatized by their association with the disease and were isolated and ostracized by their community.

Although polio at midcentury typically struck only one member of a family, the terrible possibility that others were exposed and possibly infected added to the worries following a diagnosis. Dorothy Horstmann found that "by the time a physician is called to see a case, virtually all other susceptible members of the family have been infected, whether or not they have symptoms."[49] For a small number of families these fears of contagion became real as polio struck more than once. Even though John Lindell's symptoms had begun a week earlier, his ten-year-old son Jimmy was diagnosed with polio a day before Lindell himself. Luther Robinson watched both of his adolescent daughters contract bulbar polio within days of one another in 1953. Anita died of a virulent form of bulbar polio and Alta was completely paralyzed and dependent on an iron lung. In the Howard family of Lodi, California, sisters Eleanor, Charlotte, Linda, and Patti all had polio; one brother, Richard, died in an iron lung; and their father, Rufus, developed polio on the day of Richard's funeral.[50]

Many families faced official quarantine or isolation by friends and neighbors.[51] Fourteen-year-old Agnes Dalton had to burn all her sister's toys and carefully wash all the bedclothes as well as care for her arthritic father while her mother accompanied her sister to the polio hospital 160 miles away in Hickory, North Carolina. Agnes would be in charge during the three weeks the family was quarantined. In Minnesota, the brothers and sisters of Arvid Schwartz were kept out of school for two weeks because of their exposure to polio. Charles Andrews learned quickly that it was easy to keep his other children isolated: "The neighbors—bless them—made very sure their children stayed miles away. They were scared to death." When Louis Sternburg came down with polio in 1955, doctors told his wife Dottie to stay away from their two children, then eighteen months and six months old, if she wanted to be able to visit her husband. As he put it, "the Sternburg family were lepers."[52] Thus at the very time when many families needed assistance to cope with this devastating illness they found themselves largely on their own, cut off from help either by official quarantine or by the fears of apprehensive friends and neighbors.

In his study of polio patients and their families in Baltimore, however, Fred Davis discovered that the family's period of being ostracized and isolated by friends and neighbors was relatively short-lived. Once the fear of spreading infection was past, and especially if it became clear that no one who had associated with the patient was coming down with polio, "neighbors and relatives rallied around the family." This support, Davis argues, went a long way toward reassuring the parents that they were not to blame for their child's illness. Relatives and friends provided not only emotional support, but also practical assistance such as rides to the hospital and babysitting with the unaffected children so both parents could be at the hospital.[53] The support of these friends and relatives was not only important at the onset of the disease, it would also continue to be important during the long period of hospitalization and rehabilitation that most patients could expect to experience.

In less than a week, these boys and girls, young men and women were transformed from healthy individuals to very sick patients diagnosed with the most feared disease of young Americans. Their comfortable worlds of play, sports, school, or work had been narrowed to the confines of the sickroom where fever, muscle pain, and sometimes an inability to breathe tortured their bodies, and a dread of polio haunted their feverish minds. A diagnosis of polio brought no immediate relief of the bodily pains and only partial emotional relief, for there was little medicine could do other than to let the virus run its course. With an accurate diagnosis you at least knew what caused your agony, but the knowledge was hardly comforting when it conjured up, as it so often did, a future filled with braces, crutches, and wheelchairs. Unfortunately, when doctors diagnosed polio they had no way of knowing how severe a particular infection would be. That became apparent only after weeks, months, and sometimes years of hospitalization and rehabilitation.

| 3 |

The Crisis of Acute Poliomyelitis

WITHIN HOURS OF BEING DIAGNOSED with a case of polio, most patients were admitted to an isolation ward or isolation hospital. Separated from parents, family, and friends, who were forbidden to visit, and surrounded by doctors and nurses garbed in white with only their eyes visible, these very sick boys and girls, men and women, experienced a psychological crisis that often rivaled the physical assault of the virus. Polio patients confronted the acute phase of the illness alone, largely bereft of the psychological and emotional support parents, spouses, and family provided in the early stages of the disease. The doctors and nurses, especially during an epidemic, were too busy caring for the substantial physical needs of patients rapidly losing control of their bodies to pay much attention to the psychological and emotional toll on the young men and women in their care.

The acute stage of poliomyelitis was a frightening, even terrifying experience. Sometimes slowly, sometimes rapidly, but always unpredictably, the body lost its ability to move as the virus invaded the central nervous system, damaging and destroying the nerves that activated the muscles. You might lose function in an arm or a leg, or perhaps one side would become paralyzed, or the paralysis might begin at your toes and work its way up, leaving you immobile below the waist or neck. If the virus attacked the nerves that controlled the muscles of breathing, you were left desperate for air unless an artificial respirator, an iron lung, was available to breathe for you. And if the cranial nerves were affected, you might lose the ability to swallow, to talk, to smile. The spreading paralysis was often accompanied by excruciating pain that was usually endured without relief from drugs, the most effective of which would have depressed your breathing, something most doctors were unwilling to risk. Beyond supporting breathing if necessary and trying to make the patient comfortable, medicine had little to offer in relief of acute poliomyelitis. Patients and physicians could only wait to see how far the virus would progress and how much damage it would do.

The terror of losing control of one's body was often matched by the fear and anxiety produced when children were separated from parents and men and women from spouses. Most polio patients were hospitalized in isolation, typically in separate wards or wings of hospitals, separated from family until the infection had run its course, which might be as long as three weeks. Children, many of whom had never spent a night away from their parents, found isolation terrifying. Always before when they had been sick their mother or father had been there to cool a feverish forehead, to offer a soothing drink, or just to hold their hands. Now perhaps their only contact was to see them at a distance, behind glass. Had they been abandoned? Had they done something to deserve this treatment? What was happening to them, and why? Adolescents and older patients also found isolation difficult. It was hard to comprehend how one could go from healthy activity on farm or athletic field to pain, paralysis, and confinement in a matter of days or even hours. Married patients found separation from spouses particularly difficult. The anxiety for older patients was compounded by the unwillingness of the doctors to offer any prognosis regarding the course of the disease.

Most polio patients received at least a tentative diagnosis at home from their family physicians. They were then taken to the hospital by parents, spouses, or ambulance. Many of these trips were difficult both physically and emotionally. Some patients suffered considerably from the increasing pain and paralysis, especially on the longer trips. Both patients and parents worried about how far paralysis would spread, what the hospital would be like, and how to deal with the impending separation of unknown duration. The trip to the hospital marked the passage from the familiar to the unfamiliar, from health to illness, and the memory of this transition from one world to another stands out in many narratives.

Once a decision had been made to take a newly diagnosed polio patient to the hospital, the next question was often which hospital. Because it was common practice to isolate polio patients in a separate ward or wing of the hospital, not all hospitals had the necessary facilities or a staff trained in the arduous work of caring for the acutely ill, paralyzed, and contagious patients. In most larger communities, particular hospitals were designated to care for polio patients. For example, in 1943 only seven hospitals admitted acute polio patients in Cook County, Illinois, which includes Chicago. By 1952 fifteen Cook County hospitals admitted newly diagnosed polio patients, and that number rose to thirty-five in 1956. During the severe 1955 polio epidemic in Boston, children were cared for at Children's Hospital and Boston City Hospital. Adult polio patients were sent to Haynes Memorial Infectious Disease Hospital and Boston City Hospital. As the number of polio patients increased beyond the ability of these three hospitals to care for them, they were also admitted to Massachusetts General Hospital and Boston Floating Hospital. Ambulance drivers knew to take polio patients to one of the designated hospitals.[1]

African Americans who contracted the disease faced the challenge of finding a hospital that was both equipped to handle polio patients and that would admit them. The era of the polio epidemics was also the era of Jim Crow segregation. Almost all southern hospitals were segregated, with larger communities having both black and white hospitals. Even some northern and western hospitals practiced segregation in these decades by refusing to admit blacks or relegating them to inferior wards in a separate part of the hospital. In smaller southern communities the only hospital was often restricted to whites, which meant that African American polio patients had to travel farther to seek treatment. In addition, most black hospitals had inferior facilities and medical equipment when compared with their white neighbors. Occasionally, however, the overwhelming demands of a major polio epidemic could temporarily override the normal segregation. In the major polio epidemic in Hickory, North Carolina, in 1944 the community quickly constructed an emergency infantile paralysis hospital on the grounds of an appropriated fresh air camp. At the height of the epidemic, "African American and white children lay side by side in hospital beds in the same ward and were attended by both African American and white nurses." This unusual arrangement, however, did not last long. As soon as "time and circumstances made separate buildings available, African American patients were moved to and segregated in Ward Eleven," which was in the basement.[2]

Some medical authorities recommended against transporting polio patients long distances because of the pain that movement and jostling brought to paralyzed muscles. However, the distance traveled depended largely on the location of the nearest hospital accepting polio patients. In larger cities that usually meant a relatively short ride across town, but for patients in small towns or for rural victims it might be a long journey across rough country roads where every bump was agonizing. Even a journey across town could be excruciating. Shirley Paul remembered her ride to Children's Hospital in Washington, DC, on a hot August day: "I kept calling out to my father, 'Daddy, Daddy! Go slower! It hurts!' Every little bump in the road was so painful to my

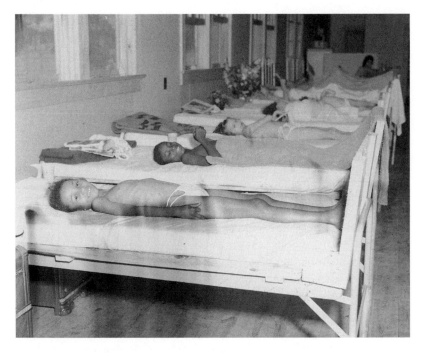

FIG. 4. African American and white children together in an acute polio ward
during the epidemic in Hickory, North Carolina, in 1944. Because of segregation,
it was unusual for black and white patients to be housed together in the South.
When the Hickory epidemic waned, the African American patients were moved to
a newly constructed segregated ward.

whole body." Charlene Pugleasa recalled "every bump, every railroad track" on
the sixty-mile ride across rural Minnesota propped up between her parents because she could no longer sit by herself.[3] During an epidemic, isolation wards
and hospitals quickly filled and it was sometimes difficult to find a hospital
that would admit another polio patient.

Although parents and spouses took many polio patients to the hospital,
others were transported in ambulances. Unlike during the great 1916 epidemic in the northeastern United States when parents often forcibly resisted
the efforts of ambulance attendants to take their children to isolation hospitals, parents in the forties and fifties often called the ambulance if they did not
themselves take their children to the hospital. Although a few polio patients
were treated at home, by the forties the vast majority were treated in hospitals
with little objection from patients or parents. Ambulances often hastened the

separation of patient and family, as family members were usually not allowed to ride in the ambulance to the hospital. The ambulance ride was often a harrowing experience. When seventeen-year-old Robert Gurney was taken to the hospital, he passed out from the pain when the ambulance attendants lifted him onto the stretcher. When his mother inquired why the attendants covered his face with a rubber sheet and blanket, they replied, "Because we don't know if he's contagious, and we don't want to take any chances." Sheila Tohn was twelve when taken to the hospital in a "'contaminated' ambulance." She remembers her "pregnant mother crying on the sidewalk and the attendants garbed in white gowns and masks." She also recalls "the unreasoning fear that I was being taken somewhere to be killed."[4]

The process of admission for some patients reinforced the fears that surrounded polio, especially during an epidemic. When the ambulance bringing Jane Needham to a San Francisco hospital in 1949 arrived, the attendants were told that that they could not use the elevator to take her to the second-floor isolation ward; they had to carry her stretcher up the narrow outside metal fire escape. She recalled that when the heavy steel door closed behind her, it shut her off "forever from the life that I had known." Charles Mee was fourteen in 1953 when he was admitted to a hospital in Elgin, Illinois. He recalls a ride in a wheelchair into the dark bowels of the hospital, where the head nurse diagnosed polio. The others in the room then moved away from the bed, and those who had touched him "stepped to the sink one at a time and washed their hands." Soon the nurse picked him up and carried him to the isolation ward. Mee recalls that he "felt a shudder of deep, deep fear . . . [and] awesome terror." He knew then that he had been "separated from the rest of the world."[5]

For other patients whose entry into the hospital was less dramatic, one incident early in their hospitalization stuck out in their memories: the last time they walked. Fifteen-year-old David Kangas's parents had taken him to the hospital at midnight after he was unable to finish marching in a parade to benefit the March of Dimes. It was his first time in a hospital, and he recalled, "I walked into the hospital, walked down the hall to my room and that was the last time I walked ever again." For others, the last steps came sometime after admission, often when they attempted to use the bathroom. Hugh Gallagher recalled that on the night of his admission he managed to walk, with great difficulty, to the bathroom and back. At the time it did not seem momentous. Only in retrospect did he realize that "those were the last steps I will ever take in this world. There should have been more ceremony attached to them."[6] Most polio patients entered the hospital expecting to walk out cured and fully recovered. Thus the last steps these individuals took usually passed without ceremony or notice at the time; it was only months, perhaps years, later that they could look back and pinpoint when and where they took their last free and unaided steps.

While still at home, families and patients had some room to negotiate a diagnosis, but once the polio patient entered the hospital any opportunity to negotiate care, treatment, even access was significantly reduced. The locus of power and decision-making shifted away from the family and the patient toward the doctor and the hospital. Young patients were often not even informed of what was happening to them, and certainly had no voice in decisions about their acute care. Older patients were often too sick to participate in decisions about their care, especially in the days immediately after admission when the infection and the accompanying fever were at their height. Too young or too sick to make good decisions and separated from the emotional support of their families, most polio patients ceded to their physicians' decisions about care and treatment. In any case, during serious epidemics when the polio wards were crowded with very sick and dying patients, physicians had little time to discuss the fine points of diagnosis or treatment.

Polio patients were admitted to hospitals for such care as medicine could provide as well as to limit the spread of the disease. Most patients admitted had a high fever as well as evidence of paralysis. On admission to the hospital, many patients were subjected to a spinal tap. This often-painful procedure provided confirmation of the diagnosis of polio. During the febrile stage, which might last several days, doctors tried to reduce the fever, to keep the patient comfortable, and to prevent the spreading paralysis from creating deformities. By the 1940s, hot packs were often used to reduce pain and to maintain muscle flexibility. Many patients had periods of hallucinations, especially if they suffered from oxygen deficiency. Although hospitalization provided little immediate relief to most polio patients, that was not true for those who suffered from paralysis of the breathing muscles. Paralysis of breathing quickly produced a crisis for the patient, who could not breathe, and for the hospital staff, who scrambled to install the patient in an iron lung. The patient's stay in the acute hospital could be as short as two weeks, or as long as several months, depending on the severity of the paralysis. Once the fever broke, and the progression of paralysis stopped, most acute hospitals in this period began the long process of rehabilitation. As soon as the patients were stable and no longer contagious, they were moved to general polio wards, to rehabilitation hospitals, or discharged home.

Typically, a spinal tap was given just before or just after admission to the hospital. Because of the risks and pain involved and because the test only confirmed a diagnosis, some doctors recommended against it in cases of "unmistakable poliomyelitis."[7] Those who underwent the procedure never forgot it. The physician who performed Marilyn Rogers's spinal tap first injected her with Novocaine so it was relatively painless. Her most vivid memory is of arriving on the children's ward, noticing that all of the other children had bandages on their backs, and thinking "Gee, I must have one too." Extremely painful spinal taps were far more typical. The doctor told Stanley Lipshultz that the spinal tap "wouldn't hurt," but it caused tremendous pain and Lipshultz still carries the memory: "What six-year-old would—or could—forget the physical pain linked with a needle in the back." For Robert Hudson the spinal tap was "like driving a wooden stake in my back." Others passed out from the pain.[8]

For many polio patients, but especially for children, admission to the hospital was marked by the devastatingly painful separation from parents and family. Most hospitals immediately placed polio patients in isolation following the admittance procedures and/or the spinal tap. Because so many families and physicians had downplayed the seriousness of the symptoms in the vain hope that it was not polio, many children were totally unprepared to be separated, often without even an opportunity for a final good-bye. As a result, they experienced an acute sense of abandonment as they were wheeled or carried through the doors leading to isolation. Their sense of abandonment was heightened by the white halls and rooms through which doctors and nurses moved, garbed in white from head to toe. Hospital policies that prohibited or severely limited visitors to patients in isolation meant that when most patients were sickest they were also the most alone.

The separation of parent and child was deeply felt on both sides of the door to isolation, but the child's agony of abandonment may have been more intense because it often came without warning or explanation. Nurses prohibited Charlene Pugleasa's mother from accompanying her daughter into the contagion unit. Pugleasa remembers crying out, "'Mom, please don't leave me here.' And they just swung those doors. My mother's face was in this little window and she was crying. . . . There were no parting, loving, kind words because they whisked me off so fast." The psychic and emotional scars of this traumatic separation were apparent to Mary Cook when she brought her two-year-old son home from the hospital after two weeks in isolation. When she and her husband picked up their son, "he did not want to come to us, and all the way home he stared at us like a trapped animal. He was a child not only physically hurt; he had been deeply wounded by the two people closest to him, who had deserted him when he most needed them."[9]

Older patients also felt the agony of separation, especially from spouses who they loved and on whom they had come to rely. Kenneth Kingery came down with polio his last day in the air force. When the doctor informed him that he would be put in isolation he wondered how he would deal with polio without his wife Fran beside him: "For a terrible moment the hospital was a quicksand of fear, swallowing me with a cold clinical detachment. . . . I was cut adrift, alone and friendless." Fourteen when he was placed in isolation, Charles Mee had "never been so alone in my life as in that bed, where I was confined for the next three weeks, feverish and contagious."[10] In their more lucid moments, these older patients understood the necessity of isolation, but that did not lessen the distress they felt at being isolated from spouses and family members.

Some facilities, however, allowed parents access to their children even during the height of the illness. Boston hospitals overwhelmed by the number of polio cases in the 1955 epidemic welcomed volunteers, including parents and spouses of polio patients. They helped with patient care and provided "recreational diversions." Some mothers stayed in Boston City Hospital during the day and "helped take care of not only their own children but also those of others; many relatives of . . . respirator patients did likewise." Grace Audet's mother was allowed to spend eight hours a day with her daughter in a Des Moines, Iowa, hospital, perhaps because the family home was eighty miles away. Other parents, however, were allowed in only during visiting hours. My mother, like some others, volunteered to work as a nursing assistant, giving hot packs on the polio wards. Her work on the ward helped ensure that all patients, including me, received the necessary care, and it enabled her to snatch a few minutes now and then to visit me.[11]

More typically, visits during the period of isolation, if they were allowed at all, were brief and not very satisfying for either visitor or patient. Visitors were gowned and told to stay away from the bed and not to touch their child. Irving Zola, for example, was isolated in a private room where his parents visited "eerily dressed in long hospital gowns and face masks." Other parents could see their children only through glass doors or talk to them from the parking lot through an open ward window. Fathers and mothers who visited didn't always stay in the doorway; "when no one was looking, parents crept across the room to kiss their paralyzed children and touch their feverish faces." For some children, a parental visit only heightened their fears. After a few days in isolation they had come to realize that "visitors were allowed only when doctors thought the patient wouldn't live much longer."[12]

Clearly, considerable variation existed regarding isolation visitation policies for parents and spouses. Smaller hospitals and those in the west seem to have been more flexible than larger and eastern hospitals. Some severe epidemics led hospitals to ban all visits, while others welcomed the families' assistance in caring for paralyzed patients. One rationale for limiting or prohibiting family visits in isolation wards was to prevent the spread of the virus. However, several studies in the early fifties demonstrated the strong likelihood that by the time a polio patient was taken to the hospital other family members were either already infected or immune. Since family members were probably already exposed, keeping close family members from visiting their son, daughter, or spouse did little to prevent the spread of the disease if the visitor observed reasonable precautions. In addition, doctors and nurses who worked daily in intimate contact with infectious patients were seldom quarantined, nor were those parents who volunteered to provide assistance during an epidemic. Furthermore, toward the end of the epidemics several studies of polio patients demonstrated a growing awareness that the psychological and emotional costs of separation were substantial and had a potentially negative impact on the patient's adjustment to hospitalization, her response to the disease, and the family's relationships.[13] Throughout the polio epidemics, however, most hospitals maintained their strict prohibitions on family visits during isolation.

Although the absence of loved ones at bedside compounded the agony of acute poliomyelitis, the physical pain produced as nerves were damaged and paralysis set in occupied the patient's conscious moments for days and sometimes for weeks. Hallucinations, nightmares, and the failure of major bodily functions often accompanied the intense muscle pain and extreme discomfort brought about by the inability to find restful positions. In their more lucid moments, these young men and women experienced directly the terror of immobility and the inability to breathe. Dorothea Nudelman recalled that her acute experience was "unspeakable—the stiffness, fever, chills and agony of being moved, even touched, for a change of bedsheets or night shirt. Total paralysis was like being trapped in a nightmare where you waited to wake up." Charles Mee remembers the fever during a hot summer and the "relentless pain, like the pain of a tooth being drilled without novocaine, but all over my body." Sixteen-year-old Irving Zola thought he was going to die because every time he was "conscious enough to appreciate what was going on, another part of my body felt immobilized."[14] Many polio patients went through the acute phase without any amelioration of the intense pains. Pain was not treated as vigorously at midcentury and many of the most effective painkillers, such as morphine, also depressed breathing, which could be dangerous for polio patients. The acute phase of the disease remains something of a blur for many polio survivors. Days of intense pain, terrible nightmares, and moments of clarity stand out, but much of the experience was lost to conscious memory.

For those whose respiratory muscles were paralyzed, the terror of being unable to breathe intensified the pain and fever. Paralysis of respiration occurred in a small minority of cases, but it was the most dramatic consequence of an attack of polio for both patient and the hospital staff. Respiratory distress could come on slowly or quickly, depending on which muscles were affected and how badly. In cases of bulbar polio where the respiratory center was affected, the onset of paralysis could be quick indeed. When Larry Alexander's chest muscles were becoming paralyzed by spinal polio he was aware of "blackness and a tearing pain in my chest, a pain so intense it numbed my entire mind and body." The iron lungs parked in the hall no longer seemed "monstrous. They were angels of salvation." When the attendants finally slid him into the iron lung, "the weight, the unbearable weight on my chest continued for a few breaths; then, as the dials were regulated, it lifted as if death itself were lifting from my body and my soul."[15]

Not all placements in the iron lung went smoothly. Hugh Gallagher was one of those who underwent an emergency tracheotomy to place a breathing tube into his lungs. The surgery was performed without anesthesia before he was placed in the iron lung. His breathing failed so quickly that the doctor operated in Gallagher's hospital room without explaining what was about to happen. Anesthesia would have depressed his breathing even further, so Gallagher watched the surgeon "slit" his throat as reflected in the doctor's glasses. When the tracheotomy was completed, the attendants lifted Gallagher and ran out of the room and down the hall to insert him in an iron lung. Gallagher fainted but he soon "regained consciousness, a prisoner of the iron lung."[16]

The iron lung was both an "angel of salvation" and a prison. The iron lung, along with crippling and braces, was one of the frightening images of the disease that most Americans of that era carried with them. Dr. Robert Eiben, who worked with many respirator patients at City Hospital in Cleveland, believed that it was "unlikely that there was ever a polio patient who was not fearful of the 'iron lung.'" Patients told him that "they thought going into the tank res-

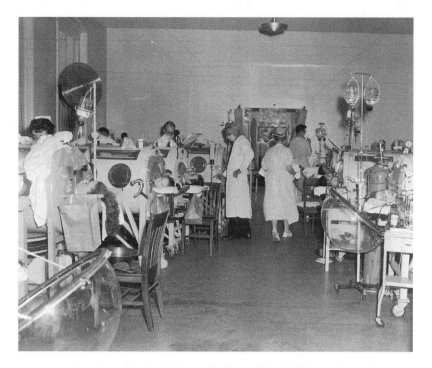

FIG. 5. Iron lungs in an isolation ward at Haynes Memorial Hospital during an epidemic in Boston, Massachusetts, August 3, 1955, illustrating conditions during the acute phase of the illness. Note the crowding, the gowned and masked doctors, and the mix of ages and sexes of the patients.

pirator meant almost certain death, and others equated the machine with a coffin in which they would be buried."[17] Patients were fully aware of the large yellow tanks standing in hallways or the corners of wards waiting for the next patient who needed one. In many hospitals polio patients could hear the rhythmic sound of the bellows moving air in and out of paralyzed lungs elsewhere on the floor. It was all too easy in one's own pain and fever to imagine the terrifying possibility of being placed in an iron lung.

In spite of their fearsome reputation, iron lungs saved many polio patients, most of whom would eventually be able to breathe on their own once again. However, sufficient iron lungs were not always available in remote locations or during severe epidemics. Then doctors faced "agonizing decisions" in choosing which patient would use the lung, "the patient with the severest disability, who possibly would die anyway; or the patient with lesser disability and a better prognosis." Louise Lake recalled that doctors had originally planned to put her in an iron lung, but decided instead to use the one respirator they had for a young mother who had just given birth. Her case seemed to the doctors to be "more hopeful" than Lake's deteriorating condition. However, in spite of the aid provided by the iron lung, the young mother died within a week. Lake survived an agonizing struggle to breathe on her own.[18] Even when available, iron lungs could not save every patient whose respiratory system was attacked. Josephine Howard saw five of her six children and her husband contract polio. Her son Richard was the most seriously paralyzed and in an iron lung. The hospital permitted her and her husband to visit their son briefly and then to sit outside the room and "listen to the pumping." Unfortunately, they were not with their son when he died. After seeing his daughter Alta placed in an iron lung, Luther Robinson spent the night in the hospital with his other daughter Anita, who died as he slept nearby. Tests after her death revealed virulent spinal bulbar polio that had killed quickly.[19]

Although iron lungs saved many lives, some polio patients died in the machines. The iron lungs worked best in cases of spinal polio that attacked the respiratory muscles, but even here almost half of the patients died. Bulbar polio that affected the cranial nerves of the throat also caused respiratory insufficiency by closing the airway, but in these cases the iron lung was ineffective. Bulbar patients were also at risk of pneumonia and of choking on secretions. Approximately 60 percent of patients with bulbar respiratory polio died. Some individuals had both types, and their prognosis was especially poor.[20]

Hospital staff generally tried to shield other patients from the deaths of ward mates, but patients quickly learned to read the unmistakable signals. Patients accustomed to the rhythmic sound of the iron lungs in the ward knew instantly when one was silenced. As Sid Moody recalled, "Part of you is alert to any break in the blanking rhythm which might jeopardize the life of someone now your friend." Iron lungs in the hall or curtains drawn around a bed or respirator in the ward were also signs that someone had died. Kathryn Black discovered that "for those in iron lungs, the death signal was the passing of a nurse down the row of tanks, turning each mirror so the patients couldn't watch while a body was wheeled out in a now silent machine."[21]

In spite of the constant presence of death on the acute polio wards, most patients survived. The paralysis of their muscles did not mean, however, that acute polio patients spent their days in restful repose. Acute polio wards were hives of activity. Virtually everything had to be done for the patients when paralysis was at its most extensive. Patients had to be fed, bathed, moved when uncomfortable, assisted in urination and defecation. Many could not cover themselves, scratch an itch, blow a nose, or wipe a tear away without help. Physicians and nurses also worked to try to prevent permanent deformities by either splinting affected limbs to keep them in a nearly normal position, or, increasingly, using hot packs to provide pain relief and to loosen tightened muscles. In addition to the physical pain of acute polio, patients had quickly to accustom themselves to a lack of privacy, and, in many cases, substantial dependence on others for even the most intimate of tasks. Polio imposed an infant-like dependence that many, especially older patients, found difficult to accept. Being an acute polio patient was hard work.

Hugh Gallagher recalled that the acute stage of his disease required "the concentration of both mind and body. . . . The struggle was intense, exhausting, and constant." Jim Marugg remembered that his body "was watched and tended as if it were an expensive and complicated machine. . . . Its air intake controlled by the faithful respirator. Its calculated amount of nourishment injected into it without the effort of chewing and swallowing. Its waste removed by enemas and catheters and throat pumps."[22]

Nursing patients in iron lungs was difficult for both attendant and patient. During the acute phase of their illness most patients needing this level of respiratory support could not breathe on their own for more than a minute or two. Access to the patient's body was through portholes along the side of the tank that opened, or the patient on his bed could be slid forward out of the tank. Opening portholes significantly reduced the effectiveness of the respirator, leaving the patient gasping for breath. Opening the tank entirely left the patient dependent on his own paralyzed muscles for however long he was out. In their early days in the respirator, unable to breathe on their own, patients were terrified when nurses and orderlies opened the portholes to give necessary care. When a nurse opened Louis Sternburg's respirator to care for him, he immediately felt "a new wave of terror" as he suddenly lost his breath. He "screamed for help, but it came out only as a faint whisper." In order to clean Sternburg adequately, they had to pull him out of the respirator, but he had no ability to breathe on his own. Having an anesthesiologist "bag breathe" him through his tracheotomy tube did not work well; nor did using the clear "plastic bubble" that fit over the head end of the respirator. Similarly, Hugh Gallagher remembered how "exceedingly difficult" his care in the lung was for the nurses and how "painful" it was for him. The rubber cuffs around the portholes through which the nurses stuck their arms never provided a tight seal. These "drops in pressure would result in shallow breaths, half-filled lungs. It was annoying, frightening, to be robbed of expected air through circumstances outside one's body."[23] Until the patients could breathe on their own, even for a few minutes, none of the options available to the staff for necessary care were good ones.

In spite of the fact that the patients' bodies were encased in a steel cocoon, all their regular bodily functions needed to be maintained and more. Nurses had to scratch where it itched, move arms, legs, and torso to more comfortable positions, cover or uncover the body depending on temperature, bathe the patient when needed, and provide urinals and bedpans. As Jim Marugg remembered, "attendants treated my bedsores, moved my limbs, cleaned my teeth, washed me, now and then shaved me and chopped off my hair around the edges." He was irritated that he couldn't change position, find a cooler spot on the bed, or itch his heels. "The indignities of bedpan and feeding wounded my spirit." During his acute crisis, Hugh Gallagher developed bedsores and, because his bowels were not working, a fecal impaction. After several days he was "raped" in a "horrible and humiliating manner" by a nurse who "reached in and ripped out the fecal matter piece by piece. She did it without warning and without explanation; she did it without sedatives or anesthesia."[24]

During the height of their paralysis these patients were totally dependent upon the nursing staff to meet all of their physical needs. Even when allowed to visit during the acute stage of the illness, parents and spouses were generally limited to feeding the patient or providing other minor care. Patients quickly learned how dependent they were on the hospital staff and the necessity of placating them and complying with hospital regulations and routine as much as possible. Jim Marugg remembered that the nurses were always "within call," and "they did the best they could," but because nursing respirator patients was so labor intensive, the nurses "had a routine to perform and the patient had to fit into the routine." It was frustrating when you could do nothing for yourself and had to "wait and wait and try to catch the attention of someone hurrying by and stop him." Arnold Beisser acknowledged "a blind rage" when attendants thought they knew better than he what he needed to be comfortable. But he generally kept his rage bottled up because "you cannot get mad in hospitals. If you do, you may be in trouble. The next time you call for something, there may be a long delay in the nurses' response, or no response at all. There is always more than enough for the nurses to do in hospitals. . . . Angry patients come last." Patients quickly learned that they got better care by adopting what Howard Brody has called the role of "the good handicapped person." By not lashing out in frustration, by accommodating themselves to hospital routine as much as possible, and by working with, not against, the staff, most polio patients learned that nurses generally responded quickly and cheerfully to their myriad needs and requests. As Hugh Gallagher acknowledged, "with the exception of an older cranky nurse . . . my nurses were a cheerful, pleasant, dedicated crew. Every one of them during the crisis worked very, very, hard." Arnold Beisser recalled that "compassionate helpers" made him "feel human again. . . . The pariah was forgiven for his crime, and felt restored to life." [25]

While none of these respirator-dependent patients would have survived without good nursing care that extended over weeks, and sometimes months or years, many of them also experienced indifferent, overworked, abusive, or cruel nurses and attendants. Because they were so helpless and dependent upon these staff members, many of the patients silently buried their rage and anger at the cruelty directed toward them. To reveal that anger in the hospital setting was only likely to bring forth even more abuse. Doctors and nurses at midcentury were accorded considerable power over patients and most patients and parents or spouses were unwilling to challenge medical power and authority. Furthermore, with visitors prohibited or severely restricted, patients had few opportunities to seek help from someone outside the hospital structure. In some cases, the behavior of the nurses reflected only indifference, or irritation at having to do everything for totally paralyzed men and women. The quality of Arnold Beisser's care directly affected how he felt about himself: "If I was cared for willingly and without reluctance, I felt good and the world was sunny. If my care was given grudgingly or irritably, in a callous way, powerful feelings of degradation swept over me." Others had more harrowing experiences. Regina Woods remembers respirator patients being "treated worse than animals, and . . . frequent displays of unbelievable ignorance and cruelty, like that of the nurse who cut the bows from some flowers I had received and taped them into the hair of a young man who, at sixteen, had lost his manhood before having a chance to gain it." Woods and other respirator patients experienced fear and rage when nurses kept them out of the iron lung too long: "Fear that they would not survive the next attempt to help them and rage that they could do nothing to strike back when the keepers went beyond the bounds of human decency, which they did quite often." One day nine-year-old Marilyn Rogers was crying because the cloth around her neck to prevent the collar of the iron lung from rubbing had slipped. When she told the nurse what was wrong, "she just told me to stop crying. She said she would turn my respirator off if I didn't stop crying. When she did I passed out immediately."

Other assistants "saddened" by the nurse's actions turned the respirator back on. Rogers recalled, "I didn't say anything because I was too afraid." After she told her mother what had happened, she never saw that nurse again, but the damage had been done, her "neck was worn away down to the bone" and it took months to heal.[26]

When family members were allowed to spend considerable time with their paralyzed child or spouse they provided additional nursing assistance and tried to protect their kin. Louis Sternburg's wife Dottie protected him "like a tigress, constantly watching the nurses and doctors. . . . She decided who were the best doctors and wouldn't let anyone else near me. She learned to help the overworked nurses by doing as much as she could for me herself." Dottie recalls spending most of every day at the side of Louis's iron lung and "did anything I could to help. . . . I emptied catheters, ran for supplies, applied hot packs to alleviate the pain of muscle spasm, anything they would let me do." Similarly, Regina Woods recalled that there were "many instances in which my family, who had practically lived in the hospital, had intervened to protect me."[27]

Patients, especially men, found the complete dependence during the acute phase of poliomyelitis very difficult to accept.[28] In their own eyes, and often in the attitudes and words of their nurses and attendants, they had been reduced to the condition of babies. Like babies, they could do little for themselves, but they never completely lost their sense of manhood, and the incongruity between their treatment and their sense of self added to their pain. Kenneth Kingery couldn't imagine why they wanted to bring him warm milk instead of coffee: "Ugh! Warm milk—trying to treat me like a baby." He also objected to talk of "weaning" him from the respirator as "blasted baby talk." Even when they acknowledged that there was some logic to the analogy, these men found it difficult to accept. Beisser found that "I had to deal with all of the overwhelming, degrading conditions of dependency that belong with infancy and childhood—at the same time that I considered myself a mature adult. . . . The baby and the man were in conflict."[29]

This agony of infant-like reversion to dependency was all the more painful when medical attendants treated these men as babies and even called them babies. Arnold Beisser's discomfort was heightened by the way others treated him: "Some seemed concerned with controlling what they considered the unruly child, while others wanted to nurture a helpless infant. Nurses and attendants often talked to me as if I were a baby. If I became soiled through no fault of my own, they were likely to say, 'Naughty, naughty,' or 'You've been a

bad boy.'" When a new night nurse grew frustrated at Kenneth Kingery's repeated requests to be turned, she exploded, "Well, you're more darn trouble
than a two-year-old, and I expect you to *grow up*." As Kingery recalled, "She
couldn't have calculated a better set of words with which to shrivel my self-
respect." Lorenzo Milam, writing years later, was still incensed at the indignity
of being forced to wear a diaper when he was nineteen: "I am the child again.
I dirty my bed, so they give me a diaper, so I can dirty that. I have no control,
filled as I am to the brimming with mineral oil, milk of magnesia. I am out
of control. Dignity gets it with the bludgeon." [30] The thoughtless comments
of harassed, frustrated, and overworked nurses and attendants reinforced the
patients' self-realization of their child-like dependency and assaulted their
fragile sense of dignity and manhood.

Nothing, except perhaps power failures, caused more fear in iron lung patients than the first efforts to have them breathe on their own again without
the assistance of the respirator. Dr. John Affeldt, who directed the respiratory
center at Rancho Los Amigos near Los Angeles, acknowledged that although
patients wanted out of the iron lungs, they were also afraid. The key to reducing fear was continual reassurance that the "staff was there to help." [31] While
compassionate staff could sympathize and work with the patients to build
trust and confidence, it was the patients who, when they were slid out of the
iron lung, experienced the heavy weight on their chest, the suffocating feeling
of insufficient air, the hard work of trying to breathe, even for just a minute or
two. And if the staff was not compassionate or careful, it was the patients who
wore themselves out attempting to breathe, or in some cases, blacked out from
lack of oxygen. The process of weaning a patient from the iron lung was a deli-
cate one. It was necessary to lengthen the stay outside the lung to give the
muscles a chance to work on their own and to get stronger. Lengthening the
stay outside, however, always meant pushing just beyond the time the patient
could comfortably breathe on her own. For the process to work smoothly, the
patients had to trust that the nurses and physical therapists would be closely
attentive to their breathing and not push the time out beyond their very limited capacity. It is, thus, not surprising that the process was fraught with terror for those who had come to rely on the respirator to keep them alive.

Initial efforts to wean patients from the iron lung did not always go well,
in part because of the patients' fear that they would not be able to breathe on
their own, or that the nurses would not return them to the security of the iron
lung in time, but also in part because doctors and nurses were not always sensitive to the different capacities of their patients. Although some of the prob-

lems appear to have been the result of applying a standard weaning timetable inappropriately, other problems stemmed from a basic lack of trust rooted in the callous and brutal behavior of some attendants. On her first day out of the iron lung, Regina Woods had spent two reasonably comfortable, but tiring, hours on a bed using a chest respirator. The nurses, however, refused her request to be returned to the lung briefly to gain strength after they took the chest respirator off and before they performed their necessary tasks. Woods passed out from lack of oxygen before she was returned to the iron lung. From then on, she was "filled with fear about leaving the lung." Kenneth Kingery discovered to his dismay that when nurses opened the lung to care for him he "had to *work* to breathe." He dreaded the opening of the lung because "there was always a helpless terror—wondering whether they'd close the tank in time." Forcing the patients to breathe on their own was supposed to give them confidence in their returning muscle strength. But, as Kingery wrote, "whatever confidence I gained from these fish-out-of-water torture trials came *after* each tank opening. Never before." While the process could never be entirely comfortable for those in iron lungs, some hospital staff seemed intent on heightening the fears of the patients. For example, one of Hugh Gallagher's therapists played a cruel game to test his slowly returning breathing capacity. If she found him asleep, "she would turn off the respirator and, with a stopwatch, time how long it was before I awoke from suffocation." Once the panicking Gallagher woke up, she would laugh and turn the respirator back on.[32]

Wards of iron lungs thumping and whooshing away and the harrowing experiences of those reliant on them represent the most dramatic images from the acute poliomyelitis hospitals. However, many patients less severely paralyzed also found their hospitalization for acute poliomyelitis to be difficult, frightening, and alienating. As the fever and pains of the critical stage of poliomyelitis receded, the challenge facing physicians was to prevent the development of deformities. Because the poliomyelitis virus was so erratic in the damage it did to the nerves that served the muscles, many patients were left with unbalanced pairs of muscles. One muscle might be largely unaffected while the opposing muscle was severely weakened or even permanently paralyzed. This could easily produce the characteristic physical deformities of polio as the stronger of the paired muscles pulled the body in unnatural ways. Post-fever acute care for poliomyelitis patients during the 1930s had come to rely heavily on the immobilization of affected limbs using splints, braces, and plaster casts designed to keep the affected parts of the body in their natural positions. The purpose of the splints was threefold: "(1) to balance muscles and thereby retain neutrality of muscle pull, (2) to protect weakened muscles, and (3) to support limbs or other parts of the body." Dr. Philip Lewin recommended a variety of devices for the immediate orthopedic care of polio patients, including splints, footboards to prevent foot drop, sandbags, pillows, fabric restraints, and plaster casts. In the view of Dr. John Paul, "the 1930s was decidedly an era when early and prolonged splinting of paralyzed limbs was carried to excess."[33]

By 1940, however, as John Paul notes, physicians had recognized that "the fashion of treating weak limbs by early and prolonged immobilization had gone too far."[34] That is borne out by the narratives, in which the only form of restraint commonly mentioned was the footboard at the end of the bed to prevent foot drop. Still, some patients in the early forties spent considerable time immobilized by various restraints. For example, Richard Owen, who was twelve when he had polio in 1940, spent nine months in "Toronto splints, which were leather covered splints that kept the knees bent, the feet pulled out a bit, and the legs spread apart." This reliance on immobilization had become so established that it took, as John Paul observed, "a vigorous personality to show that the prevailing system of rigid and prolonged fixation of paralyzed limbs was not having the desired effect, and could be harmful."[35] That vigorous personality was, of course, Sister Elizabeth Kenny.

Elizabeth Kenny was an Australian nurse who had developed a method of treating paralyzed polio patients with hot packs of wet wool and "the development of muscle power by reëducation, or the re-awakening of impulse." Kenny came to the United States in 1940 to push for the adoption of her treatment methods just as physicians were beginning to question the value of intensive and prolonged immobilization. She condemned immobilization because it prevented her from treating the effects of the disease and failed to prevent muscle spasms and permanent deformities. In addition, immobilization often produced psychological problems in patients.[36]

The Kenny system of treatment involved the use of hot wool packs to reduce pain and muscle spasm, the stretching of contracted muscles, and the therapist-guided reeducation of paralyzed muscles and limbs. Kenny was particularly concerned to reduce muscle spasm, a condition she conceived. "Spasm" involved a "series of contractions" that were "rapidly repeating" and were exacerbated by attempts to relax the muscles. She believed that untreated spasm could result in permanently contracted muscles. Hot packs were to be applied early in the patient's hospitalization, while the stretching and reeducation generally began after the acute stage of the disease had passed.[37]

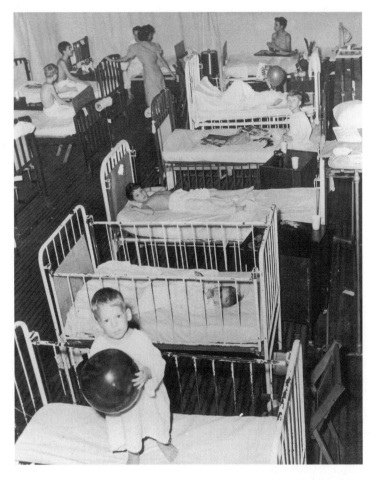

FIG. 6. Polio patients in a makeshift ward in the Evangelical and Reformed Church, Akron, Ohio, September 16, 1947. The nearby Children's Hospital created a ward in the church gymnasium to handle the overflow during an epidemic. The young boy with the ball is Kenneth Lute, age 2, of Mogadore, Ohio.

Kenny's relationship with the American medical establishment was a difficult one. Most physicians eventually rejected her theory of poliomyelitis, that it was a muscle disease not a nerve disease, even as they adopted her methods of treatment. John Paul concluded that "Sister Kenny's ideas and techniques marked a turning point, even an about-face, in the aftercare of paralytic poliomyelitis." Through her persistence, "she helped to raise the treatment of paralyzed patients out of the slough into which it had sunk in the 1930s." Paul felt that her methods also had significant psychological benefits. As he observed, "there was little use in exhorting a patient to exert himself physically if he was in a plaster cast."[38]

Beginning in the early forties, patients with paralytic poliomyelitis could expect to be swathed in wet wool hot packs as soon as their fever broke. Recollections of the smell of wet wool is a constant in narratives from the forties and fifties. Hot packs, and the often painful stretching of stiff muscles, was part of the rite of passage from illness to recovery. The hot packs, or "foments" as Kenny called them, were typically made of old wool blankets because wool retained the heat well and was less likely to burn the patients. The wool pieces were cut individually for each patient in order to fit properly. They were heated in a tub of very hot water, removed with tongs, run through a wringer twice, and placed carefully on the patient. During the height of the crisis, the hot packs were used twenty-four hours a day and were replaced hourly. Once the crisis passed, they were applied from 8:00 A.M. to 8:00 P.M. at two-hour inter-

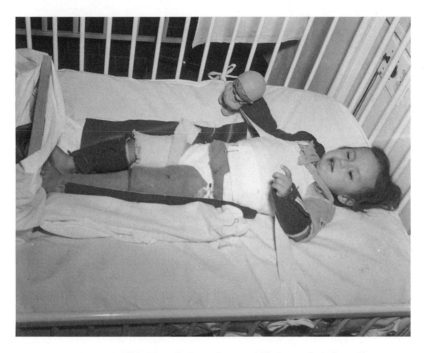

FIG. 7. A young child, Consuela Garza, is wrapped in hot packs in her crib at Shannon Hospital, San Angelo, Texas, June 1949.

vals. The packs quickly lost their heat, but Kenny argued that the alternating hot and cold temperatures stimulated recovery of muscle function. The hot packs were often covered with other layers in an attempt to retain the heat as long as possible. Kenny recommended continuing the hot packs as long as the muscles exhibited spasms.[39]

Hot packs were both welcomed for the relief they brought to tight, painful muscles, and dreaded for the smell of wet wool, for the ever present threat of being burned, and for the itching that accompanied the packs as they cooled. The packs themselves brought a forced immobility, for there was little one could do while wrapped in pieces of hot, wet wool. The ritual was the same day after day, until the muscle spasms subsided. Margaret Benbow recalled that when measured for her packs she had little inkling of what was to come. The nurse cut three sets: "army blankets," "some kind of cellophane or plastic," and "cotton blanketing." The wet wool was placed on the body first, followed by the plastic, and then "the cotton blanket was pinned on to hold everything together." Even though the hot packs provided some relief, they were dreaded, even hated, by many patients. Charles Mee remembers hot packs as "such a bizarre, disgusting procedure that no one who had polio in those days has forgotten what seemed like a punishment for having gotten sick. The blankets itched, of course, and were either so hot to begin with that they scorched and burned—mere warmth was never considered sufficient—or else they got cold and clammy in short order." Like many others, Dorothea Nudelman dreaded the sound of the treatment cart. Few hospitals at midcentury were air conditioned, so that during the warmer months, when polio was at its height, the heat and humidity intensified the discomfort. As Sharon Kimball recalled, "the combination of the sultry August weather and those hot, moist blankets was very uncomfortable."[40]

Beyond dreading the discomfort of being wrapped in hot, but rapidly cooling, wet wool all day, polio patients feared being burned. The wool was heated in boiling or near-boiling water and the nurses usually removed it from the water with wooden sticks or tongs. Sending the wool pieces through the wringer twice was supposed to reduce the chance of scalding the patient, but it didn't always work. Dorothea Nudelman still remembers children on the ward screaming, which "usually started when someone got burned, scalded by a piece of wet wool." When she was burned, she "sobbed out loud, wore myself out with it. The shock was as bad as the pain. I knew it could happen again." At those times, "terror was alive in the ward." Whatever their anxiety about the procedure, most patients learned to accept the hot packs, not that they had much choice. Nudelman and others quickly learned they were at the mercy of the attendants applying the packs. "If you screamed in terror when you heard the treatment cart at the foot of your bed, you were called a 'whiner.' You got scolded. If you 'cooperated' with the treatment, you got more care. Even tenderness, occasionally, when there was time." In spite of assertions that "hot packs were 'nothing to be afraid of,'" patients, nonetheless, feared them.[41]

Although hot packs had largely supplanted immobilization by the mid 1940s, some forms of restraint continued to be used. In order to combat the characteristic foot drop of poliomyelitis, many patients were required to use a footboard to keep their feet at the proper angle. Many patients recall being forced to lie flat on the mattress, often without a pillow, with their feet pressed against the footboard at the end of the bed. Robert Hall tried to keep his feet "absolutely flat on the footboard," but "it was not easy. It took will power to keep them flat." As his hamstrings tightened, the pain increased and it was "easier to curl up my legs and forget the footboard so the pain would go away." Two men on his ward who couldn't keep their feet flat "had their feet strapped to their footboards. . . . They were in much pain as they writhed back and forth across their beds with their feet anchored to their footboards." Even into the 1950s some physicians still combined the older method of immobilization with the newer hot pack procedures. For example, Joyce Ann Tepley, who had polio in 1952, wore "metal and felt-lined splints all the time so that my leg muscles would not draw up," and twice a day she was draped in strips of hot wool blankets.[42] As with many medical treatments, the older procedures retained adherents, even as the new were widely adopted.

Splinting and hot packs were orthodox treatments for acute poliomyelitis, but other unusual treatments existed. Both Barb Grile and Grace Audet remember a series of daily penicillin shots while in isolation. Sharon Kimball recalls not wanting to take either of the "vile kinds of red and green liquids" she was given. Robert Gurney's physician gave him a shot of vitamin B1 every morning, telling him, "We don't know if it is going to help, but we know damn well it isn't going to do any harm!" Edmund Sass, who received injections of curare, remains puzzled that his physician injected his "already paralyzed muscles with poison to paralyze them even further." A number of doctors, however, used curare to lessen the tightness of muscles in order to facilitate stretching and to prevent the characteristic deformities of polio without using casts or braces.[43] Some physicians seemed to be prescribing these medicines with little evidence of efficacy and little confidence that they would alter the course of the disease. But perhaps the point was to convince themselves, their patients, and their families that everything possible was being done.

As the fever, pain, and delirium of acute polio receded, patients began to take inventory of their bodies to see what still worked and what remained paralyzed. They tried to move toes, fingers, legs, and arms, and were relieved when bladder, intestines, and sexual organs began to function again. Once out of the isolation ward, Charles Mee lay in bed "getting used to the idea that I hadn't died and taking stock of my body parts." Initially he found he was able to move the fingers of his left hand, and soon after that, his wrist. For Mee, "a very big event, a moment of freedom" came when he could turn over in bed by himself: "If you can turn over in bed, you are no longer entirely immobile."[44] In these little victories over their paralyzed bodies these young men and women measured their efforts to recover.

An important measure of recovery was the return of normal urination and bowel movements. Acute poliomyelitis often temporarily paralyzed muscles in the urinary and intestinal tracts. Until urinary function returned, patients had to be catheterized, itself often painful, especially if it lasted any length of time. When Robert Hall's roommate was finally able to use a urinal by himself, he "let out a whoop and announced to the world at large" his "glad tidings." Paralysis of abdominal muscles and the lack of movement by paralyzed and bedridden patients also led to bowel problems. Many, if not most, polio patients experienced a failure to move their bowels and suffered the energetic efforts of nurses to bring about a bowel movement. Nurses used a variety of laxatives, including milk of magnesia and mineral oil, as well as frequent enemas, often leaving the patients with a deep sense of shame and disgust at their inability to perform such a natural bodily function. Robert Hall recalled that they "had to fight it out with an enema" every other day. Like the others, nineteen-year-old Lorenzo Milam struggled with his bowels and with the shame and embarrassment of losing control. Nurses attacked his impacted bowels by filling him repeatedly with "mineral oil, castor oil, [and] milk of magnesia" until "the bowels turn to water." Bedridden, he often soiled himself and the bed when the nurses didn't respond in time. After the nurses pinned a diaper on him, Milam lay in his "own dismal dirt, moveless, speechless, hopeless, a foul babe again, without hope, with no reason for existence."[45]

This unwelcome reversion to behaviors of infancy was made all the worse because it was so public. In spite of his troubles with urination and defecation, Robert Hall managed to find some humor in the lack of privacy. It seemed inevitable that just as he or another of his ward mates began to use the urinal a student nurse would "come bouncing in." At first, this stopped "production," but Hall soon learned to dispense with modesty. Many patients, however, found the lack of privacy emotionally wrenching—Lorenzo Milam, in particular. When a medical student pulled back the sheet, revealing Milam's naked body, he remembers thinking, "I don't want them looking at me without my clothes, not at all." But he soon realized he had no choice: "No one is listening to me. My body is no longer my own." As his bowel problems mounted, Milam discovered to his dismay that "there is no way to go to the private world of toilet which is our heritage from the age of child on. No privacy, no freedom, no exit." Arnold Beisser echoed these feelings when he realized that his "most private and personal functions rested in the hands of others." He felt "exposed utterly and completely . . . vulnerable to everyone and everything. Nothing was private; there was only wordless shame for what I had become."[46] Here, again, the psychological anguish, the sense of violation, only heightened the physical pain of polio.

For young men paralyzed by polio the inability to achieve an erection and to masturbate caused considerable anxiety that could not be easily shared even with ward mates. Although poliomyelitis rendered many patients temporarily impotent, the problem seldom lasted longer than a few weeks. Like many others, fourteen-year-old Charles Mee was "terrified" when he first "tried to masturbate, and failed." He tried to put the failure in perspective, since he was still terrified at the prospect of dying, but the failure was dismaying nonetheless. Shortly after leaving isolation, while reading an article on the recently published Kinsey Report in *Life* magazine, he was relieved that he "could feel the stirrings of an erection. And so I could check that off the list I hadn't known I was making in my head: My ability to have sex was intact." Irving Zola's impotence lasted several months until one morning he woke up with an erection: "I wanted to shout, 'Look at this!' to my friend in the next bed but was too embarrassed." It took him another week before he could successfully masturbate. As Zola acknowledged in retrospect, he was "trying to reclaim my sexuality, my sense of control, and with it part of my selfhood."[47]

As the fever, pain, and delirium of acute poliomyelitis lessened, patients became more cognizant of their surroundings. When they were no longer contagious, many were moved out of isolation to a polio ward elsewhere in the hospital. Here they soon made new friends and were integrated into life on a polio ward. Transfer out of isolation was a sign of progress and most polio patients found their spirits lifted in their new quarters. After a disinfecting bath,

Robert Hall was taken to the convalescent ward where he joined friends who had been moved earlier. As he remembered, "there was something symbolic about moving into that new ward." He found the routine in the new ward "so much more enjoyable." Nurses no longer wore masks, patients took warm baths instead of being covered in hot, wet wool, and visitors were allowed twice a week.[48] Although convalescent and rehabilitation wards would pose their own challenges in the weeks and months to come, the initial experience was a welcome relief from isolation and the terrifying and painful experience of acute poliomyelitis.

Although the convalescent polio wards were generally less restrictive than isolation wards, the limited visiting policy of many midcentury hospitals was a source of continuing irritation and even anger. Where some hospitals had permitted unlimited visits when the patients were sickest and in danger of dying, they reverted to once or twice weekly visits once the patient was moved out of isolation. For patients who were still very ill, and whose emotions were fragile, the limits on parents or spouses visiting was very difficult. For example, Kenneth Kingery was devastated after moving out of isolation to the "slightly-more-cheerful world" of the polio ward. The nurse told his wife she would have to leave and, since Kingery was better, she would now be allowed to visit only twice a week. He wondered whether he had "committed a crime in contracting polio." Other hospitals were more flexible about visiting. Dottie Sternburg was able to spend most of every day with her husband in his iron lung even after his acute crisis had passed. Part of the reason may have been that she quickly became another pair of hands to help care for someone totally dependent on others. Whether it happened every day or only once or twice a week, these boys and girls, men and women soon learned to listen for familiar footsteps. Charles Mee observed that everyone "has one memory vivid above all others: the sound of their mother's high-heeled shoes in the hallway—utterly distinct from the shoes of anyone else's mother—when she came to visit."[49]

Although not all hospitals severely restricted visitation after patients were out of isolation, those that did seem to have done so to facilitate control over the patient. As Fred Davis put it in his classic sociological study of fourteen polio families, "a prime prerequisite for structuring and defining the child's recovery orientation in the hospital is the loosening of his affective ties with home and his immersion into the hospital's subculture of illness." So long as the child continues to miss his parents desperately, "his incorporation of hospital routines and values is mechanical at best." When parents visited frequently, they served as a counterforce to the authority of the physician and the hospital, and from the point of view of the medical staff, the child was less likely to cooperate. Davis acknowledged that this immersion was aided by the reduction of parental visits, by hospital staff assuming a parental role, and by their creating a more home-like atmosphere on the ward through "familiar activities and diversions" (television, games, picture and comic books, group play, etc.)[50] Clearly the situation was more complicated with adolescent and adult patients who were capable of assuming greater responsibility for dealing directly with the physicians and hospital staff. Yet, I suspect that something similar operated with adult or nearly adult patients who were restricted to only weekly or biweekly visits. Many of them came out of the polio crisis very fragile psychologically, lacking in self-confidence, and dependent on the staff for almost everything. At this vulnerable point, the absence of any regular visitor, such as a parent or spouse, who could become an effective advocate, left many of these older patients with no real choice but to cooperate, accepting and adapting to the routines of the ward and the habits of the staff.

While the vast majority of polio patients were hospitalized, at least for the acute stage of the disease, a much smaller number were never hospitalized and were treated at home. In most instances, these were relatively mild cases that did not require skilled nursing care. Some doctors decided that during a serious epidemic such mild cases could be better cared for at home.[51] At home the patient would likely get the full attention of the parents and the home care would free up a bed and nursing staff to care for those more severely stricken. Dick Weir's family physician wanted to send him to the nearest polio ward sixty-five miles away. His parents didn't want their son to be so far away and insisted they could care for him at home in spite of paralysis in both his legs and arms. His father's sister, who had had polio thirty years before, came to help, and they had the assistance of a nurse trained in Sister Kenny's methods. The local Lions Club purchased a hot pack machine which the family used, along with regular rubdowns with Ben-Gay, to treat the six-year-old.[52] Treating an acute polio patient at home had a significant impact on family life. The family might be quarantined until the danger of infection had passed, and the necessary care could be onerous. But even when the family member was hospitalized, the impact on the family was often significant and long lasting.

Polio struck families as well as individuals. Parents or spouses spent long days at the hospital waiting anxiously for the crisis to pass or, in some cases, helping to care for a son or daughter, husband or wife. The family members left at home had to fend for themselves and were sometimes quarantined for several weeks. Even when families were not formally quarantined by public health authorities, neighbors and friends fearing infection often shunned families in which polio had appeared. Families also bore emotional and psychological costs due to polio. Siblings sometimes resented the attention that their brother or sister received or felt abandoned by parents who spent all their time at the hospital. Finally, there were financial worries. Somebody was going to have to pay for the costly hospitalization, and parents and spouses worried how they were going to afford the expensive care at a time when most Americans lacked adequate health and hospital insurance.

Many families tried to station a family member at the hospital during the acute stage of polio. If the hospital permitted, she might stay in the room, or just outside, but she remained in a waiting room if hospital regulations kept her from the bedside. Parents and spouses were anxious to provide reassurance and emotional support, to assist in care in any way they could, and to learn what they could from the doctors and nurses. Hugh Gallagher's parents, for example, were allowed to visit him "once or twice a day for a few minutes," but he also remembers them standing in the rain outside the screened window of his isolation room. He later learned that his mother "spent the two weeks of the crisis seated on a straight-back chair in the small lobby of the quarantine building, 'awaiting developments.'" Grace Audet's mother spent days by her daughter's hospital bed reading to her. Her mother's voice was soothing to the eight-year-old girl and helped her rest. Some family members were able to provide more than just emotional support. Dottie Sternburg spent most of her days at the hospital, where she quickly became a valued adjunct to those nursing her totally paralyzed husband. She interceded when she thought he was being badly treated and soon learned basic nursing skills to relieve the burden on the staff.[53] While it was not always easy to gain access to polio patients in isolation, some parents and spouses who waited daily at the hospital succeeded. Perhaps because of their own assertiveness, an understanding and flexible physician, or a shortage of staff, some families found ways to provide comfort and reassurance and, occasionally, to help care for their acutely ill child or spouse.

Family members who remained at home were also affected by a case of acute poliomyelitis. Most significantly, several studies demonstrated that a case of poliomyelitis significantly increased the risk to other members of the family. In spite of the increased danger, multiple cases of paralytic polio in a single family were relatively rare. A study of the 1949 epidemic in New York revealed that over 95 percent (2,235) of the families had only one case, 4.2 percent (98) had two cases, and just 0.2 percent (5) had three cases. While rare, multiple cases had a devastating effect on a family. Ann McLaughlin and her husband Charles both had polio in 1955, which they probably caught from their nine-month-old son who had a "mild case." Both McLaughlins were seriously affected and spent months in hospitals before being reunited with their young son. In 1953, polio struck both thirty-three-year-old Ted Hoover and his two-year-old daughter Penny. Ted died during his first night in the hospital and Penny survived with significant paralysis.[54]

Even in families with only one case of paralytic polio, the lives of those unaffected were significantly altered. When a parent had polio, provision often had to be made to care for the children, especially if the spouse was spending long hours at the hospital, and older children were expected to take on greater responsibilities in the household. While some families successfully coped with the intense emotions surrounding polio, others fell apart. John Lindell remembered that his "whole family was in turmoil" as a result of his own and his son's simultaneous polio. His wife, Ruth, continued to teach to provide an income for the family, and then drove an hour to visit either her husband or her son. Their fourteen-year-old son came home to an empty house, and the two younger children went from school to a nearby orphanage to wait for their mother to pick them up after her hospital visits. Dottie Sternburg was not allowed to see her two very young children for a month after their father contracted polio and entered the iron lung. She spent long days at the hospital and left her children in the care of a nurse. The nurse's family, fearing polio, would not allow her to visit them on her days off, so she cared for the Sternburg children without a day off for several months.[55]

Polio and the permanent crippling of a close brother or sister could alter sibling relationships. James Carroll, who was about four when his seven-year-old brother had polio, found the roles of older and younger brother reversed: "I did everything asked of me, and more than was expected. Yet my every success, since it came at Joe's expense, would feel like a failure." Carroll came to see his brother's illness as "the radioactive mushroom cloud" hanging over this Irish Catholic family's complex internal dynamics. Kathy Vastyshak remembers that her polio had a "large impact" on her family. Her brother, who was two years older, "was left pretty much to fend for himself at a young age," and although her parents had wanted more children, they decided against it because they were "too busy" caring for their daughter.[56]

Although the official quarantining of families in which polio occurred was much less common in the forties and fifties than it had been earlier, family members were often advised to limit their outside contacts for several weeks. Sometimes they had no choice; neighbors and more distant family members shunned close relatives of a polio patient. When my mother took my younger sister and a friend for a walk after I had been hospitalized, one of the neighbors called the city health department, which sent a nurse to talk to my mother. The nurse, who knew my mother, told her that she could safely take my sister for a walk, but my mother, nonetheless, felt ostracized. When Charlene Pugleasa had polio in northern Minnesota in 1953 her family was quarantined for two weeks. Only her father was allowed to leave the house to go to work in the mine, where he had to shower before going into the mine, as well as upon leaving. The school informed Pugleasa's parents that they had burned her desk, everything in her locker, and all her school books before disinfecting her locker. Given the contagiousness of polio and the uncertainties about how the virus was acquired, the fears of neighbors and friends were understandable. Most families, however, soon discovered relatives or friends who would help out with child care, making meals, and running errands regardless of the risk.[57]

In addition to the psychic and emotional toll that polio exacted from families, many parents and spouses grew anxious as the staggering costs of a severe case mounted. Most families in this period lacked health insurance that covered the extended hospitalization and round-the-clock nursing needed by extensively paralyzed polio patients. For men like Kenneth Kingery and Larry Alexander, who were the major breadwinners in their families, the financial cost of their illnesses was a major worry as they began to assess the magnitude of their severely altered lives. In both cases, they were relieved to discover that the National Foundation for Infantile Paralysis (NFIP) would pay their hospital and medical bills. As Kingery observed, "financial relief was [as] welcome as bodily relief." Arvid Schwartz's father, who was a farmer without health insurance and without the resources to pay his son's sizeable medical bills, was happy to discover that the March of Dimes paid about 90 percent of the bills. Such assistance was commonplace during the early 1950s when the NFIP gave assistance to an average of more than 72,000 individuals a year at an annual cost of more than 26 million dollars.[58]

Although it was widely believed that the NFIP provided assistance in every case of polio, that was simply not true. In many mild cases where the medical bills were small, there was no need for outside assistance. Those who sought assistance from the NFIP had to be evaluated and approved by local chapters. Guidelines from the national headquarters suggested that financial aid was to be given to "any family which would have to lower its standard of living by paying the total costs of medical and hospital care." Although many families clearly met this standard, not all did. Even those who qualified sometimes found the process demeaning. Rosemary Marx's mother still vividly recalls the qualification interview with the local March of Dimes representative. Marx's parents were separated and interviewed individually, "apparently to be sure that they were being truthful." Her mother was reluctant to divulge the family's finances in the absence of her husband. The March of Dimes representative finally told her, "Look, if you don't want to answer these questions, then just take your crippled child home." Although the March of Dimes paid for Marx's hospitalization, not every family who applied qualified. Edmund Sass was discharged from the hospital after only three or four weeks. His stay was shorter than many because the family had exhausted their insurance and the NFIP refused to pay his medical expenses. His father, a carpenter, had "to work side jobs, at night and on the weekends, to pay the medical bills."[59] The NFIP and the March of Dimes did provide substantial financial assistance, especially to those most seriously paralyzed by polio, but the financial burdens of polio were not reduced or eliminated for all families.

A polio patient's stay in the acute care section of the hospital might be as short as a few days or as long as several months. The length of contagiousness, the severity of the paralysis, the readiness for rehabilitation, the need for acute care beds in a serious epidemic, and the availability of beds in an appropriate rehabilitation facility were all factors in the decision to release a patient from isolation wards and acute care. By the early fifties physicians knew that individuals with polio could shed the virus in their feces and thus be contagious for as long as seventeen weeks following the onset of the disease.[60] However, most patients were isolated for much shorter periods, typically no more than two weeks to a month. Once their fevers had returned to normal, the spread of paralysis had ceased, and their conditions had stabilized, patients were usually moved to convalescent or rehabilitation wards, sent to a rehabilitation hospital, or discharged home. Patients in iron lungs were likely to have the longest stays in an acute ward, as the extent of their paralysis and the difficulty of their care limited the options for moving them. Although most acute facilities began the process of weaning iron lung patients from the respirator, it was often not completed until they had been moved to a rehabilitation facility or respiratory center. When they left acute care most polio patients were weak and still partially or fully paralyzed. Ahead lay long months, perhaps years, of hot packs, painful muscle stretching, and physical therapy to rebuild damaged muscles and to compensate for the muscles permanently paralyzed by the virus's attack on the central nervous system.

Covenants of Work: Recovery and the Rehabilitation Hospital

MOVING OUT OF ISOLATION to a convalescent polio ward or to a rehabilitation hospital represented a significant milestone in the recovery from acute poliomyelitis. The patient was beginning to feel better, his temperature had returned to normal, and he was no longer contagious. Parents and spouses often had greater visiting privileges, and they were no longer gowned and masked when they visited. Muscles served by damaged nerves slowly began to function once again. Patients became more aware of their surroundings, and, in the larger wards, began to make friends among their ward mates. While this move was clearly evidence that recovery had begun, it also initiated the long and arduous process of rehabilitation. Patients, with the help of physicians and physical therapists, had to discover what muscle function remained, what could be recovered through physical therapy, and what was lost forever. Rehabilitation was not simply a matter of reconstructing the body out of the wreckage left by the virus, it also meant coming to terms with one's new body, discovering how to compensate and how to rebuild a satisfying life. Although patients and health professionals tended to focus on rebuilding the body, psychological and emotional considerations often came into play. Patients were generally encouraged to be compliant, work hard at the tasks set them, and hope to recover and be released sooner rather than later. Being a good patient meant repressing as well as one could feelings of confusion, fear, anger, rage, hopelessness, and despair. While physicians, surgeons, physical therapists, and nurses focused on rehabilitating the body, the polio survivors of whatever age were largely left alone to deal with the significant emotional and psychological responses to physical crippling and extended rehabilitation and hospitalization. The cost was tremendous.

To the dismay of many polio patients, recovery from the acute phase of the disease did not mean recovery from polio. Unlike the many childhood diseases with which these patients were familiar, polio patients who had more than an

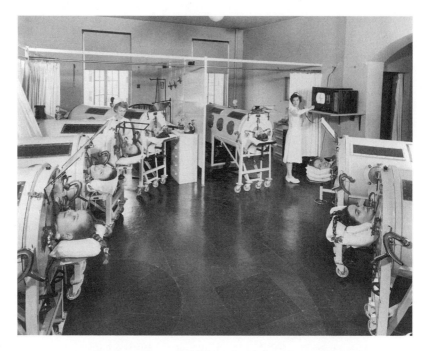

FIG. 8. Respirator Center at Children's Hospital, Baltimore, Maryland, October 1948. Conditions in respirator centers were more orderly than in the acute-care wards. Hospital staff were not gowned and masked, although there was still a mix of sexes and ages. Here we see an early television to entertain the patients.

abortive or inapparent case were not cured when the fever broke and the infection ended. Most polio patients endured months of painful physical therapy as therapists used hot packs to relax contracted muscles before stretching them to restore the full range of function. Long hours would be spent exercising weakened muscles to restore their functioning so they could carry the crippled bodies out of the hospital. Where adequate muscle function could not be reestablished, bracing allowed many to sit, stand, and move by themselves. Later, surgeries sought to restore mobility by transplanting tendons and muscles and to strengthen torsos and limbs by fusing bone to bone to make up for weak or absent muscles. Polio rehabilitation involved more than the hard labor of physical therapy. Just as they were reconstructing their bodies during the months and years of therapy and repeated surgeries, polio sur-

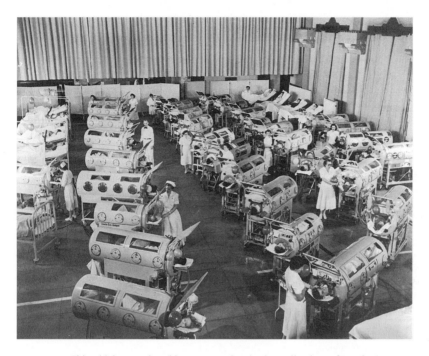

FIG. 9. This widely reproduced image was taken in the auditorium of Rancho Los Amigos Hospital in Downey, California, on December 26, 1952. Patients in iron lungs and on rocking beds were moved from their normal wards to the auditorium solely for this picture. The photograph was used in National Foundation for Infantile Paralysis and March of Dimes publicity.

vivors had to fashion a new identity consistent with their rebuilt bodies and altered range of possibilities.

Polio patients underwent rehabilitation in a wide variety of institutions and hospitals. Many states and some counties and cities supported public rehabilitation hospitals for their children and adults with disabilities. For example, the New York State Reconstruction Home north of New York City and the Gillette Children's Hospital in St. Paul, Minnesota, had been established decades earlier to care for and rehabilitate crippled children whatever the cause. Others, such as the well-known Rancho Los Amigos Medical Center in Downey, California, had been established by the county to care for local residents. There were also facilities, such as the Kenny Clinic at the Wilmington General Hospital in Wilmington, Delaware, that were associated with general hospitals. The Kenny Clinic was established at Wilmington General because it was the only infectious disease hospital in the state that treated acute and contagious polio cases. There were also private rehabilitation institutions such as the Elizabeth Kenny Institute in Minneapolis, Minnesota, and, of course, the Georgia Warm Springs Foundation. Private foundations, patient fees, and the National Foundation for Infantile Paralysis (NFIP) supported these facilities. The Shriners also established a number of hospitals that treated disabled children from low-income families who could not otherwise have afforded expensive hospitalization and rehabilitation. The quality of care at these facilities varied widely. Some, such as Warm Springs and Rancho Los Amigos quickly gained reputations for providing the best in polio rehabilitation, while some state institutions were grim, forbidding places lacking modern facilities and treatment. Where one underwent polio rehabilitation was dependent on geography and the availability of local facilities, on family income that could perhaps support a private institution or if low enough gain admission to a Shrine hospital, and on race, because many facilities, especially in the South, were segregated.[1]

With the exception of facilities dedicated to polio rehabilitation such as Warm Springs and the Kenny Institute, many of these hospitals had been established to treat children and adults with a wide variety of disabling conditions. However, during the polio epidemics of the 1940s and 1950s their rehabilitation wards filled with the many victims of the disease. Surrounded by others similarly afflicted, polio patients became part of a community that generally supported one another and helped them endure separation from family and friends, painful procedures, hospital regulations, and sometimes callous or indifferent care. Ward mates also encouraged and pushed one another to succeed at the hard tasks of rebuilding their bodies and their lives. Although it took far longer than most polio patients expected, physical therapy and surgeries eventually came to an end.

Polio rehabilitation at midcentury was rooted in the Protestant work ethic as well as in the techniques of physical therapy and reconstructive surgery. Cultural expectations shaped responses to polio, and medical professionals sought to inspire their patients by appealing to the widespread notion that hard work inevitably brought rewards. Once the acute phase of polio ended, it was difficult to determine precisely how severely the nerves had been damaged or destroyed. The work ethic coupled with physical therapy enabled patient, therapist, and physician to discover what nerves and muscle function remained, to build toward maximum physical recovery, and to regain some sense of purpose, some sense of self, in a life shattered by disease. The appeal to the work ethic was no accident. As Fred Davis wrote in his study of recovering polio patients, "the paralytic polio treatment procedure is of the quintessence of the Protestant ideology of achievement in America—namely, slow, patient, and regularly applied effort in pursuit of a long-range goal."[2] Although the work ethic psychologically and emotionally helped sustain patients, families, and therapists in the long, arduous task of rebuilding a polio-ravaged body, the ultimate outcome often fell short of a complete recovery. An important part of rehabilitation was learning to accept gracefully the successes achieved and to compensate for and to learn to live with the disabilities that remained.

In addition to the Protestant work ethic, polio rehabilitation in the forties and fifties was shaped by an emerging philosophy of rehabilitation that put the emphasis on "normalizing" people with disabilities so that they could become productive members of society rather than being warehoused in institutions. Promoted by prominent rehabilitation physicians Howard Rusk and Henry Kessler, this theory argued that "disabled people must compensate for their physical or mental impairments with their whole minds and bodies to gain entrance into the work force." This theory required "that disabled people accommodate society rather than have society accommodate them." An individual's rehabilitation from polio would ideally be directed by a rehabilitation team that included "a psychiatrist, a physician, social workers, occupational and physical therapists, [and] vocational rehabilitation experts" whose job was "to make such people fit in with society." Much of rehabilitation was to be directed toward "diminishing what made [disabled people] different from the rest of society." In addition, "rehabilitation was to help disabled people maximize their potential by compensating for their problems." Rusk and Kessler replaced an emphasis on an "anatomical model of the mind and body" with a "functional" one. "That is, rehabilitation medicine no longer concentrated on what disabled people could not do but what they could do. This 'can do' perspective became known as the 'whole man theory' of rehabilitation." These physicians also stressed "building strong and healthy egos" because they were convinced that "people suffered more from the so-called emotional maladjustments or personality defects that accompanied their physical impairments than from the impairments themselves." For these advocates of the new rehabilitation, "people with disabilities, unlike 'normal' healthy people, particularly needed to develop their potential, because a 'sick' individual led to a 'sick' society.'" This rehabilitation doctrine was especially apt in the conformist years following World War II when fitting in politically, socially, and economically was highly valued. In the context of cold war fears, anxieties about postwar prosperity, the flight to the suburbs, and the baby boom, the pressure to appear "normal" and not "sick" was powerful.[3] As applied to polio rehabilitation, as we will see, the burden was on the polio survivor to work hard to recover physically and mentally, to conform to societal expectations, and to make whatever accommodations were necessary to fit in.

What neither physicians, therapists or polio patients realized when they adopted the "can-do" attitude and the Protestant work ethic in the forties and fifties was that these values would set up problems later in life. Many polio survivors so successfully internalized these values that they became touchstones for life. As we will see, by embracing these attitudes most polio survivors returned to home, school, and work, had reasonably successful careers, married and had children. However, some twenty to thirty years after they acquired the disease many polio survivors began to experience disturbing symptoms of muscle weakness, fatigue, and pain that produced new disabilities. By the mid-1980s these symptoms would be collectively recognized as post-polio syndrome. To their dismay, polio survivors learned that the very values that had carried them so far had helped produce the new symptoms and disabilities. In struggling with post-polio they would have to unlearn the lessons of their initial rehabilitation. Instead of "use it or lose it," they would have to make "use it and lose it" their new touchstone. But those problems lay in the future; the more immediate problem was recovering the use of weakened or paralyzed muscles and returning to the life so dramatically interrupted.

It is difficult to specify precisely when rehabilitation from an attack of acute poliomyelitis began. As we saw in the previous chapter, nurses and physical therapists began to work with most patients applying hot packs and moving limbs passively to maintain range of function as soon as the fever receded, the acute pains had lessened, and the patient was again conscious and coherent. Dr. John Affeldt, a physician at the rehabilitation hospital at Rancho Los Amigos near Los Angeles, argued that during the acute phase "all activity must be rigidly disciplined and centered on life saving, forcing curtailment of many desirable and long-range activities that are at that time secondary." That did not mean, however, that no steps could be taken to try to prevent permanent crippling. Traditional orthopedic treatment recommended complete bed rest with the muscles "kept in a position of neutral muscle pull." Deformity was preventable if muscles were "protected from stretching and fatigue," which was achieved through individualized splints. Sister Kenny and physicians who employed her methods also believed that it was important to start treatment during the acute phase of polio. Dr. Miland E. Knapp argued that "rehabilitation of the poliomyelitis patient commences during the acute stage of the disease. Treatment with the eventual rehabilitation of the patient in mind should be started as soon as the diagnosis is made." He had found that "the prevention of contractures," and thus the prevention of permanent deformities, could not "be done as efficiently later in the course of the disease." [4]

Polio rehabilitation almost always required physical therapy. Fortunately, by the time of the epidemics of the forties and fifties physical therapy had emerged as a profession, and trained physical therapists were in greater supply. The two world wars of the twentieth century along with the polio epidemics helped spur the growth of physical therapy because of the large number of war casualties and polio victims. At the time of the First World War, the practice of physical therapy was virtually unknown in the United States, although in a number of European countries physical rehabilitation was more advanced. With over 100,000 disabled soldiers returning from Europe, the War Department began a program to train aides in physical therapy to facilitate the soldiers' return to productive civilian life. The large 1916 polio epidemic in the northeastern United States created another large contingent of individuals with disabilities. Dr. Robert Lovett, an orthopedic surgeon and expert on poliomyelitis at Harvard University, trained a number of young women to administer "muscle training, corrective exercise and massage" to recovering polio patients.[5] Both of these developments were aided by changing views regarding the treatment of individuals with disabilities. Physicians and others involved with the disabled began to argue that with proper rehabilitation many of these individuals could be reintegrated into society as productive citizens instead of being warehoused in institutions.

Alice Lou Plastridge was one of the young women trained by Dr. Lovett. After she had worked in Chicago in private practice for several years, Dr. Lovett in 1926 recommended her to Franklin D. Roosevelt, who was recovering at home in Hyde Park, New York. She worked with FDR for a year before returning to Chicago. In 1929 she accompanied a patient to Warm Springs, where she was soon named director of physical therapy and where she remained for twenty years. In that position she trained many other physical therapists.[6] Following Sister Elizabeth Kenny's arrival in the United States, Plastridge, like many other physical therapists, received training from the Australian nurse in her new methods of treating the disabilities of polio. Kenny's methods, as we will see, fostered a more active role for the patient, and the successes associated with her methods strengthened the role of the physical therapist in rehabilitation. In the early 1940s the NFIP made a number of grants to the University of Minnesota to study the effectiveness of Kenny's methods and to train over one thousand doctors, nurses, and physical therapists to use them on polio patients. In addition, a new emphasis on the idea of "total rehabilitation" used the particular skills of a variety of medical specialties—physical therapy, occupational therapy, physiatry—to enable men and women with disabilities to be fully reintegrated into normal society.[7]

Whether one was rehabilitated by traditional or by Kenny methods, or perhaps by a mixture of both, months of physical therapy lay ahead before bracing or surgery were even considered. The greatest potential for muscle recovery came in the first ten to twelve months, but polio patients could continue to recover muscle function for up to eighteen months after the acute attack. As one physician observed, "recovery in musculature is variable as to amount and time," which meant that "at the start of the disease one cannot judge accurately the potential recovery of the muscles." The only reasonable approach, for physician and patient, was to assume that "the involved muscles will recover, until the subsequent course indicates that they will not."[8]

In the thirties and early forties, the orthodox treatment of post–acute polio patients employed splints to prevent contracture and deformities. The deformities resulted from the selective destruction of motor neurons by the poliovirus. Dr. Philip Lewin, in his *Infantile Paralysis* (1941), made the case for early immobilization to prevent permanent deformities. Immobilization was designed to "correct existing deformities or to maintain normal positions and to keep the joints from becoming over-stretched." The affected muscles were to be kept immobilized for eight weeks, followed by a muscle test. If improvement was noted, this pattern of immobilization followed by muscle tests could be continued for as long as eight months. Once muscle soreness and tenderness ended, Lewin recommended physical therapy that included x-rays, electrical stimulation, massage, and exercise to "actively promote the return of function to weakened or paralyzed muscles."[9]

Some physicians continued to rely on rehabilitative splinting even after the Kenny method became widely accepted in the 1940s. As Dr. William Green of the Harvard Medical School wrote in 1953, "in a considerable percentage of patients, splints of various types are of great assistance." However, Green advised that the splints or casts be designed to go on and off easily so as not to interfere with exercise or treatment with hot packs. These splints and casts were to be used "intermittently." Unlike Lewin, Green cautioned that "continuous immobilization is never desirable." [10]

A dozen years before Sister Kenny challenged rehabilitation orthodoxy in the United States, Franklin D. Roosevelt's decision to establish a facility dedicated to the rehabilitation of polio victims at a failing resort in Warm Springs, Georgia, pointed toward more humane and successful treatment of those disabled by the disease. The story of Roosevelt's discovery of the restorative powers of the warm spring water at the Georgia resort is well known.[11] Several features of Warm Springs made it distinctive in polio rehabilitation. Rather than splinting and immobilization, treatment at Warm Springs began with hydrotherapy in pools of the warm (88–90 degree) spring water. Equally important, Warm Springs put as much emphasis on the social rehabilitation of the polio patient as on his or her physical recovery. Once the warm water had freed the patients' tight spasmodic muscles, they received "the physical therapy treatments necessary to maximize muscle recovery" and learned "the techniques necessary to allow functioning in society to the maximum extent possible." More, perhaps, than any other rehabilitation facility, Warm Springs became "a community of the handicapped." At Warm Springs the extensive social life which developed around the hydrotherapy and exercises "provided a way for polio patients to relearn their social skills." Many of the techniques of physical therapy and innovative bracing developed at Warm Springs were later adapted by other therapists and rehabilitation facilities, but of no other polio rehabilitation facility could it be said that it "was a cheerful, active, lovely resort in the country."[12] Unfortunately, treatment at Warm Springs, which rehabilitated about 100 patients at any one time, remained only a lovely dream for most polio survivors.

While white polio patients dreamed of being treated at Warm Springs, the dream was denied African Americans, who were never admitted during the years of Jim Crow segregation in the South. The Georgia Warm Springs Foundation established the policy in 1937 following inquiries about providing such treatment. Henry N. Hooper, administrator of the facility, laid out the reasons for supporting such a policy in a letter to Basil O'Connor, chairman of the foundation's executive committee. Hooper simply assumed that if blacks were to be treated at Warm Springs the facility would be segregated. He cited the cost of constructing separate housing and treatment facilities, the unavailability of "colored graduate nurses" and "colored graduate physical therapists," the cost of treating what he assumed would be charity cases at over $2,000 per year for each one, and the likely inability of families to provide adequate care following treatment at Warm Springs as the major reasons for recommending against treating African Americans at the facility. Hooper did note that Warm Springs had treated on an out-patient basis "colored victims of infantile paralysis" who had been referred by local physicians. He also recommended that the Georgia Warm Springs Foundation provide assistance to "an institution already equipped for the care of colored people." In his letter to President Roosevelt, O'Connor concurred with Hooper's recommendations.[13]

The Georgia Warm Springs Foundation, and later the NFIP, did help establish an Infantile Paralysis Center at the Tuskegee Institute in nearby Alabama to serve African American polio patients. They provided some funding as well as an opportunity for the Tuskegee physicians to train with Warm Springs physicians and surgeons. According to Dr. John Hume, an orthopedic surgeon at Tuskegee, the entire staff of the center was black except the brace maker. This facility, he asserted, "was the only place [in the South] where all of the necessary care was available to black children." Tuskegee also provided other black physicians with information regarding polio treatment and it trained black physical and occupational therapists. In addition to Tuskegee, the Meharry Medical School in Nashville provided care for African American polio survivors. Where blacks were admitted to facilities that treated whites, they were segregated. Clara Yelder remembers that when she was treated at the Montgomery Clinic the children were all on the same floor but divided by race. As she put it, "the white kids were way down the hall and it was like another world. I don't know what went on in their section."[14]

The arrival in the United States in 1940 of the Australian nurse Elizabeth Kenny transformed acute and post–acute polio treatment for the vast majority of patients. Sister Kenny originally developed her method for treating poliomyelitis in the acute stage of the disease, but soon extended it to the convalescent or rehabilitative phase. In opposition to the orthodox physicians who argued that polio was a disease affecting the nerves, with important consequences for the muscles, Kenny's theory treated polio as "primarily a disease affecting the peripheral structures and muscle fibers." The most common symptom was muscle spasm, to be treated with the hot packs. In addition, polio caused "alienation," the inability of the nerve impulse to reach the muscle for "some unknown reason . . . possibly due to some physiological block." Spasm and alienation, if left untreated, eventually produced "incoordination" due to the "misdirection of the motor impulses." Alienation and incoordination were treated through the "establishment of mental awareness by means of passive movements," and, eventually, through active movements, or exercise, by the patients. Kenny and her followers argued that early treatment and "meticulous adherence" to her principles and procedures prevented stiffness and deformities, and reduced crippling.[15]

One advantage of the Kenny method of rehabilitation was that it involved the patient more fully in his or her own recovery. Dr. Miland Knapp in his description of Kenny-guided polio rehabilitation advised therapists to set rehabilitation goals that patients could meet in a relatively brief time. He suggested three-month goals because patients were likely to cooperate that long, and if progress was evident then, the patient's cooperation in future plans was easily secured. He urged therapists to always be sensitive to "the psychologic problems and the morale of the patient." Good morale was necessary to keep the patient working hard at the difficult and sometimes painful process of rehabilitation. Knapp always withheld a poor prognosis. Such information often depressed the patient and usually discouraged cooperation with the program of rehabilitation. Knapp argued that patients who were committed to the arduous task of rehabilitation regularly exceeded the physician's original expectations regarding the extent of recovery.[16]

Polio patients treated with the Kenny methods often faced a lengthy stay in the rehabilitation facility. As her methods began to be adopted in the early forties, several physicians who supervised Kenny facilities evaluated the treatments. Studies at three different Kenny hospitals involving a total of 98 patients revealed that the shortest stay was one week and the longest was by a ten-year-old girl still receiving treatment after forty-six weeks. The average length of hospitalization for these patients was just under ten weeks. Some of the patients were discharged as "recovered" or as normal without residual effects. Others were released substantially improved, walking with crutches, or manifesting continuing muscle weakness.[17] Discharge did not necessarily mean the end of physical therapy and rehabilitation; all of these facilities provided out-patient treatment to those who had not yet reached the maximum possible level of recovery.

By the early 1950s many physical therapy programs had adopted significant features of the Kenny method even if they did not accept her concept of polio as a disease of the muscles. Jesse Wright, who specialized in physical medicine and rehabilitation at the University of Pittsburgh, argued that the first goal of physical therapy was to relax tight muscles to permit "complete range of motion in the joints." Therapists could use hydrotherapy, hot packs, and curare for this purpose. Hot packs, however, should be used only intermittently as extended continuous use did not help at this stage and interfered with active physical therapy. Passive motion—therapist movement of affected limbs—was accompanied by efforts to have "the patient sense the location of the muscle for anticipated active effort." Once active function was restored, the muscle was strengthened through an individually prescribed set of exercises. The therapist guided the patient in careful stages from the passivity and dependence of acute poliomyelitis to active participation in "a practical program" of rehabilitation. Each patient, Wright argued, eventually reached a point in his or her recovery when "one has a vision of the future possibilities." At that point, nearing the end of rehabilitation, "definitive treatment becomes less important than making the best functional use of residual power, helpful body mechanics and assistive devices."[18]

Once physical therapy had achieved maximum muscle function, rehabilitation physicians evaluated the patients for braces and/or surgery to compensate for permanently paralyzed muscles. Doctors distinguished between splints and braces. Splints were temporary devices used early in the convalescent phase "to maintain neutral muscle position, to prevent later deformity, and to diminish pain." Braces were used later in rehabilitation to support "structures which no longer have sufficient muscular control to allow satisfactory function." In some cases, braces were a temporary expedient until orthopedic surgery could permanently correct the deformity. However, even then, braces might still be necessary. Physicians were cautioned not to prescribe braces too soon. Braces were "not a method of treatment" and could "handicap recovery" if used too soon.[19] In effect, when a physician prescribed braces for a polio patient he believed that maximum recovery had been achieved through physical therapy and surgery. Once braced, patients could expect little if any additional recovery, and they needed to begin to learn how to function and live encased in the heavy steel and leather braces of the period.

Orthopedic surgeons performed a variety of procedures to provide structural support and to restore function but only after physical therapy had done all it could. Dr. Philip Lewin recommended that no surgery be attempted within a year of the initial attack or on children younger than ten or twelve. Dr. William Green recommended waiting at least two years after onset in order "to permit full recovery of the muscles to occur and then to allow a further period so that the functional state may be evaluated more adequately."[20] These recommendations, which seem to have been generally followed, meant that children who had substantially recovered from one lengthy hospitalization for acute polio and physical therapy sometimes faced additional hospitalizations, painful procedures, and additional physical therapy during their teen-aged years.

Orthopedic surgeons were confident in their ability to "completely change the functional capacity of the patient." They believed that the right operation could enable the patient "to do things that he could not otherwise do, . . . to discard braces," and "restore lost muscle function." In addition, surgery could give a patient better control of an affected limb and, in some cases, "correct deformities and remove deforming factors." Typical procedures included tendon transplants to restore function, surgical lengthening of tendons and muscles, arthrodesis or the "surgical obliteration of joints" to correct deformities, surgery to stop the growth in a limb, and spinal fusion to correct scoliosis.[21]

Polio rehabilitation was marked by uncertainty, both regarding its length and its ultimate outcome. Fred Davis's studies of fourteen young polio patients and their families in Baltimore in the midfifties reveal how they slowly came to terms with the uncertainties of rehabilitation. He found that most families had initially expected a relatively short stay in the hospital. However, within weeks of the onset of the disease, both the children and their parents began to lengthen their time perspectives and to alter their expectations of the eventual outcome. Davis tellingly quotes one physiotherapist: "When they come in here, the children think in terms of days. Very soon they're thinking in terms of weeks and not long after that in terms of months." Davis argued that it was important for the physician to find ways to convey to the parents the notion that the uncertainties in their child's case derived from "the nature of the disease itself and not from therapeutic incompetence or an unwillingness to speak the truth." Some parents, unwilling to accept the initial doctor's assessment, shopped around for other opinions that they hoped would promise quicker and more certain success. Talking to other parents or patients only reinforced the unpredictability of the disease and of recovery from it. Most parents eventually accepted that "much is unknown and only time will tell."[22]

Davis found that physicians and institutions managed expectations in part by restricting parents' visits to once or twice a week. On their infrequent visits, parents saw very little change, and soon understood that recovery took time. Parents were repeatedly cautioned not to expect to much too quickly, although they were also encouraged to remain hopeful. Periodic reports, especially muscle checks at six-week intervals, and the "ordered sequence of physiotherapeutic exercises" had the effect of "directing the parents' expectations to points in the future."[23] It was important to gain the parents' confidence and support so that they would both encourage their children to work hard at their therapeutic programs and not interfere with the work of the physicians and therapists.

As important as it was to gain the parents' acquiescence in the lengthy process of rehabilitation, it was perhaps more important to gain the confidence and willing participation of the children in their own recovery. In addition to loosening a child's ties with home and immersing her in the "subculture of sickness," institutions established "a reward and punishment system both formal and informal," which sanctioned "good behavior and cooperative attitudes." This process was aided by the simple fact that a hospital is "a milieu in which sickness is the norm rather than the deviation and which permits the child to relate in a more thorough and structured fashion to a common universe of special meanings, goals, and evaluative rankings." [24] In reality, patients' responses to their hospitalization and rehabilitation were seldom so neatly managed. Some children adapted quite easily to hospital routines and to the polio community on the wards, but others, as we will see, resisted conforming to hospital norms and in that resistance found the strength to rebuild muscles, to find ways to function, and, ultimately, to come to terms with living with a disability.

Davis argued that lengthening the time perspective of the polio patients had certain important "latent functions," encouraging patients to focus on achievable short-term goals such as sitting, moving one's limbs, feeding oneself, or using a wheelchair. Focusing on goals that could be achieved in days or perhaps weeks as opposed to long-term goals, such as walking or returning to athletic competition, helped sustain morale and participation in the program of exercises. The lengthened perspective assisted hospital staff in "blocking repetitive and incessant questioning" by patients and parents regarding progress and likely outcomes. Families who accepted the idea that recovery was "slow and full of uncertainty" generally ceased pestering doctors and other staff, thus freeing them to devote their full energies to "diagnosis, prescription, and treatment." Finally, the lengthened time perspective enabled both patients and families to begin to accept the very real possibility that the polio survivors would leave the hospital with a "residual disability" that would have a significant lifetime impact.[25] Physicians and hospitals, however, were never completely successful in managing patient and family responses to extended hospitalization and rehabilitation. There was always tension between the patient's and family's desire for a quick and complete recovery and medicine's slow, steady progress toward full rehabilitation.

The hospital staff's attempted manipulation of the patient's and family's re-sponse to the lengthy hospitalizations typical of midcentury polio rehabilita-tion often imposed emotional and psychological scars to accompany the phys-ical crippling inflicted by the virus. Limiting visits to once or twice a week was painful for both patients and families. These policies were not medically nec-essary: some very good hospitals had very liberal policies; assertive parents and spouses could usually gain frequent bedside access; and exceptions were sometimes made. The hospitals that restricted visitors seem to have done it mainly for their own convenience. Similarly, other policies, such as revealing little about prognoses or lengthening the time perspective of patients and families, seem to have been adopted to discourage questions and to keep decision-making about rehabilitation and recovery firmly in the hands of the physicians.

Therapists continued to use hot packs during rehabilitation so long as the patients' muscles experienced spasms and contractures. Except in very mild cases, this generally meant weeks of having the hot, wet, smelly wool blankets wrapped around affected muscles. Many polio patients described the muscle stretching that followed hot packs as torture. The patient was more comfort-able in the contracted, deformed position because stretching the muscles increased pain. If the muscles were not forcibly stretched and were allowed to remain too long in the contracted position, "the part [became] fixed in the de-formed attitude, and it [was] difficult or even impossible to return the muscle to its original length." [26] When adequately prepared by their doctors or thera-pists, polio patients could accept the necessity for stretching their muscles, but the pain of the procedure surprised even these patients. Unfortunately, in too many cases, the patients were not adequately prepared for or warned about the pain, and in some cases, the therapists seemed to have gone out of their way to increase the suffering.

Even when done correctly, stretching was inevitably painful because the procedure was designed to force the muscle to stretch beyond what was com-fortable each time until full range of motion was achieved. Skillful therapists earned the respect of their patients, who recognized that each day's pains meant gains in the struggle to recover. Arnold Beisser compared stretching to "the rack," but he and his ward mates were fortunate to have in Rita a thera-pist who "gave no quarter when she stretched, taking a stretch to the limit of the patient's tolerance," but who also knew "just the right point at which to stop." Rita, a pretty young woman working in a ward of thirty men, inspired the men to joke that "'the definition of mixed emotions is being stretched by Rita,' implying that the pleasure of seeing her was mixed with the pain of stretching." [27] Stretching was painful no matter who did it, but it was clearly easier to endure with compassionate therapists.

Some polio patients, however, were cursed by having therapists who were insensitive to the pain they inflicted or who were perhaps touched by sadism. The attitude of some physicians and therapists seemed to be not just that the pain had to be endured, but that it was a positive good, a conviction not shared by most patients and families. For example, when Lorenzo Milam's therapist forced his legs "into certain positions which are as close to elaborate and exact fainting painfulness as possible," he compared it to being put "through the tortures of the damned," but without any redeeming cause. He was tortured not as a martyr for a "noble cause," his god, or his country, but simply because he "chose to continue living." Hugh Gallagher acknowledged that "even with the closest cooperation between patient and therapist, even with the greatest patient confidence in his therapist, the process will be arduous, painful." His therapist, however, did not prepare him for the pain and soon lost his confidence. From his perspective, she "did her job in a sadistic way." She pushed the limb to the "threshold of extreme pain," and, then, instead of releasing the limb at the count of 10 as promised, she attempted "to inflict just a little more stretching, just a little more pain." [28]

Stretching at the hands of a physical therapist was effective only early in polio rehabilitation. If too much time had passed and the contractures had become fixed, they could be loosened only with stretch or wedge casts or, ultimately, surgery. The leg or arm would be put in a full cast with a slot at the joint, where wedges could be inserted to slowly force the muscles to release and the joint to move. Ed Keohan recalled that every day the physicians would check his cast, and they frequently put in a bigger wedge. This "wedge routine was an extremely painful ordeal 24 hours a day for six weeks" until his knee achieved full extension. David Henson had a similar experience with a wedge cast for his ankle when he was eleven. He still remembers the "intense pain" twenty-four hours a day for weeks. The only relief the physicians offered was two aspirin a day.[29] What is striking in all these accounts is the physicians' apparent indifference to the suffering they inflicted with these procedures and their inability or unwillingness to relieve the pain they caused. There is no doubt that stretching by therapists and by casting restored increased or full range of motion to many polio patients, but all too often it was done brutally with little sensitivity to the pain and agony it caused.

Once the full range of motion had been restored, patients could begin active exercise to strengthen remaining muscles. Physical therapy often filled the day, taking hours to loosen and properly exercise all the affected muscles. As Irving Zola remembered, "time did not drag. Every day—in fact, almost every minute—there was something to do." Following stretching by the physical therapists, the nurses "prodded" Zola and his ward mates to exercise. With therapy, Charles Mee's "big events" included being able to have his head propped up on a pillow, wiggle the fingers of both hands, and raise one arm off the bed, which gave him hope that he would have "something, at least one arm, to use to remake some sort of independent life." As Wilfred Sheed recalled, "the small triumphs that are almost guaranteed in the early stages were of the kind that caused Roman emperors to close the city for parades and Wall Street to bury itself in ticker tape. Hey, I can sit up without help—well almost. Well, I did it once."[30] It was out of such "big events" and "small triumphs" that recovery was built.

Patients and therapists both confronted the difficult task of maintaining morale and engagement in the exercise program over the weeks and months of hard work. Good therapists found ways to motivate their patients, especially when progress was so slow as to be barely perceptible and pain was a constant companion. However, until results became evident, patients often scorned the encouraging words of the therapists. Robert Hall, for example, initially resented the therapist's exhortations to do more than try to move his leg. But when he moved his big toe after two weeks of therapy, Hall "yelled and yelled with delight. 'Hey look! I can do it!'" Edward Le Comte also detested his therapists' "moralizings," especially when they pointed to the example of others who could already perform an exercise. Le Comte recognized that the ability to move certain muscles was not simply a matter of will; it was often a matter of how much damage the virus had done. But even he recognized that, as was "likely to happen with incessant propaganda, some of it stuck." Perhaps there were borderline cases where belief and willpower did make a difference.[31]

As Fred Davis recognized, the Protestant work ethic when shared by patient and therapist effectively stimulated patient cooperation and participation in the therapeutic program. Along the way toward the goal of "optimal motor functioning" there were numerous interim goals that contributed to the idea of progress emphasized by the therapists. The moral at the core of "the physiotherapy regime" was deeply embedded in American culture.[32] Because the work ethic was so much a part of American culture, patients could adapt it to their exercise regime almost unconsciously. Wilfred Sheed, for example, took pride in the "small accomplishments" that made him feel "like one of the world's winners." Irving Zola "needed little pushing. My recovery became a series of large and small goals—the first time I could wiggle a toe, keep my arm up for five seconds, stand unaided." As Kenneth Kingery spent more and more time out of the iron lung breathing on his own, "there was a clear connection between work and reward. Now the recollection of an old lesson: that true pride comes only from accomplishment, and accomplishment only from effort." The pervasiveness of the work ethic and its applicability to polio rehabilitation meant that many polio patients felt compelled to conform publicly even if they privately dissented. For example, Charles Mee carefully kept up the outward appearance of "a well-balanced, emotionally stable all-American boy." The façade, however, was maintained by "sheer will," for underneath was a seething cauldron of repressed emotion in which the "damaged" and "wounded" boy repressed the urge "to kill."[33] The Protestant work ethic was thus a double-edged sword; its promise of reward for steady, hard work helped sustain and inspire polio patients during their lengthy and arduous rehabilitation, but if recovery slowed or stopped short of the hoped-for goals, it fostered feelings of guilt and unworthiness that made adjustment to any remaining disability more difficult. In addition, as Charles Mee suggests, the public embrace could hide feelings of anger, rage, and despair too dangerous to bring into the open.

Although the poliovirus could kill or damage any of the body's nerves, it seemed to have a special affinity for the legs. Many of the narratives recount the difficult struggle to learn to walk once again, and the fund-raising posters of the March of Dimes often portrayed a youngster in braces and on crutches. Even Franklin Roosevelt went to great lengths to create the illusion that he could walk.[34] The inability to walk thus became the iconic polio disability at midcentury. Conversely, learning to walk again became the primary objective of many polio patients with weakened or paralyzed legs. Learning to walk took weeks, sometimes months, of exercises to strengthen weakened muscles, and was marked by excruciatingly slow progress. First, there were braces to be fitted. Then one could stand, haltingly at first, between parallel bars or propped up on crutches. Finally, the first small step forward. When learning to walk these boys and girls, men and women, also had to learn to fall safely, since falls were inevitable. In some cases, learning to fall proved almost as difficult as learning to walk. With luck and salvageable muscles one might walk out of the rehabilitation hospital and eventually discard braces, crutches, and even canes. Not everyone, of course, could walk again. No amount of willpower could substitute for permanently paralyzed muscles, but the emphasis placed on learning to walk made it all the more difficult to accept that walking was impossible and that wheelchairs would have to provide mobility.

Walking was sometimes held up to polio patients as the Holy Grail of recovery, a view many of them shared. Jan Little, who never was able to walk, remembered "the pressure to learn to walk. Walking was proof that you had worked hard and overcome your disability. Wheelchairs were associated with old or sick people." She tried braces and months of outpatient physical therapy but without success: "Usually I imitated a tree. I'd sway back and forth a few frantic moments, then crash to the ground, maintaining a straight position until I hit the ground." The family received lots of unsolicited advice about her failure to walk, including from one aunt who suggested that if her father set the house on fire she would learn to walk so she could get out. Like Jan Little, Charles Mee recalled that "the goal was to be a real person who could walk. Walking was the whole deal." It was a goal that Mee and many of his ward mates shared: "The common dream—and it was my dream, too—was that one day we would just get up and walk again, like a real miracle, like making a pilgrimage to Lourdes and being cured by the holy waters there."[35] Unlike Little, Mee did learn to walk with braces and crutches, but it was something less than a Lourdes miracle.

The first step in learning to walk again was the ability to stand after weeks and months lying in bed or sitting in a wheelchair. Even with weeks of physical therapy, muscles were still weak, and many polio patients could initially stand only with the aid of braces and crutches. The first attempts were not always successful, as patients had to regain control over atrophied muscles and overcome the disorientation of a newly elevated perspective. Charles Mee recalled pulling himself upright out of his wheelchair by grasping horizontal bars attached to the wall. He tried to stand holding on, his "midsection swaying from side to side" and his "knees giving out from time to time." He had to learn a "new equilibrium, a bizarre, jury-rigged system of muscular checks and balances that could not be taught. The body had to learn this on its own through days and days of trial and error." Leonard Kriegel first stood on crutches. After fitting him with his first set of braces, the brace maker put crutches under his arms and stood him up. He felt "suddenly light-headed and brittle, afraid that I would topple over like a glass vase to a stone floor." It was supposed to be a moment of triumph, but as he stood there, unsteady, propped up, and unable to move, the word "cripple" was all that came to mind. Not all patients waited to stand until the therapists had decided they were ready. Ray

Gullickson learned to stand after surreptitiously reading in his chart that he would never walk again without a brace. Determined not to wear a brace, Gullickson began by lowering himself off his bed after the lights were out: "It was like my feet were asleep, and I was being pricked by hundreds of tiny needles. I broke out in a cold sweat, and I started to shake." He managed to get back into bed, and every night he repeated the exercise. After ten days he took his first step and in another few days he could walk around his bed and still have enough strength left to get back in it.[36] With standing, as with so many other facets of recovery from polio, what was possible, with or without braces, and with what speed was largely determined by what muscles were still enervated. And standing, of course, was only a prelude to walking.

While the first steps marked progress on the long road to recovery, their difficulty, encased in steel braces and supported by parallel bars or the arms of the therapists, only highlighted how slow progress was and how much further they had to go. Edward Le Comte recalled that his first shuffling steps between the parallel bars left him feeling an "incredible feebleness and utter weariness." Instead of exhilaration at his first steps in months, he became depressed: "The road ahead was longer and rougher than my worst imaginings, the mirror at the end of the parallel bars hopelessly distant; and reaching that—sometime in the fifth month—would only be the beginning of the beginning." Charles Mee took his first steps in his leg brace held up by four therapists. A few days later his therapist had him working on the parallel bars. His "assignment was to throw myself forward, holding on to the bars, and drag and fling and scuffle my feet forward a little at a time, and in this way lurch from one end to the other." The first time he took only a few steps this way before the therapists lowered his "wobbling, exhausted, jellylike body back into the wheelchair," accompanied by much praise and encouragement. Once his therapist began him on crutches, a few weeks of practice enabled him to "scuttle . . . crablike . . . down the smooth, polished floors of the corridor."[37]

Learning to walk again took lots of practice. Every day after he began to walk Edward Le Comte was "expected to do something terribly dangerous— such as going four steps further." His therapists "called it progress: that was the iron rule." But progress could be agonizingly slow. Robert Hall "put in hundreds of hours between those parallel bars in front of that full-length mirror." As his physical therapist reminded him, "It won't come easy. You have to work and work at it, but it will come." A few, however, walked more easily. For example, Robert Gurney had spent nearly eleven months in the hospital when his physical therapist decided he was going to walk. Gurney didn't believe it

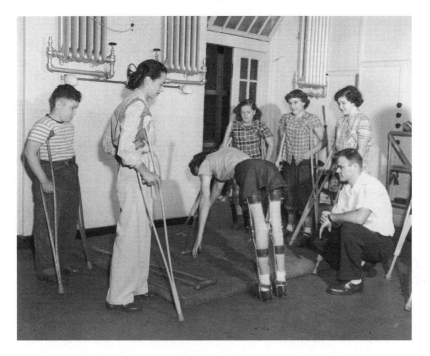

FIG. 10. Ruth Judd Ellis (second from left) instructs Rita Gillan how to use her crutches to get up from the floor. Erbert F. Cicenia, director of physical therapy at the New York State Rehabilitation Hospital, watches. Others in picture are, left to right, Herman Friedman, Arlene Hendrickson, Christine Schwed, and Sandra Franhel. August 31, 1950.

was possible, but at the end of the day's exercises he walked around the exercise table several times and then to his room. He soon improved enough to walk out of the hospital.[38] Whether walking came easily or only after weeks of grueling practice depended more on the state of one's muscles than on the power of individual will. A strong will might keep you at your exercises and practice, but only newly strengthened muscles could provide the power to move by yourself.

If you learned how to walk, you also had to learn how to fall. In the early stages of learning to walk with braces and crutches polio patients fell frequently. Their muscles were still weak and their sense of balance and equilibrium had to be reestablished. Using braces and crutches effectively was an acquired skill. The new walkers had to learn how to fall properly so they would not hurt themselves. Charles Mee's therapists coached him how to fall just as

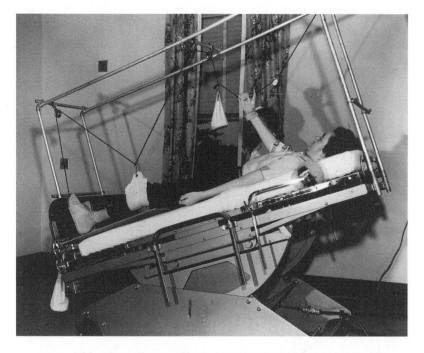

FIG. 11. Miriam Dartnell on a rocking bed practices "walking" with the aid of the
frame above the bed. D. T. Watson School, Leetsdale, Pennsylvania, 1951.

they had taught him to walk. He learned how to turn as he was falling so he
could catch himself with his arms and roll with the fall. For him, it was reminiscent of learning to fall in football. Robert Hall learned to fall in the corridor
leading to the physical therapy room. One morning his therapist made him
walk to therapy instead of wheeling in his chair. He fell thirty-six times before
he reached the exercise room. Angry and embarrassed at his inability to walk
without falling, Hall, nonetheless, soon "learned how to fall in a relaxed manner and roll with the flow of the fall." By the time he reached physical therapy
he "had the feeling of accomplishment." It took Leonard Kriegel more than
a month to learn how to fall. Although he claimed to have been a "dutiful
patient," who did all the exercises, he could not fall: "The prospect of falling
terrified me." His therapist repeatedly "pleaded, ridiculed, cajoled, threatened,
[and] bullied," all to no avail. Then one day, "the terror simply evaporated."
When the therapist yet again asked him to let go and fall, he did. It was a sweet
feeling, "a new start, a new life." In learning to fall freely he learned how "to
fall into life in order not to be overwhelmed."[39] Having learned to walk, and to

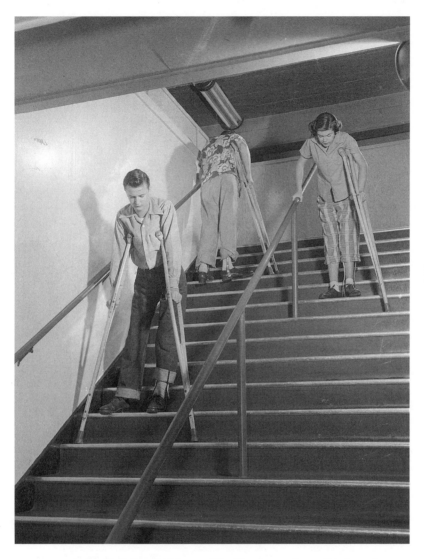

FIG. 12. Robert McClellan, Jim Watt, and Vera Vaughn practice negotiating stairs.
May T. Morrison Center, San Francisco, California, 1951.

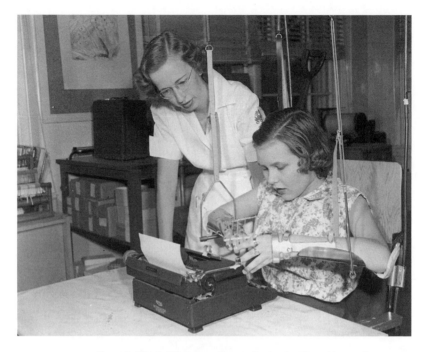

FIG. 13. Sammie Ward of Texas practices typing under the guidance of occupational therapist Cornelia Watson. Springs attached Ward's arm supports to an overhead frame so she can use her arms in daily activities. Georgia Warm Springs Foundation, July 23, 1951.

fall, these patients were ready to confront the even more challenging world outside the hospital.

While many polio patients faced the agony of stretching and extensive physical therapy, those in iron lungs confronted the even more difficult and frightening task of being weaned from dependence on the respirator. Whatever their initial apprehensions about the iron lung, many quickly became both physically and psychologically dependent upon it. Physicians wanted to lessen dependence on the tank respirators as soon as possible for both comfort and safety. If a patient could breathe on his or her own for even a few minutes, caring for their paralyzed bodies was much easier, and in the event of a power outage they could survive until emergency power kicked in or until staff could pump the machines manually. Ideally, weaning began as soon as possible after placement in an iron lung. Dr. Richard Field outlined the proper method, which began with "opening the tank for a length of time consistent with comfort." From a few seconds at the beginning, both the time out of the lung and the frequency of attempts were then gradually increased. If done correctly, "no individual should be kept out of the tank to the point of great discomfort." To keep a patient out of the lung too long, Field argued, was "not only dangerous, but cruel." Staff should always remember that "the paralyzed person in a respirator is totally helpless and wholly dependent on, if not at the mercy of, his medical attendants."[40]

Some patients also learned the difficult technique of glossopharyngeal breathing, or "frog breathing," which used neck muscles rather than paralyzed chest muscles to force air into the lungs by "gulping like a frog." Although patients could not do it in their sleep, the technique provided an additional margin of safety.[41] Once the patients had gained sufficient ability to breathe on their own, they could be transferred to rocking beds for a brief period and then for gradually longer periods. The rocking beds were like large seesaws and used gravity to force air in and out. The speed and depth of the rocking could both be adjusted to suit the patient's needs. The rocking beds provided some respiratory support, though less than the iron lung, and they had other advantages. The mattress was a real bed mattress rather than the hard pallet of the iron lung, and the rocking motion provided a "kind of exercise, reducing stiffness and contracture." In addition, the patient had a wider perspective now that vision was not restricted to what could be seen in reverse through the mirror on the iron lung. Some patients were also able to use a chest respirator, which was a shell fitting over the torso with a hose connecting it to a pump. The pump used air to push the chest down and then release it, forcing air out and allowing it in. Although they seldom fit properly and were often uncomfortable, they allowed the patient to sit on a bed or in a wheelchair and offered some respite from incessant rocking. In the early stages of using rocking beds and chest respirators patients often slept in their iron lungs or returned to the lungs for longer periods if they ran into any kind of respiratory difficulty such as a cold.[42]

Some of the most seriously paralyzed respirator patients were eventually moved to one of the regional respiratory centers established with help from the NFIP in the late forties and early fifties. In the early fifties, these centers could care for about 230 of the estimated 1,000 patients dependent on iron lungs. The fifteen centers ultimately established included the Mary MacArthur Respirator Center outside Boston, the Northwest Respirator Center in Seattle,

Rancho Los Amigos near Los Angeles, and others in Baltimore, Houston, Ann Arbor, and Buffalo. They were designed to provide better care and rehabilitation than could generally be achieved in hospitals with only one or two long-term iron lung patients. The centers worked to free patients from dependence on the iron lung so that they could go home. They also conducted research on the problems of rehabilitating respirator-dependent patients. These regional centers generally provided a more pleasant, less restrictive atmosphere in which the patients could develop friendships as well as encourage and motivate each other.[43]

For many of the patients sent to the respiratory centers, the change in facilities marked a major step forward in the long process of recovery. Louis Sternburg remembered that whereas "the polio ward had been a torture chamber in Bedlam," the Mary MacArthur Respiratory Center was "hospital heaven." There was sufficient staff to care for the patients "calmly and thoroughly," a measure of privacy, and a world outside the windows to enjoy. Plus, "the best thing about life in the rehab center was the companionship that developed among the patients." Regina Woods, who was sent from a Nashville hospital to the center in Houston, also remarked on the "family atmosphere" of the place. The Houston center encouraged a "sense of relationship to others" and she found the whole experience "wonderfully helpful."[44]

For those whose respiratory muscles were most extensively paralyzed, the process of reducing their dependence on the iron lung was particularly difficult and frightening. Initially, many had no ability to breathe on their own, or, at best, they struggled to take a few breaths before their weakened muscles gave out. As Dr. John Affeldt recognized, fear was the prevailing emotion among these utterly dependent patients. Many, of course, wanted out, but they need constant assurance that staff would help them. The patients wanted to believe the reassurances of the doctors and therapists, but it was difficult even in the best of circumstances. Larry Alexander recognized their psychological dependency on the iron lung: "The idea of leaving it would always make our hearts beat a little faster and bring an anxious lump into our throats. We were incomplete embryos in a metal womb." When the time came to be moved out of the protective cocoon of the iron lung, Louis Sternburg wondered how he could trust his therapist: "Trust? I couldn't even trust myself. Look how my own body had failed me."[45] Only by conquering their fear, by working with their therapists, could these patients begin to work toward freeing themselves from dependence on the iron lung.

The process of learning to breathe on one's own again was slow and protracted. Many iron lung patients were like Hugh Gallagher, "reasonably comfortable" in the iron lung and "not anxious to alter my circumstances." Thus the process also required therapists who pushed patients to breathe longer and longer on their own until they could spend ten minutes, an hour, several hours, and, finally, the whole day out of the lung. For Gallagher the process began several weeks after the acute attack, when his "Prussian therapist" put him on a schedule that "seemed, quite simply, impossible." She began by turning off the respirator for thirty seconds. At the beginning, Gallagher had no ability to breathe on his own. Over the course of a week or more, he "learned to take a breath, perhaps two." Soon the therapist doubled the time to a minute, and, when he could breathe for a minute, to two minutes. Once he could breathe for ten minutes on his own, the pallet on which he lay could be pulled out of the lung to care for him. When he could breathe for an hour on his own he was placed on an ordinary bed outside the lung for the first time in weeks. In spite of his continuing panic, "the driving schedule, just one more painful and frightening event in the day, went on inexorably. Somehow the muscles that were responsible for breathing were able to meet the challenge." But he still had a long way to go; the exertion of breathing for only an hour was such that when he was returned to "the warmth and comfort" of his "familiar prison," he slept for hours.[46]

Louis Sternburg also found that leaving the iron lung was slow, painful work. His first real sign of progress was being moved to a rocking bed. Although skeptical that it would work and afraid of getting seasick, he was surprised to discover that he was "breathing . . . a more natural type of breathing." He had to admit it was "a triumph. Another way to breathe, another choice." The next step was to use a chest respirator. When he could use the rocking bed and chest respirator he was "finally weaned from the womb of the iron monster," but there was yet one more step, learning to frog breathe, so he would not be totally dependent upon mechanical assistance. He recalled that all the work at the respiratory center was "hard and often painful and frustrating, but this was the worst." In learning to frog breathe he drew upon the "fighting spirit" he remembered from his days as an athlete. Over twelve "agonizing weeks" he "learned to breathe for longer and longer periods without a machine." He could eventually frog breathe for as long as fourteen hours, but he never really got used to "the strain and anxiety of it." Sternburg and his friend Bert, who was learning at the same time, "made up a game—'frog challenge'"—in which they each tried to outperform the other. They even found some humor in the situation: Bert suggested they could get jobs in "a summer camp, teaching a bunch of frogs how to man breathe."[47]

In spite of and partly because of their success in ending their dependence on the iron lung, many of these respirator patients experienced a severe psychological crisis just as they began to see some improvement. The crisis was often precipitated by a patient's recognition of just how little progress had been made since the acute attack and by discussions with their doctors regarding their prospects for continued improvement and ultimate recovery. They had assumed that through hard work and persistence they would recover and return to something close to their pre-polio lives. Now they were being told they would never walk again, or, perhaps, never breathe on their own for very long. One day after he moved to a rocking bed, Louis Sternburg asked his physician when he was going to walk out of the respiratory center. After a long, painful pause, the doctor told him that not only would he never walk again, he would also probably never breathe again without assistance. Sternburg heard himself scream, " 'You sonofabitch, you're lying!' It can't have been a loud scream, but its resonance in my head was loud." The doctor left him depressed and questioning the "meaning and purpose for my life." Breathing on his own had initially boosted Larry Alexander's confidence in his eventual recovery, but a conversation with another patient sent him into a downward spiral. He had started to believe he could fight his way to "a cure": "*If you have the strength to do it, you can do it. If you really want to get well you can fight polio.*" The realization that he was permanently paralyzed ushered in one of his "blackest periods": "All the promise of my increased breathing, all the confidence of a cure, seemed to vanish completely." He felt that he had "no logical reason to go on living" and that he would be "better off dead."[48]

Like those of Sternburg and Alexander, Hugh Gallagher's psychological crisis came with the full recognition that he might remain paralyzed. He had borne over two months of painful illness and grueling therapy. He had come to accept the treatments because they were the means by which he would get well. He could not imagine that his paralysis was permanent. During one of his physical therapy sessions he bluntly asked his doctor about his condition and prospects. The doctor was "direct and kindly," and answered Gallagher's questions. He told Gallagher that he would never walk without assistance. At that point, Gallagher was forced to acknowledge that his life had forever changed: "I would never again be beautiful, innocent, secure in health, strong in body, confident in mind . . . and I would be forever crippled." Gallagher's initial reaction, when the physician had left and his father and the therapist returned to continue the exercises, was to become hysterical, but the hysterics soon subsided into an emotional shutdown. Although he became again "the cheerful patient, the dutiful son," emotionally he "retreated into a private place" where he gave up "all feelings" to protect himself.[49]

Respirator patients were not, however, the only polio patients to experience a psychological crisis during their lengthy rehabilitation. Most of the polio patients who remembered having a period of deep depression or a psychological crisis were older at the time of hospitalization. They were adolescents and adults who had a sense of how polio would forever alter their lives, of what they had lost besides the ability to move their muscles. For fourteen-year-old Charles Mee, the low point came when he was out of isolation and the hot packs were being applied. This was when he began to cry: "This was the moment I thought this process of recovery was going to fail, that it was much too slow, that I never would be better, that I was forever—that dreaded word—crippled, that all my strategies for denial and fighting back and outsmarting all my feelings by some heroic act of understanding were pathetic and worthless; that I might as well quit, give up, sink down, be taken care of; that I was, without recourse, a ruined child." This was his "moment of deepest anguish," and it recurred day after day as the hot packing continued.[50]

Young men were not the only ones to experience despair and depression during the long rehabilitation. Louise Lake had a young child to care for. Even though she was making progress using a wheelchair, she was continually "haunted by the fear" that she was "doomed to physical disability." Joan Hardee was twenty-one when polio struck. While under the oxygen mask, she had "a very strong, conscious wish to die." Her deepest despair, however, came shortly after the mask was removed and she could breathe on her own again: "I knew that I would not die, and could not, even though I wished it. I slumped into a great depression with no positive wish or will about anything."[51] All of these individuals found ways to overcome despair or to repress the emotions, but their achievement was often a temporary one. Because living with a permanent disability was more difficult than most initially imagined, some polio survivors found that the black clouds of depression never entirely dissipated.

Leading rehabilitation physicians in the post–World War II era argued that the psychological dimension of recovery from a crippling illness or accident was as important as the physical. Prominent figures in rehabilitation, such as Drs. Howard Rusk and Henry Kessler, had developed the "whole man theory of rehabilitation," in which a team of specialists including a psychiatrist or psychologist would work together to rehabilitate individuals with disabilities to "restore them to 'normalcy.'" Borrowing "a set of ideas, values, and beliefs from a distinctly American version of psychoanalysis called 'psychodynamic therapy,'" developed by leading American psychiatrists such as Rusk, Kessler, William Menninger of the famed Menninger Clinic in Topeka, Kansas, and like-minded rehabilitation specialists portrayed the disabled as "malformed and maladjusted" and in need of experts in order to become "normal." Rusk argued that "the prognosis of rehabilitation does not depend as much on the severity of the handicap as it depends on the patient's psychological adjustment to his disability." The idea was that the disabled child or adult could learn to compensate psychologically for whatever impairments and disabilities re-mained when physical rehabilitation was completed. The goal of this psycho-logical compensation or adjustment was "perpetually striving toward nor-malcy." Ideally, with the proper psychological therapy, the disabled could learn to fit in and to achieve the "dream" of being "accepted by American society." [52]

Rusk was one of many rehabilitation specialists who stressed the psycho-logical component of recovery from acute poliomyelitis. He acknowledged that "no two cases are the same either physically or emotionally." For him, "psy-chologic adjustment and acceptance" were two of the broad goals of rehabili-tation. He recommended that medical staff acknowledge that the patient had been seriously ill and that no one could say for certain how much recovery was possible. Staff should emphasize what the patient could do, and the impor-tance of working hard to increase the level of recovery. Rusk argued that this approach was generally "accepted with equanimity, and gratitude" and as physical gains were made "motivation was accelerated." [53] Rusk, however, was too optimistic regarding the grace with which polio patients came to terms with their paralysis. While many polio patients eventually came to accept their disabilities on some level, acceptance usually came only after a long struggle to reconcile self-image with the new reality of a permanent disability.

Dr. Harold Visotsky and his colleagues at the Respiratory Center of the Uni-versity of Illinois Medical College developed a more sophisticated understand-ing of the psychological dimensions of polio recovery based on their study of eighty-one patients at the center. The researchers wanted to understand the "coping behavior" of polio patients. Coping behavior included "keeping distress within manageable limits; mobilizing hope; maintaining a sense of personal worth; restoring relations with significant other people; enhancing prospects for recovery of respiratory and motor functions; and increasing the likelihood of working out a favorable situation after maximum physical recovery has been attained." They were impressed by how "resourceful" many patients were, "even in the face of a catastrophic situation." Most eventually "showed an impressive resiliency and ability to work out new patterns of living."[54]

Psychological adjustment to severe polio was a process that often lasted months or years and that was usually marked by setbacks as well as by progress. In spite of considerable variation, these researchers were able to discern a series of stages through which most polio patients passed. Patients first tried to "minimize the impact of the event" through "extensive denial of the nature of the illness, its seriousness, and its probable consequence." These defense mechanisms protected the patient from "being overwhelmed" and permitted a "more gradual transition to the exceedingly difficult tasks" of rehabilitation. As patients came to have a more realistic sense of the situation, they often became depressed. As the researchers put it, "as the denial diminishes, depression increases." Coping was more effective if the patients had "a firm sense of belonging in highly valued groups" including, most importantly, "(1) the ward group, consisting of some of the other patients and some members of the staff; (2) the family; and (3) some aspects of his home community." Patients had to feel "needed in one or more reference groups—a sense that one's presence is not only valued by significant other people but is virtually indispensable to them." Another coping mechanism was to avoid focusing on ultimate goals that might be unreachable, such as walking, and to emphasize, instead, intermediate goals which had a relatively short time-frame, were directly tied to the patient's immediate physical condition, and which were possible to attain. Reaching these goals was "intrinsically rewarding," stimulated further effort, and strengthened "a self-concept encompassing capability of change." Most patients in the study, however, had to settle for less than a full recovery and to accept "severe limitations of motor and respiratory function" even after "several years of treatment, effort, and suffering." Acceptance came only through a "slow transition from a self-concept of physical vigor to one of physical limitation." In the view of the doctors, "Having accepted the possibility of a modest limitation, it later becomes less shocking to consider the possibility of an additional limitation."[55]

If polio patients saw psychologists or psychiatrists during their stays in rehabilitation hospitals, few of them commented on that fact in their narratives. And, when they did talk to psychologists or psychiatrists, the outcome was not always positive, at least in the short run. Hugh Gallagher's hysterical episode began when the neurologist/psychiatrist told him that he would never walk again. The response of the doctors and nurses to his hysteria was to treat it "as something shameful, embarrassing, something to be hidden, to be throttled as quickly as possible." Gallagher was soon given "a shot of something, which produced an almost immediate and beatific calming result." He was, however, given no assistance in working through his raw emotions, either by the medical staff or by his father, who had witnessed the episode and who was "repulsed by it, repelled by it." Later at Warm Springs, the resident psychologist told him, "You don't adjust at Warm Springs. . . . That comes afterwards, when you leave." When, the psychologist might have added, you are on your own. Gallagher was not the only one to have a difficult encounter with a psychiatrist. The confrontational approach of some psychiatrists seems particularly inappropriate for totally paralyzed men and women still dependent on an iron lung. For example, Louis Sternburg first saw a psychiatrist shortly after moving to the Mary MacArthur Respiratory Center. Dr. Howard Blaine's first question to Sternburg, who had yet to take a breath on his own, was "How's your sex life, Louis?" Only nine years later, did Sternburg find a psychiatrist with whom he could begin to deal with his depression, fear, and anxiety. When Kathryn Black's mother was having a "difficult time emotionally," she was seen by the consulting psychiatrist. Her father, however, remembers the visits as unhelpful. He found his wife crying one evening after the psychiatrist had asked her, "How does it feel to know you'll never hold your children again?" [56]

Not all hospital staff were so insensitive to the psychological fragility of their polio patients. Hugh Gallagher, for example, remembered a young night nurse, who, when he was still in the iron lung, hovered over his head talking and sharing dreams. He was grateful to her, even though there were many things he could not tell her. Two of Larry Alexander's therapists, Claire and Kelly, helped him to choose to resume his therapy, to recover to the extent that he could, and to live as fully as possible. In the midst of his depression he had become convinced that the only choice was between death and a kind of living death in the iron lung. He drew "comfort and strength" from his talks with them and ultimately decided that he wanted to live and that the only way he could was "by accepting the situation." He was then determined to accept his paralysis and limitation and "build something around it." [57]

Very often it was a family member whose unfailing support helped pull the polio patient through the psychological ordeal. Louis Sternburg's wife, Dottie, "comforted and cheered" him "through the bad times of despair." It wasn't always easy. She recalled that after Lou had been told he would never walk again, she "felt sick," but she soon "went back to the ward and started to try to rebuild Lou's optimism." Similarly, Larry Alexander's wife, Norma, supported him emotionally as he worked to get out of the iron lung and to find some meaning in a life devastated by polio. Near the end of his narrative and after he had returned home, Norma acknowledged that "this isn't the kind of thing you can grin and bear, not if you're going to be realistic. . . . It was hell for both of us." Not all family members were capable of being as supportive as these two. Louis Sternburg's father "tried to help," but he couldn't deal with his son's illness and withdrew "more and more into himself." And Kathryn Black's father was never able to accept his wife's illness or to take on the dual role of father and mother to their two children after she died.[58]

However supportive family members were, they generally did not spend all day, every day, in the rehabilitation hospital with their spouse or child.[59] Polio patients spent the day on the ward and in the exercise rooms with other patients. In many cases, these polio wards became supportive communities in which the patients helped one another through the physical and psychological challenges of polio rehabilitation. Louis Sternburg remembered that "the best thing about life in the rehab center was the companionship that developed among the patients. Like survivors in a life boat," they "grew dependent on each other and very close." While the hospital concentrated on rehabilitating their bodies, they "were restoring each other's souls." For Robert Hall, "an invaluable part of our recovery program at the V. A. Hospital was the fact that we were a group." They were "all there to pick each other up, and that went on constantly. . . . In the pain, we were there for each other."[60]

In spite of these sources of assistance and strength, some polio patients discovered that they could cope only by repressing their emotions, by creating a public persona that obscured their deeply wounded psyches. Dorothea Nudelman was only nine when polio struck, but she remembers that she and the other children received no help in dealing with their fears and anxieties: "We weren't allowed to feel sorry for ourselves. There wasn't time for that." She went through physical therapy in a "culture of denial and suppression. No one wanted to acknowledge the pain which was omnipresent. It was too much to bear." Children who "showed pain too much" were "ostracized as 'babies' by other kids." Nudelman soon learned to "be ashamed of herself if she expressed pain" and even to feel ashamed simply "to have these feelings." Charles Mee soon discovered that he could not buy into the cultural values of the time: "This culture made me feel, as a boy, that I needed to keep my chin up, reassure my parents about how well I was doing, never be sad, look to the future, be optimistic, perform a can-do persona even if I felt no connection to it." As he remembered, it made him "live a lie" to protect himself from the unrealistic expectations of his priest, his football coach, and his parents, all of whom had bought into the notion that a strong will and determination were all that was needed to recover.[61] It is no coincidence that these adolescents would experience severe depression as adults. All the emotions and feelings they had buried—fear, anxiety, guilt, anger—eventually came to the surface and blossomed decades later. While their bodies had been rehabilitated as adolescents, it was only as adults, years removed from the events that triggered those emotions, that they began to confront and work through the psychological legacy of polio.

| 5 |

Straws on the Ceiling: Life on the Polio Wards

IN THE FORTIES AND FIFTIES many polio patients experienced rehabilitation communally. Private and semiprivate hospital rooms were the exception; most polio rehabilitation centers housed their patients in wards of four to twenty or more beds. Hot packs, painful stretching, and passive exercise as well as all the activities of daily life—eating, sleeping, studying, playing, receiving visitors—took place in public on the wards. There was little privacy, perhaps only curtains separating beds, and even customarily private activities—enemas, defecation, urination, preparation for and recovery from surgery—became semipublic affairs. In addition, once the patients had recovered sufficiently to begin an exercise program they spent a large part of their day with the other patients in the gymnasium, swimming pool, or other rehabilitation facilities of the institution. Here, too, one's progress, or lack of progress, in rehabilitation was obvious to all.

Polio communities developed on the rehabilitation wards in part because of the lengthy stays typical of the forties and fifties. Many of the narratives describe hospitalizations ranging from several months to a year or more. While new patients were always being admitted and others were going home, an individual might spend most of his or her hospitalization with the same core group. In addition, while hospital routine, hot packing, therapy, and exercise took hours out of each day, patients spent a lot of unoccupied time on the wards. In most cases, patients had to find ways to entertain themselves. Some facilities did provide play space, or toys and games that could be played in bed. Radios were relatively common on the wards; television appeared on the wards only toward the end of the polio epidemics. Many hospitals tried to provide occasional treats, such as weekly or monthly movies or visiting athletes or entertainers. Children of school age were often given the opportunity to keep up with their education. Patients of all ages played, talked with one another about what they would do when they got out, contrived and launched pranks on one another and on the hospital staff, cooperated with and sometimes confronted the staff, resisted hospital regulations, and, in general, acted like children, adolescents, and young adults.

Physicians and hospital staff established the institutional structures and policies, such as age- and sex-segregated wards, visitation policies, ward regulations, and rehabilitation procedures that shaped polio rehabilitation. The patients, however, quickly developed a polio patient subculture that both reinforced and subverted the hospital regime. The patient subculture reinforced the hospital authority and program of rehabilitation by providing patients with emotional and psychological support, by fostering competition in exercises to recover muscle function, by encouraging reluctant or resistant patients, and by providing an outlet for patient frustrations. Creating and participating in the community on the polio wards made both their stay in the institution and the pain of extended rehabilitation more bearable. However, even as it reinforced the hospitals' plan of rehabilitation, the patient subculture subverted it. The friendships developed on the wards gave patients a source of emotional and psychological support outside of official channels. Visits from family and friends provided a continuing link to the outside world. When it applied derogatory nicknames to cold, distant, difficult or abusive staff or plotted and sometimes carried out acts of revenge, the ward community asserted its own identity and independence and helped rebuild the shattered self-confidence of those involved. When the polio community facilitated the play of children and adolescents, created opportunities for young adults to explore their returning sexual impulses, and fostered post-rehabilitation planning by adults, its members could escape, for a brief time at least, the more confining aspects of the hospital. Thus, the ward community was an important bridge to resuming life outside the hospital. It encouraged its members to become once again an independent human being instead of a dependent polio patient.

These polio ward communities developed in part out of a shared need for companionship during the many unstructured hours in the day, in part out of a recognition of shared experience, and in part because once the acute phase of polio had passed, these patients were not in any real sense sick.[1] Patients admitted to rehabilitation facilities were past the active and infectious stage of poliomyelitis. They no longer had a fever, delirium had ceased, and paralysis had reached its fullest extent. To be sure, some had continuing pain, many had paralyzed muscles and limbs, and most needed to rebuild and strengthen weakened muscles, but in many ways these were healthy children, adolescents,

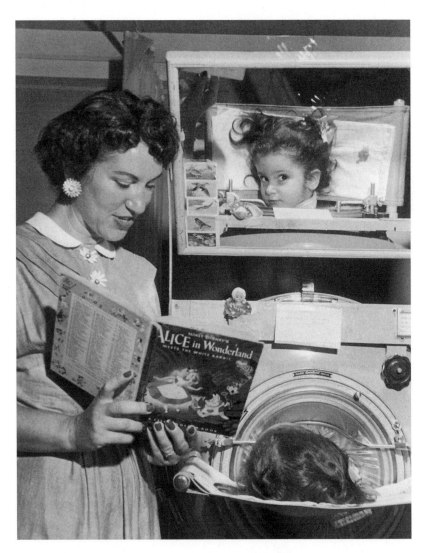

FIG. 14. Corrine Gold, a volunteer at Rancho Los Amigos Hospital in Downey, California, reading *Alice in Wonderland* to Debbie Stone. 1955.

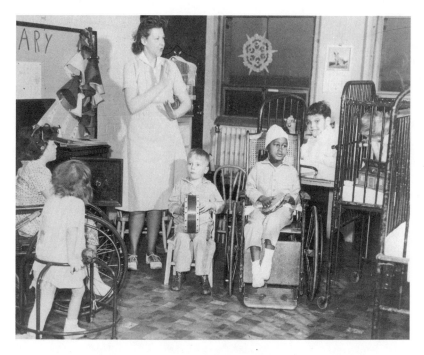

FIG. 15. A wheelchair musical band provides entertainment on a polio ward.
Location unknown, 1950.

and adults. Their cognitive and social skills were unimpaired and the unparalyzed parts of their bodies were slowly regaining strength and usefulness. These communities introduced a touch of normality and even levity into what was otherwise an alienating and often painful experience.

Older patients usually welcomed the move to a rehabilitation ward because it marked progress toward recovery and because it significantly expanded their social horizon. In some hospitals outside visitors had greater access to the rehabilitation wards than to the isolation wards, and in almost all hospitals the new patient was quickly welcomed into a flourishing polio community. Larry Alexander was encouraged by the atmosphere in his new six-patient ward at the Kenny Institute in Jersey City, New Jersey. He remembered "a comforting feeling in the presence of other men, in the constant talk, the arguments and the horseplay. Even the view . . . was better." Because it felt less like a hospital, it was "a step back toward the land of the living." In some cases, polio patients endured several hospital regimes before they found one that helped heal the mind and soul as well as the body. Hugh Gallagher, like many others, found the ideal rehabilitation setting in Warm Springs, Georgia: "The difference between life as a patient in the old hospital and rehabilitation at the beautiful resort, deep in the Georgia pines, was as great as the difference between Kansas and Oz." At Warm Springs he discovered he "could have fun again."[2] Few if any other facilities could match the atmosphere at Warm Springs, but most polio patients found the ward communities a welcome change from the isolating and dependent experience of the acute hospital.

Of course, not everyone remembered his or her introduction to the rehabilitation wards so positively. When the young Don Kirkendall was left at a state children's hospital in Minnesota for corrective surgery he woke up on "the Small Boys Ward with the ego-smashing sensation that I had become a blob" and "overcome with homesickness and fright." Lorenzo Milam's first experience with a rehabilitation ward was, if anything, less successful. Still weak, confused, and in pain, the nineteen-year-old Milam was one of the oldest and sickest of thirty-five boys on the ward. He didn't want to be "in a football-field-length medical ward with noise from 6:30 A.M. to 9:30 P.M. non-stop. Noise: babbling, calling out, yelling, whistling, stomping, running, singing, crying." Fortunately, he, too, would later discover the "paradise of Meriwether County, Georgia." Not everyone, however, found Warm Springs to be a paradise. John Swett, who at age five spent seven months at Warm Springs, remembered nothing pleasant about the experience. He felt abandoned when his family returned to their Florida home, and he "cried for about a week not knowing when I would see them again."[3]

Young children, especially those too young to understand fully what was happening to them and why, often had difficulty adjusting to a new ward community. For children at Gillette Children's Hospital in St. Paul, Minnesota, and at many other rehabilitation facilities, "the bad experiences were separation from parents, loneliness, surgery and pain, food, the behavior of hospital staff members, and going home to strangers. The good experiences included seeing and learning new things, making friends with other children, being treated well by staff members, eating good food, and going home." Many youngsters felt the terror of being abandoned by their parents, especially when the parents lived some distance from the hospital and because of distance or the lack of transportation could visit only rarely. Gail Bias was one of the children who had a bad experience at Gillette. Admitted for reconstructive surgery when she was six, she remembers it as a "very lonely time." Because of limited visiting hours and farm chores, her parents could visit only on Sundays. She cried before, during, and after her parents' visits and when they had gone she was left with "such an empty, empty feeling being there all alone."[4]

Other children adjusted more easily to life on the polio rehabilitation ward, even if they missed their parents, family, and friends. Coming out of isolation, they were feeling better and, if apprehensive about the new situation, more open to the possibilities of making new friends. Twelve-year-old Arvid Schwartz worried about moving to a new place "where there were again a sea of beds." When he saw "all those strange faces, all young boys approximately my age, ten to fifteen," he thought "I don't know anybody in here." Soon, however, a young boy introduced himself and Schwartz began to be integrated into the life of the ward. When he was admitted to a children's hospital in Maine, nine-year-old Larry Fournier was apprehensive since his family spoke French. Fortunately, a boy in his ward spoke both English and French, "and suddenly, things were better." Like the others, Joyce Ann Tepley, who was also nine, quickly integrated herself into the ward community. She recalls that she "adjusted well to group living with my peers." She eagerly anticipated her parents' weekly visits, but she "didn't have time to be homesick," and rehabilitation was "mostly a good experience."[5]

For children, whether or not they had a good experience in the rehabilitation ward seems to have been dependent more on their emotional and psychological readiness to regard the experience as positive than on the conditions on the ward. Children who were ready quickly made friends, and together they endured the pain, discomfort, boredom, and loneliness of lengthy hospitalization and rehabilitation. Children who were emotionally and psychologically unready to become integrated into the ward life and its consolations generally had a worse experience.

The polio community on the wards provided adolescent and adult polio patients emotional support and reassurance that they could recover. Irving Zola, for example, recalled that his "spirits rose almost immediately" upon his entry into the rehabilitation ward. Not only was he "welcomed as the 'new polio,' but it felt good to see others in my situation." Even more reassuring, "was seeing some patients actually move about; it made me hope that I too might recover." Norma Duchin remembered that the sense of a community developed slowly but it brought benefits to all. "The feeling of wanting not to be less brave than the person in the next bed was followed by the feeling of honestly wanting to be considerate and helpful. Then, slowly and mercifully, humor and affection grew. We became friends." At Warm Springs, and no doubt elsewhere, the polio community refused to let newcomers wallow in self-pity. As

Hugh Gallagher put it, "the new patient, surrounded by many in the same situation and some in a worse situation, casts off his self-pity or soon has it forcibly torn from him by his neighbors, who will tolerate practically anything but pity or despair."[6]

For older patients the opportunity to talk about their fears and hopes with somebody in a similar situation was particularly comforting. Ward mates were not trained counselors, but it still helped to unburden oneself to someone who fully understood your predicament. Louis Sternburg's discussions with his friend Bert Fern as they rocked in adjoining beds helped them to come to terms with their almost total paralysis. Adapting their conversation to the rhythm of their rocking beds, the two men "had long talks about our past lives and our possible futures, trying to discover the meaning of the random disaster that had hit us." These conversations among ward companions were often more helpful than those with friends and family, with whom there were often barriers to communication and understanding rooted in concern and anxiety. As Robert Hall observed, family and friends were "anxious to help, to share our feelings which we usually found difficult to express. But, because they didn't know what we had been through, they could only imagine what it was like." Worry often showed in their faces and "it was their silent looks that so often raised barriers between us."[7]

Humor, often dark and sardonic, was another vehicle for coping with rehabilitation. At the Northwest Respiratory Center in Seattle where Kathryn Black's mother was treated, "patients joked among themselves and with the staff, often with the dark humor common in difficult situations. Quips about the power going off and about bedpans and urine jugs, enemas, and visits with the consulting psychiatrist bounced around the rooms." The men on Arnold Beisser's ward found humor in the food, sex or the lack of it, and even in stretching. After a pretty nurse had been on the ward, one of the men often commented in frustration, "I'm ready, willing, and *unable*." Underlying much of the joking and banter was affection for newly found friends sharing a difficult situation. Shared laughter not only helped cement friendships, it also helped both to reinforce and to subvert the hospital regime. By making it easier for the patients to tolerate painful therapy and restrictive hospital procedures, humor deflected any sustained challenge to medical or hospital authority. But laughter could also be subversive by fostering a sense of solidarity among the patients at the expense of the hospital and its medical personnel. The secret, Bentz Plagemann learned from his more experienced friends at Warm Springs, was "submission, with laughter to take away its edge."[8]

Most hospitals were short of staff to care for paralyzed and bedridden patients who could do little for themselves, and ambulatory patients often helped in ways that both provided comfort to friends and eased the demands on an overworked staff. Robert Hall remembered that there was a "good group" of nurses but there "were not enough of them." Once he was able to get around in a wheelchair he frequently assisted one of his ward mates "when he needed to have an arm shifted or turned over" or when he wanted to "smoke a cigarette in his holder." After nine-year-old Dorothea Nudelman began to use a wheelchair she met Joanne, who was still confined in an iron lung. As their friendship developed, Nudelman would feed Joanne the sandwiches her mother had brought. She also helped Joanne in other "more private ways" by opening the portholes of the iron lung and "stretching to scratch her itchy places" or covering and uncovering her paralyzed body. Patients in iron lungs found it difficult to raise their voices to call a nurse, and their paralysis made it impossible to use a call button. Those who could whistle or make loud clicking sounds to attract attention would do so for neighbors who were unable.[9]

For patients who were less severely paralyzed, the attention and assistance from other patients could lighten the difficulties of rehabilitation in a variety of ways. For example, when Charlene Pugleasa was initially on the rehabilitation ward, one of her older ward mates encouraged her and helped her try to lift her legs. Later, when she could get around, the thirteen-year-old Pugleasa visited the younger children. After seeking permission, she taught them how to chew bubble gum and blow bubbles, thereby strengthening their face muscles. Ray Gullickson remembers being asked by Sister Kenny to encourage another patient. Gullickson had worked hard at his exercises, but the other patient "was not cooperating with his treatment and had just been lying in bed, feeling sorry for himself ever since he was admitted." Gullickson talked to the young man, but the other patient was not persuaded and soon went home, his recovery unfinished. At Warm Springs, and no doubt elsewhere, new members of the community learned from more experienced residents. This was especially true in developing functional skills, such as getting on and off toilets, or transferring from a wheelchair to a car or a bed, and back again. It was often easier to do something after seeing it done by someone with a similar disability than after having it explained by a therapist.[10] This patient-to-patient assistance was no substitute for adequate staff, but it often provided useful aid and gave pleasure and comfort to both giver and recipient.

Like older patients, younger children often relied on newly made friendships to help them endure hospitalization and rehabilitation. John Swett recalls moving his bed together with his neighbor's so they could "visit after the lights went out." Unfortunately, the nurses didn't approve, and when Swett persisted they first put him in "the isolated bathroom with no light" and then they put him in a straightjacket and bed restraints. Like Swett, Richard Foley and the boy in the next bed "used to lay and talk a lot, talk about things in school, things we'd like to become and just sympathize with each other. When he . . . had a lot of pain we'd pull our beds together and I'd just lay there and hold his hand and talk to him when he cried and stuff because of the pain."[11]

Irving Zola discovered the benefits of undergoing rehabilitation on a ward with patients of similar age and disability following an auto accident four years after having polio. During his polio rehabilitation he was "surrounded by fellow patients in varying stages of a struggle, each cheering the others on." Following his auto accident, Zola spent most of his recovery "imprisoned" in a cast in his bedroom alone at home while his parents worked. "There was no endless stream of doctors, nurses, physiotherapists. There was no need for individual effort, no daily challenges to be met, no triumphs to report. Nothing! And that's what I experienced—a vast emptiness." Recovering from the car accident was "far more difficult psychologically" than his rehabilitation from polio.[12] Zola's dual experience suggests that those who could adjust to life on the ward derived substantial psychological benefit from undergoing rehabilitation as part of a community of similarly disabled individuals.

If many polio patients drew strength and comfort from their compatriots on the ward, there is also some evidence that the very public life of the ward could be coercive as well as supportive. Joyce Ann Tepley quickly learned that "there was little room for feelings of frustration, anger, or fear," and that "being good and brave was a tall order for a little girl." Still, she "did a great job of suppressing any 'bad' feelings." Like Tepley, Dorothea Nudelman remembers "a culture of denial and suppression." Staff and patients alike made clear the unwritten rules with injunctions such as: "Don't be a baby!" "This isn't too bad. Look at how lucky you are compared . . ." When Charles Mee encountered the coercive culture of the polio wards, he outwardly conformed to what was expected of him, but inwardly resisted the pressure to take a positive approach to his rehabilitation and prospects for the future.[13]

This "culture of denial and suppression" often facilitated the work of the rehabilitative staff, even as it created psychological problems for some who fell under its influence. When patients denied the painful reality of polio re-habilitation and suppressed their complex jumble of emotions, the medical and rehabilitation staff could focus on the challenge of physical recovery. They pushed their patients to exercise through pain—"No pain, no gain"—and de-ferred any recognition and treatment of the psychological costs of polio. Per-haps it made sense at the time, given the numbers involved, the challenges of physical rehabilitation for severely paralyzed individuals, and the limited re-sources of most facilities. But there is no question that this culture added a psy-chological burden to the physical disabilities polio had already imposed.

Each individual's experience of life on the polio wards was uniquely shaped by the extent of his or her paralysis, age, and emotional makeup, as well as by the other patients, the conditions and regulations of the hospital, and the personalities of the staff. However, certain features of the ward experience re-curred in many if not most hospital settings. Patients had to find ways to oc-cupy their abundant free time. Children and adolescents needed to expend some of their excess energy, especially once they became mobile. There was always something to complain about. There were holidays to celebrate, at home if one was lucky, in the hospital if one was not. There was school to at-tend, or lessons to keep up with. There were visits from family and friends to anticipate, and their departure to dread. And, finally, one could look for-ward to being discharged and returning home after weeks, perhaps months, of hospitalization.

Rehabilitation hospitals tried, not entirely successfully, to structure and control the polio patient's immersion in the ward culture. Institutional regu-lations and practices had, as we have seen, the central goal of encouraging the patient to "assimilate the hospital's universe of special meanings, goals, and evaluative rankings." [14] However, rehabilitation facilities were never com-pletely successful in structuring, regimenting, and controlling the ward life of their patients. The individuals who lived on the wards accepted many of the hospitals' regulations and procedures, in part because they had no real choice, but also because cooperation with the hospital staff, on some level at least, was the key to recovery and getting out. Nonetheless, like other dependent groups, these polio patients repeatedly tested the limits of authority. Through their play, their pranks, their complaints about hospital rules, food, and staff they created a subculture that was antagonistic to the hospital and its staff even as it contributed to rehabilitation by making the lengthy stays more bearable. Forty and fifty years later, polio survivors still have vivid memories of the fun they had and the games they played, as well as the abuse and punishments that they suffered.

Some of the most vivid memories are of the nurses who ran the wards and provided the ordinary care and comfort the hospital provided. Most of the nurses were compassionate, caring women who did all they could to ease the recovery of their patients. Except in some of the smaller, more specialized facilities, such as the regional respiratory centers, there were often too few nurses for the number of patients, many of whom in the early stages of their rehabilitation were bedridden and incapable of doing very much for themselves. It is no wonder that some polio survivors remember nurses who were harassed, who didn't respond quickly to their needs, or who sometimes forgot them. It is also clear, however, that nearly every institution had one or two nurses who terrorized the patients and, in some cases, abused them. The many good nurses helped ease the long process of recuperation; the few bad ones left lifelong scars.

Caring and compassionate nurses figure in many of the narratives. These women not only understood the physical needs of their paralyzed patients, they also understood the emotional and psychological ones. They understood the frustration of not being able to move, to breathe easily on one's own, or to go to the bathroom by oneself. Their care and encouragement was an important element in the determination of so many of the polio patients to persist in their difficult rehabilitation. "Ma Hunley" reminded the teenaged Bill Van Cleve of "an aunt or grandma perhaps; firm, but kind and caring." Arnold Beisser, who was almost totally paralyzed and thus very dependent upon his nurses, recalled that "the responsiveness of these compassionate helpers" made him "feel human again": "With them I felt returned from exile. The pariah was forgiven for his crime, and felt restored to life." [15]

Not all nurses, however, were so caring or empathetic, and many polio survivors encountered nurses who were cold, distant, unhelpful, and sometimes physically or psychologically abusive. David Oakley had "the unpleasant experiences of knowing a couple of women who had no business calling themselves nurses. They were cruel, nasty, and abusive of most everyone." The boys on Larry Fournier's ward agreed that the night nurse, "Miss Cross, had been aptly named. She was extremely short-tempered." Mark O'Brien described one of his nurses as "more of an adversary" than an ally. Kenneth Kingery discovered what a difference a nurse could make when the "regular night nurse, a kindly Tennessean in her sixties," was replaced by a "chill-voiced Amazon" who treated this World War II and Korean War air force veteran like a two-year-old.[16] The number of cruel and abusive nurses was small, but they did considerable damage to highly dependent patients who were already emotionally and psychologically vulnerable.

A major challenge for all patients was fighting the tedium of long hours spent confined to bed or the ward. Dorothea Nudelman remembered that "in the beginning, mostly we were bored. We were just a bunch of kids together who couldn't move and couldn't get out of bed. Not sick or anything. Time dragged." Similarly, Addie Flowers recalled that "when things got dull" the patients would use "their imagination and their grit" to liven up their days. One day, listening to the radio, the whole ward joined in the "Polio Jitterbug": "Eyeballs moved from left to right. Eyebrows shot up and down. Noses twitched and lips twisted—first left, then right. A chin poked upward, foreheads wrinkled. Fingers danced on white bed sheets. Heads dipped and swayed." The girls on Nudelman's ward "made up songs that mocked the hospital, the nurses, the physical therapists." They could also laugh at themselves, mocking their "bodies that no longer worked right": " 'Breathe like a polio!' some kid would shout. Then we'd all gasp and gulp air in a strange, labored way. Everyone laughed, even the iron lung kids!" No target was too sacred. Once their rehabilitation had progressed, "walking jokes" became commonplace. Nudelman's specialty was "imitating the poster child for the National Foundation for Infantile Paralysis—hunched over on sprawling crutches with the perfect sappy grin for begging dimes."[17] In this era before television, patients were dependent upon their imaginations to fill their time. That was easier to do in the company of others.

In some wards radio provided entertainment, but one had to listen to whatever station was playing. Sometimes, as in the case of the "Polio Jitterbug," listening to the radio inspired the imaginations of the patients. In other hospitals, radio supplied almost the only diversion. Clara Yelder, who was hospitalized in the all-black Infantile Paralysis Center in Tuskegee, Alabama, remembered that they passed the time by talking and that eventually they "had a radio. The center of our day was listening to the radio. There were no televisions." On Sundays in Larry Fournier's Maine hospital the children "listened to the radio that was piped into all the wards," unless they had "behaved badly, which resulted in such privileges being denied." While the radio generally entertained, it also brought news of the outside world. Leonard Kriegel remembers sitting in his chair "listening to the radio my grandmother had sent" when "the announcer, in a somber choking voice, told me of the death of God."

President Roosevelt had died. As Kriegel's experience suggests, some patients had their own radios if families could afford them and hospital policies permitted them. Robert Hall, however, was shocked that the Veterans Administration hospital where he finished his rehabilitation would not allow him to bring his own radio. Each bed, however, had "a headset with earphones plugged into a wall plug offering four local stations." If radios were common on the polio wards, televisions were relatively rare. Louis Sternburg recalled that in the late fifties at the Mary MacArthur Respiratory Center in Boston the adult ward had a better television than the children's. In the evenings "some of the children were brought into the ward to see the 'Mickey Mouse Club,'" which meant, of course, that the adults in their respirators and rocking beds had little choice but to watch it as well.[18] Some patients saw their first television in the hospital.

Because hospital stays were so long, many rehabilitation facilities provided some opportunities for children to continue their schooling. Joyce Tepley, for example, started fourth grade in the hospital school. Grace Audet remembers "lying on my stomach under my hot packs and doing my school work." The Sister Kenny Institute in St. Paul had a school that Arvid Schwartz attended for about ninety minutes a day. He recalled that they had "an elderly lady for a teacher and a very strange classroom." Nonetheless, he learned enough to have his hometown school accept the instruction as the equivalent of his seventh grade. Some patients were taught either by teachers provided by the local school district or by private tutors. David Kangas got through his sophomore year of high school, taught by a visiting teacher while confined to the Hibbing, Minnesota, hospital. Similarly, Irving Zola was "tutored three times a week by a retired Boston school teacher, Mrs. Nichols."[19] These educational opportunities were important in two respects. First, they were a productive use of the patients' time and gave them something more to do and think about. Second, keeping the patients up with their in-school classmates eased their eventual reentry into the classroom by avoiding the stigma of being held back.

As their physical therapy progressed, many patients became increasingly mobile, either in wheelchairs or on crutches. Mobility increased the opportunities to visit other patients, to explore hospital corridors, perhaps to go outside, and to get in trouble. For patients long confined to beds by paralyzed limbs, getting a wheelchair was liberating, not confining. Wheelchairs gave them the ability to move by themselves and were the first real sign of freedom and independence since they had become sick. Len Jordan remembers that he and his friends were "sort of 'roust-abouts.' We would run around in our

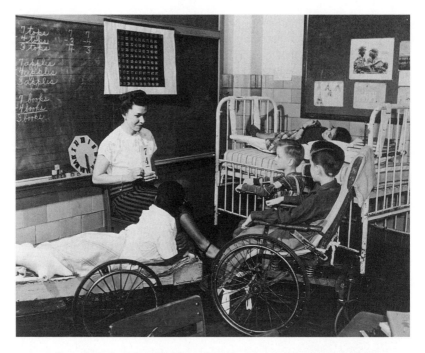

FIG. 16. Classroom instruction for polio patients in rehabilitation at the Toledo
Society for Crippled Children, ca. 1940s.

wheelchairs after hours, causing problems and chasing the nurses. . . . When
you're hospitalized that long, you have to do something to break the monotony." At Larry Fournier's Maine hospital, the children played "wheelchair
pool" and croquet. During the summer they "wheeled out on the lawn or onto
the hospital roof to enjoy a little sun." Many narratives mention wheelchair
races, which seem to have occurred wherever and whenever there were at least
two to race. Girls were as likely to race their wheelchairs as boys and young
men. Gail Bias and her friends would take "the old wooden wheelchairs" and
"race down the hall as far as we could go." Sometimes they would "catch hell"
from the nurses, but, as Bias put it, "we were just kids trying to make the best
of our situation and have a little fun." The men at Robert Hall's Veterans Administration Hospital treated their wheelchairs like the cars they would have
driven under more normal circumstances: "In a minute, we could be almost
anywhere else in the hospital in our wheelchairs. They were speedy, and we
worked on them to make them even more speedy. We constantly bugged the
crew in the maintenance room for oil or graphite for the axles so the wheel-

chairs would roll with less friction." In his rehab hospital Leonard Kriegel preferred the wheelchair to learning to walk with braces and crutches. Standing encased in steel and leather braces and expected to drag his paralyzed limbs along, Kriegel could only think of himself as a "cripple." But then there was his wheelchair: "With the braces and crutches, I faked it; with the wheel chair, I lived."[20]

Even without wheelchairs, patients, especially children and adolescents, found ways to have fun, often by playing pranks on each other or on the hospital staff. The pranks directed at each other or at no one in particular seem to have been carried out largely in the spirit of play. Some, however, were clearly directed at particular nurses, especially older ones who had the reputations of being mean-spirited "battle-axes." The youngsters made do with the materials at hand. One activity that seems to have occurred to many was to stab the paper cover of their straws into butter and then blow hard to stick the straw to the ceiling of the ward. David Graham recalled that his four-bed ward "had hundreds of them hanging there. Many a nurse went home with butter stains

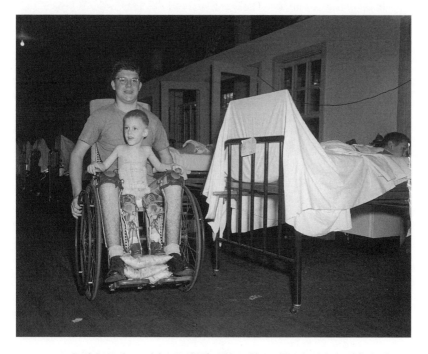

FIG. 17. Paul Conrad, 17, giving David Hensley a ride on his wheelchair while both were undergoing rehabilitation in High Point, North Carolina, in 1948.

on her back." Larry Kohout's sixteen-bed ward adjoined another of similar size. When the divider between the two wards was pulled back, "you looked across a huge expanse of ceiling that bristled with a growth of straw wrappers." Arvid Schwartz and his ward mates entertained themselves with spitball fights. After acquiring a hoard of rubber bands, the boys made "giant slingshots to shoot spitballs at each other, and those spitballs would really fly." Many of the spitball wars occurred after lights were out, and invariably the patients would get in trouble with the nurses. Sometimes, patients played pranks on one another. David Kangas remembers "high jinks" with other boys on the ward. They would "torment each other. If one was in bed and one was in a wheelchair, we would sort of play tricks on the guy in bed, knowing that he was virtually helpless."[21] These relatively harmless stunts provided a constant source of amusement on the wards and helped both perpetrator and victim, if there was one, forget the pain and boredom of polio rehabilitation. Plotting pranks, even if never carried out, exercised one's imagination, and if one had been a victim, revenge was, of course, sweet.

Not all of the mischief on the wards was so innocent. Leonard Kriegel's account of his two years at the New York State Reconstruction Home describes an active ward culture among the eight-to-thirteen-year-old boys that mimicked the rough-and-tumble culture of the playground and schoolyard. The ward culture had its leaders, who included Kriegel, and its outcasts, who became the target of jests and pranks. The boys taunted one another, made fun of each other's weaknesses, and occasionally settled their differences by fighting. Once Kriegel and his ward mates were given wheelchairs, they explored all the corridors and corners of the hospital and its grounds, and even conducted an "invasion" of the candy store in the nearby town. There was an adolescent fascination with sex and at least one instance of a sexual assault. While the nurses occasionally intervened to punish the more outrageous stunts, this boy culture seems to have operated largely outside the attention of the adults, just as it might have on the streets of Brooklyn. Caught up as they were in this flourishing ward life, these boys and adolescents occasionally forgot their disabilities and their painful struggle to recover and return home.[22]

Some illicit behavior was more dangerous. Older patients sometimes tried to smoke cigarettes when the nurses weren't looking or were on break. On one ward, "if a nurse returned sooner than she was supposed to, cigarette butts got stuck down bed posts. It's incredible that no bed ever wound up leaking the smoke." The teenaged boys in one ward at Warm Springs managed to fashion "a 'cannon' using a plugged aluminum tube about 4″ long." Match heads and cigarette lighter fluid provided the "gunpowder" to fire the device. For their ingenuity, the entire ward was grounded for two weeks, except for physical and occupational therapy. Girls also got in trouble in the pursuit of fun. Joy Hillhouse remembers the time she and her roommate were playing with their dolls and "made porrage for our babies by mixing Baby Powder with water." They then tried to cook it on one of the bed lamps. Soon it started to "smoke and stink." [23]

Some pranks were directed at particular staff members, especially nurses, whom individuals or the ward regarded as their tormentors. These activities made the staff members an object of ridicule and thereby chipped away at the authority they had wielded so imperiously. In some cases, the trick challenged their medical knowledge. When Bill Henderson's wife handed him a bouquet of dried flowers to look at more closely, "hundreds of tiny seeds dropped into the hair" on his chest. He "immediately planned a way to harass the nurse." When the nurse next came to take his temperature, he was "madly scratching and told her that something was bothering my skin. She pulled the sheet down and gave a gasp saying 'Oh my god' and hastily pulled the sheet up and tore out of the room." David Olsen remembers a similar game that involved the root beer "Fizzies" popular at the time. Olsen and his roommate would "put several of these fizzies into the bedside urinal . . . and then use the urinal." The nurse would check the urine for color and amount before emptying them. Olsen "will always remember hearing her gasp . . . and then her moving VERY QUICKLY out of the room to report her terrifying news about the state of our urinary systems." Some pranks, however, had a harder edge and were plotted to badly embarrass the nurse, if not actually hurt her. David Graham remembers how his four-bed ward of twelve- and thirteen-year-old boys got back at the nurse they called "Ol' Battle Axe," who woke them every morning by "throwing a damp wash cloth" in their faces. One morning they managed to move "a bed-side stand . . . in front of the entry door. On the edge we had placed a full water pitcher. At the 7 AM hour she came through that door with a full head of steam. Water and pitcher went everywhere. Needless to say she found us all fast asleep." These more serious escapades did not, of course, fundamentally alter the power relationships in the hospital, but they did subvert, however briefly, the authority of the staff and the regimen of the institution. For a brief time the perpetrators of the pranks were not passive and dependent. As Robert Hall observed of the campaign he and his friends waged against "Old Crotchety": "No one ever complained about her tactics, but it was war forever, undeclared war, against her. Whenever we could, we made life miserable for her. I really believed all of this added to our determination to get well. Her presence stimulated a constant, added adrenalin [*sic*] production."[24] Although the stunts could create problems for the staff, it is clear that patients who had recovered enough to plot and carry out such activities had already begun to rebuild the self-esteem and self-assurance they would need outside the hospital.

Getting into mischief was not, of course, the only social activity on the polio wards. Although wards were generally segregated by sex, the increasing mobility achieved through rehabilitation provided opportunities to build a social life that included both sexes. Although both men and women undoubtedly felt the return of interest in sex, male narratives are much more explicit in this regard. For many young men, the first question they faced was whether they would be able to perform sexually, as polio had made them temporarily impotent and unable to achieve an erection. Both fourteen-year-old Charles Mee and sixteen-year-old Irving Zola were greatly relieved when they were able to masturbate for the first time following polio. Sometimes the erections that signaled the return of sexual interest and function were not entirely welcome. Louis Sternburg recalled that bed baths on the rocking bed "became quite a sensuous pleasure." He regularly got "aroused" when his nurse Doris gave him "a fast, skilled wash and massage." Although he was "half in love with Doris," what he really wanted was "to be moved away from the nurses' station to a more remote cubicle" where he could be alone with his wife. Michael Davis also remembers the embarrassment of an unwanted erection. At the Kosair Rehabilitation Hospital in Louisville, Kentucky, "male patients wore only cotton g-strings, and every evening . . . were given cooling sponge baths and 'changed.'" One evening Davis "suddenly developed an erection during this process. Aside from acute early-adolescent shame at this unwanted display, I remember thinking, 'Well, there's at least one muscle that still works.'"[25] These sexual impulses and desires, which appeared as patients began to feel better physically, were a signal that in one important respect, at least, they would be normal, regardless of the results of their rehabilitation.

For many young men, the presence of a largely female nursing staff, many only a few years older than their patients, was both a pleasure and a temptation. Add to this the need for these young women to be in intimate contact with their paralyzed patients and you have the ingredients for sexual tension on both sides. Irving Zola recalled the "student nurses, often only a year or two older, who were a constant stimulation and encouragement for my budding sexuality." Similarly, on his later hospitalizations Don Kirkendall discovered his emerging sexuality watching "the younger nurses, rosy-cheeked and laughing . . . the way their breasts curved to fill their starched white uniforms." Arnold Beisser remembered that on his ward of "thirty severely disabled male polio patients," women and sex were missed more than anything else. As a result, "any unsuspecting young woman who entered the ward was likely to be the subject of elaborate fantasy and discussion." Beisser, in fact, would eventually marry Rita, the young and beautiful physical therapist whose efforts to stretch the men's muscles had produced such exquisite pain and pleasure.[26]

These sexually charged encounters between patients and staff did not usually lead to illicit sexual activity, but on occasion patients were subjected to unwanted sexual overtures or even sexual abuse from hospital staff. Billie McCabe remembers a young male doctor who repeatedly came into the room where she and her roommate, both teenagers, were taking their "therapeutic hot baths." After complaints to the nurse failed to stop this behavior, the two girls devised a "bubble-bath solution." The "bubbles were enormous and lasted through the ½ hr. or hour we had to stay in the tub." With the girls' modesty protected, the doctor stopped checking on them. Ed Keohan was disturbed by being repeatedly chosen to be seen naked for an exam by the new student nurses, who were only a few years older than he was. He felt that older or younger patients "would not have been as much fun for the girls." He also wondered why, when he "had to have hair removed between my legs for an ankle operation it was always a female within a year or two of my age (less than 21) that did the shaving." In some cases, the sexual abuse was even more direct and disturbing. Don Kirkendall was repeatedly fondled by a young nurse who came into the ward at night, stood by his bed, and "reached under the cover to touch me and excite me and terrify me."[27] However infrequent, these instances took advantage of the patients' dependence and immobility, embarrassed them, and in some cases awakened deep-seated feelings of guilt and shame in individuals already struggling to come to terms with their sense of sexuality in a disabled body.

Because polio paralyzed and withered limbs and twisted torsos, young men and women had to find ways to surmount their internalized sense, as Irving Zola put it, that they were "de-formed, dis-eased, dis-abled, dis-ordered, ab-normal and, most telling of all, . . . in-valid." Lorenzo Milam put it more bluntly when he wrote that the problem was their "belief that no one in their right mind would want (we think) to engage in an act of congress with a spinal case, a certified quadriplegic, a multiple-spastic scoliosis-and-iron lung crip— e.g., a patient." As Hugh Gallagher later recognized, the social life of a rehabilitation center "served a purpose greater than simple morale building. It provided a way for polio patients to relearn their social skills."[28] The protected environment of the rehabilitation hospital helped polio patients to reestablish their social skills without fear of rejection because of their disability. Where disability was the norm, they were the normal ones.

Although many narratives testify to the importance of the polio community in the social and emotional recovery of polio patients, the narratives of rehabilitation at Warm Springs contain especially warm memories of the social life at the facility. Warm Springs always retained something of its resort heritage even as it became a first-rate rehabilitation facility in the thirties and forties. Many of the patients treated at Warm Springs had already spent time in rehabilitation hospitals before being sent to Georgia. Their often unhappy prior experience with polio rehabilitation made them skeptical of the Georgia institution and of its glowing reputation. For example, after a year of physical therapy at Providence Hospital in Washington, DC, Hugh Gallagher had a "closed, safe, little world." He had no desire to go to Warm Springs and he "did not want to be around other paralyzed people" or "to associate with 'cripples.'" He soon changed his mind; "Warm Springs was the best thing ever to happen to me."[29]

The social life at Warm Springs set it apart from the usual rehabilitation hospital, at least in the minds of those who also had experience with more traditional facilities. Warm Springs, according to Hugh Gallagher, "provided an opportunity to meet people, undertake joint activities, make friends, date, fall in love. The whole range of normal social activities went on at Warm Springs, much the way it does elsewhere in the world." Lorenzo Milam concurred: "We are freed for the first time, really free of the nightmare that had gripped us just months before." He would always be grateful to those who "invented joy on earth for those of us fortunate enough to get out of the claws of the doctors in the small grey hospitals around the country and into that wonder."[30]

The memories of time spent at Warm Springs are bathed in a golden haze of appreciation that no doubt obscures moments of loneliness, the pain of physical therapy, and a fear of the future. Still, for young adults who had recovered sufficiently to participate in the extensive social life of the foundation, Warm Springs became a "paradise island set up by master Roosevelt and his merry crew." Hugh Gallagher recalled that "the parties, dinners, and activities at Warm Springs gave new patients the opportunity to exercise their skills, traits, and habits they developed and used in interpersonal contact before their illness." In the accepting atmosphere of Warm Springs, where handicaps were the norm, these young men and women discovered that they were "as attractive, as witty, and had the same positive and negative traits as before." Like Gallagher, Lorenzo Milam credited the social life at Warm Springs with restoring his sense of self: "For we are reborn. We have come born again out of the ashes of shared horror, and have come whole again." In spite of the pleasant social life, the patients and staff could not totally ignore a "current of uncertainty, of uneasiness" that ran underneath the gay surface. However normal their lives seemed within the gates of Warm Springs, everyone knew that it couldn't last. Normal was the larger world outside where graduates would have to adjust to being disabled, to being outsiders. The only proper response was to "have parties and do mad things, drink moonshine, and go to the movies." It was easier to "push the future into the distant indefinite," than to confront directly the post–Warm Springs possibilities.[31]

Warm Springs may have represented a kind of rehabilitation paradise, both for the quality of its therapeutic programs and the glories of its social life, but most polio survivors did not experience therapy in its resort-like setting. Most writers of polio narratives had some good experiences in rehabilitation, but many midcentury rehabilitation hospitals also provided ample cause for criticism. Some complaints are not surprising—institutional food has never received many accolades, and holidays away from home are never easy—but there were more substantial concerns as well. The repressive rules and regulations, and the nurses and administrators who sometimes enforced them with a rigid authoritarianism, were frequent targets of patient and family anger. Both patients and their families, for example, were especially distressed by the extremely limited visiting hours that sometimes separated family members for weeks and months. While long hours with little to do probably fostered many complaints, there is no doubt that many of the criticisms leveled against the policies, practices, and personnel of midcentury rehabilitation hospitals were deserved.

Complaining about hospital food was one of the ways in which patients entertained themselves, although many complaints had a solid basis. As Arnold Beisser observed, "food is mentioned to complain how bad it is." Millie Teders, who was nine at the time, remembers that "the bad food never stopped." Although most hospital food was bad in the estimation of those forced to eat it week after week, particular foods sometimes stood out. Teders recalled that "the jello was so rubbery, we used to play catch with it." Rancho Los Amigos near Los Angeles was remembered for its "hideous green hot dog weenies" and hamburgers that were "flat, sorry, tasteless, little things." At Larry Fournier's

Maine hospital, "not eating all the food on our plates was a punishable offense but then, sometimes, so was the food." Sometimes a little fantasy helped make eating more palatable. The children, aided by the staff, pretended they were "having a picnic at Old Orchard Beach." They ate their "hot dogs and hamburgers, and played our games along an imaginary shore." Dorothea Nudelman recalled a hot summer evening when the girls on her ward "built an elaborate fantasy meal that sounded delicious. We dreamed of salads, a huge icy watermelon, and tons of ice cream." At the suggestion of one of the girls, the parents of the patients agreed to fulfill the fantasy and brought the food into the ward. As she so rightly observed, "regular people-food tastes wonderful when you're in the hospital." For a little while, the girls "laughed and felt normal again."[32]

Parents and other family members often tried to bring favorite foods into the hospitals on their visits, sometimes smuggling them past vigilant nurses. One woman remembers that she and her roommates put "a long thin rope out our window on Wed. and Sun. nights so our husbands could send up meals we ordered them to get for us when they came to visit that day." When Joyce Ann Tepley's grandmother accompanied her parents on their weekend visits "she would bring her wonderful fried chicken. They would wheel me outside in my iron-barred bed, and we would have a picnic." During a long hospitalization for a spinal fusion, my parents occasionally brought me a lobster tail dinner from our family's favorite restaurant. Candy was a special treat, especially for youngsters, but some hospitals barred anything not on the official diet while others required that any food brought to a patient had to be shared with everyone on the ward. The Sister Kenny Institute in St. Paul banned candy, but parents continued to smuggle it in: "Parents knew they weren't supposed to be doing it and the kids knew they weren't supposed to be getting it, but it was this great undercover operation that worked." After the visiting hours were over, the kids had to find a place to hide the contraband. Periodically the "nurses would have a raid after visiting hours" and confiscate all the candy they could find. Letters reminding parents of hospital rules would be sent to the parents, and the smuggling would cease for a few weeks only to resume again. Arvid Schwartz eventually came to the conclusion that "the nurses knew what was going on all the time, but they kind of let us get by a little."[33]

Unlike the Kenny Institute, the Gillette Children's Hospital in St. Paul didn't ban food, but if "somebody brought you something good to eat when you were on the ward, you were expected to share it with everybody, and it would be given out at 2:00 P.M. with orange juice." Gail Bias recalls that when parents brought you something like candy, "you didn't always want to share it because there probably wasn't enough for all 25 or so girls on the ward." After an Easter visit from her mother, Bias hid the candy in her bedpan: "That seemed like the safest place to put it. After all, who in the world would ever go looking for something to eat in a person's bed pan?"[34] Patients found outside food a welcome break from the monotony of hospital food and a reminder of the good things one could look forward to upon discharge. Parents and spouses liked bringing food to their loved ones because it brought the patients pleasure and because it enabled them to be nurturing. Smuggled food was especially tasty because it challenged the authoritarianism of the hospital and because it united parents and children or spouses in a common cause against the institution.

Complaints about food are almost universal in any institutional setting. Complaints about enemas, however, may have been more common on the polio wards than anywhere else. Polio patients had particular problems with their bowels, especially if the virus had damaged or destroyed the nerves that served the abdomen. Paralyzed or weakened muscles were often incapable of moving material through the intestines. In addition, the long hours spent lying flat in bed combined with the lack of exercise contributed to the problems of constipation. Nurses typically insisted that patients have a bowel movement on the schedule devised by the hospital. While regular bowel movements are necessary, the nurses' insistence on a rigid schedule, the very public nature of using a bedpan on a crowded ward, the frequent and regular reliance on enemas, and the perception that enemas were sometimes used as punishment made bowel movements into a contest of wills between nurses and patients.

Nurses invariably won the contest, but in the process they sometimes exacted a heavy psychological toll. Don Kirkendall recalled that one of the hospitals where he had surgery required all children to attempt to move their bowels between seven and seven-thirty every evening. Those who missed two days in a row were punished by being denied the Tuesday evening movie, "banished, bed and all, to the large ugly main bathroom down the hall," where the offender remained "for the duration of the show." One of the Shrine hospitals had a regular schedule of escalating treatments designed to produce a bowel movement: "They always kept a chart and if you didn't move bowels within a two day span you had prune juice, three days and it was milk [of] magnesia, four days and it was prune juice and milk [of] magnesia together, five days and you had something called . . . cascara with a prune juice chaser and after six days it was the ENEMA." Patients were particularly embarrassed when nurses announced their bowel status in front of everyone on the ward. David Graham and his teenaged roommates were "embarrassed about the whole procedure," but the nurse continued to "announce the event hours ahead of time for all to contemplate."[35] The efforts of nurses to induce bowel movements were some of the most unpleasant aspects of the long hospitalizations associated with polio rehabilitation.

Enemas were not the only hospital practices that embarrassed polio patients. Many recall the embarrassment of being virtually naked and on display as doctors examined them or explained surgical procedures in front of an audience. They also resented being treated merely as an object of scientific interest. Shortly after his spinal fusion, Edmund Sass found himself in an auditorium in front of what he assumed were medical students. His physician explained the surgery as he changed Sass's dressing. For Sass, "lying there naked on that table while a physician talked about me like I was a scientific exhibit was a humiliating experience for a 14-year-old to endure." Because the incision was on his back, at least he did not have to look at the audience. Girls also suffered from being treated as objects for medical display. Roxann O'Brien remembers that when she was ten, the cast to straighten her scoliosis was "applied during the filming of [a] medical school instructional film." She was "naked, scared and very embarrassed."[36] In the face of medical authority, patients, especially children and adolescents, felt they had no alternative but to endure the experience. Challenging the physicians or questioning the need for such public display was unthinkable.

Perhaps the most disliked of all hospital policies were the restrictions on visitors. It was common to limit visiting to several hours on Wednesday and again on Sunday. As Dr. Steven Koop put it in his history of Gillette Children's Hospital, "the rare visits by parents or family were one of the biggest causes of loneliness." Every polio survivor "wished they could have seen their family more often" when they were hospitalized.[37] In some cases, the parents' weekly visit, as welcome as it was, also forcefully reminded the children of the many lonely hours facing them in the week ahead. Even adult polio patients, to their dismay, were often limited in the frequency with which they could have visitors. Kenneth Kingery was appalled when he learned that the visiting hours on the convalescent ward in his Wisconsin hospital were severely limited. As the nurse informed his wife, "now that your husband is better, you'll only be able to see him twice a week." What's more, his children were not allowed to visit at all. Shocked at this development, Kingery wondered, had he "committed a crime in contracting polio? Why else prison visiting rules? I must have sinned."

When he protested, the nurse only reiterated the hospital rules; she offered no justification of the policy.[38]

It was not only hospital regulations that limited the frequency with which families visited during rehabilitation. Distance from the hospital, lack of transportation, and bad winter weather were all impediments to frequent visiting. While she was at the facility for African Americans at Tuskegee, Alabama, Clara Yelder's parents visited her weekly, but they were the exception. She speculated that the parents who didn't come lived farther away, or were poorer. One Virginia patient's mother had to take a bus 130 miles from Danville to visit him in a Richmond hospital. She would catch a bus on Saturday, ride for several hours, visit her son and then return home by bus on Sunday so she could go to work on Monday. The family had "no car, no health insurance, almost no money." Arvid Schwartz's father had never driven to the Twin Cities before his son contracted polio, but all during the time Arvid was in the Sister Kenny Institute his parents made the "seven hour round trip . . . every Sunday with the exception of one time when they got caught in a snowstorm."[39]

Some hospitals, however, went beyond the norm in restricting visits from family and friends. For example, the San Francisco Shrine Hospital allowed parents to "visit once a week on Sunday, and then for only half-hour each, and they couldn't come in together." The Shrine Hospital in Philadelphia allowed visits only every other Sunday from April to October. In addition, all gifts had to pass through an autoclave to be sterilized. That meant "no pictures, nothing made of plastic or wood." Books that made it though would fall apart as soon as they were read. Kathy Vastyshak recalls that at the Alfred I. DuPont Institute in Wilmington, Delaware, visiting hours took place in the auditorium: "The kids would line up in chairs or beds, whatever they were in, wheelchairs. Then they would have two folding chairs in front of each child. We'd all come in and we'd all get in our places. The bell would ring, they'd open the doors, and the parents would come in. We'd visit for two hours or whatever it was. The bell would ring, they'd file out." When he was hospitalized, Ed Keohan's parents often did not have the money to pay bills, and the family received no help from the March of Dimes. The result, as Keohan recalled, was that "the hospital would never let my mother in to visit me (only one visitor was allowed for one hour per week) unless my mother had some money to pay toward my bill." Initially Iva Grover's parents could visit daily from 2:00 to 4:00 P.M. and again from 6:00 to 8:00. But after they "challenged some rule" the hospital restricted them to one hour at 10:00 A.M. and one hour at 7:00 P.M.[40] There was no medical necessity for such regulations.

Perhaps the most extreme instance of reducing, indeed eliminating, parental influence was the scheduling of surgeries without informing parents. Several accounts from different hospitals suggest that this practice, if not commonplace, occurred repeatedly throughout the period. Larry Fournier recalled that he was particularly lonely when he had one of his many surgeries, but his "parents had no car—had no way of knowing when the operation was scheduled." "During or after surgeries" at the Shrine Hospital in San Francisco "parents could not visit." Jana Weston could not "even talk to them on the phone." In addition, all of the patient's "out-going or in-coming mail was read by the staff. If they felt that any of it was 'inappropriate,' they would censor it." At the Philadelphia Shrine Hospital, one young woman's "parents were never notified about surgery until it was over." The family eventually "developed a code so that I could let them know ahead of time." At this hospital they could write home only on postcards that were censored by the nurses.[41] In these instances the physicians and hospitals usurped the right of parents to make decisions regarding their children's treatment.

In the context of postwar attitudes about physicians and hospitals, such occurrences were not necessarily aberrations. Doctors and hospitals had taken it upon themselves to decide what was best for the patients in their care. Fred Davis, in his study of Baltimore polio patients, observed that some physicians were reluctant to discuss treatment possibilities and outcomes with parents because it was "time consuming, difficult to handle, and disruptive of their tightly scheduled routines." In addition, he suggests that when someone other than parents was paying for the care, as would have been the case with the March of Dimes and in state institutions or Shrine hospitals, doctors "may have felt themselves to be under less compulsion" to consult with parents than under the "more usual fee-for-service arrangement." Furthermore, doctors seem to have assumed that some parents, at least, lacked the necessary knowledge to make informed decisions regarding their children's rehabilitation. Perhaps that helps explain why parents who challenged the prevailing system were likely to be labeled as uncooperative. For example, after Janice Knight's parents questioned the treatment their daughter was receiving at the Pennsylvania State Hospital for Crippled Children, one of the hospital staff wrote in the case notes, "The parents of this child are extremely uncooperative."[42] Given the respect most parents felt toward the medical establishment in postwar America, and the fear that their inquiries might result in diminished care for their children, not many parents were willing to be labeled as "uncooperative."

If many rehabilitation hospitals severely limited their patients' visitors, other institutions allowed family members, and sometimes friends as well, almost unlimited access to recovering polio patients. In his Boston hospital Irving Zola's visitors helped fill the long days. He "never felt deserted by friends or family. Every day was filled with a variety of visitors, and with them came endless books and forbidden goodies (the hospital canteen did not supply corned beef sandwiches, cheesecake, or liquor)." Gus Petitt remembers that at the hospital in Birmingham, Alabama, "friends, distant relatives and children were not permitted to visit but parents, grown-up brothers and sisters, spouses and fiancees were allowed willy-nilly."[43] These hospitals recognized that a more liberal visitation policy was compatible with effective rehabilitation.

Although visits were welcome any time, they were especially important around the holidays. Patients of all ages hated being stuck in the hospital at Christmas, Easter, or on one's birthday. Most facilities attempted to create a festive mood for those patients unable to go home for the holiday, but holiday decorations, special meals, and extended family visits were no substitute for being home. At Larry Fournier's Maine hospital the Salvation Army provided presents for the patients. Fournier was surprised to receive the camera and harmonica he had wished for when "Santa Claus appeared on Christmas Eve, overwhelming us with his generosity and good cheer." In spite of the fancy gifts, Christmas left Fournier in "the grip of despair." He would have "gladly traded everything for one of my family's 'fruit and candy' Christmases, or even the company of my parents who were simply too far away to visit." John Swett was particularly happy that his parents were able to make the long journey from Tampa to Warm Springs to see him at Christmas, since they had been unable to come for Thanksgiving. For adult patients, holidays often sparked gloomy reflections on polio's high cost to them and their families. The staff at the Jersey City Medical Center tried to give Larry Alexander's room an "air of cheerfulness," but "the tree seemed only to exaggerate the bare tile and cold, hospital look." Lying in his iron lung, with his wife by his side, Alexander felt "a sudden sense of loss" sweep over him. For both of them, uncertain of what lay in the future, the holiday was something to be gotten through rather than enjoyed.[44] No matter how much hospitals tried to create a festive mood at holidays, and no matter how much patients might appreciate the effort and extra attention, almost all would have traded the holiday in the hospital for a few hours or days at home.

Some rehabilitation hospitals allowed patients who were sufficiently advanced in their recovery to spend time at home over major holidays if the distance was not too great and the home could be adequately prepared. While eagerly anticipated by both patients and family, the actual visit was sometimes more difficult and less satisfactory than anyone hoped. In 1952, Arvid Schwartz had a two-day pass at Christmas from the Sister Kenny Institute in St. Paul. Because the staff had made a "superhuman effort," most of the patients enjoyed Christmas with their families. He remembers sitting outside the small church in the family car listening to the congregation sing "Silent Night." Christmas was a "happy one," but there were few presents for the children, and Schwartz began to realize how much his illness was costing his parents. Schwartz's mother made him all his favorite foods, even though they were "absolutely the wrong thing to eat." When Schwartz and his ward mates returned to the hospital after their two days of freedom, they came back "sick with the flu, diarrhea, and everything else, and parents were scared that they did something they shouldn't have, and we were scared." Unlike Schwartz, Jim Marugg still needed a chest respirator when he went home for Thanksgiving. He had been using the Monaghan chest respirator for only a couple of weeks and he still felt fragile and uncertain away from the ward. As he put it, "I felt like a glass man that might break or come apart at a touch." The excitement of the adventure made it difficult for him to breathe and he spent "a good part of my two hours at home in bed, with the Monaghan clasped to my bosom." Although he was relieved to get back "to the safe and ordered routine of the hospital," the brief trip had convinced him that he "could do it again and that each time it would be easier. And that eventually it would be for good." Marugg's Christmas visit went more smoothly than his Thanksgiving one had, even though it took him more than a week to recover once he returned to the hospital. He remembers that Christmas as "the happiest of my life."[45]

Not all polio patients were able to spend holidays at home, but many hospitals allowed patients to take brief excursions home before they were finally discharged. These brief visits allowed both the patient and his or her family to discover what still needed to be done before the patient completed his therapy or her recovery from surgery. Were modifications to the home necessary to accommodate a wheelchair, a rocking bed, or an iron lung? Who would oversee the continuing program of exercise and therapy? Were parents or a spouse ready to assume whatever continuing care was necessary? Had the patient broken the psychological as well as the medical dependence on the hospital and its staff?

The trial visits home were an opportunity for both the patient and the family to get reacquainted after months of separation. As might be expected, however, not all of the initial visits home went smoothly. Louis Sternburg was finally able to make a trip home when he could use a chest respirator and had learned to frog breathe. However, the first trip went so badly that he concluded that it "wasn't worth it." Sternburg did nothing but worry "all the time about power failure"; his wife "was too anxious to sit down"; and other members of his family were "so nervous that they couldn't enjoy this longed-for visit." Subsequent weekends home went more smoothly, as everyone began to adjust to having a respirator-dependent father in the house. Sternburg also felt an overwhelming sexual longing for his wife. He was determined that when he was "home for good we'd have to find some way to make love." Like Sternburg and his family, Jim Marugg and his wife began to rediscover one another on the weekend visits. After a particularly good weekend, Marugg concluded that "Sylvia and I were people again." For married couples, weekend visits home gave them the opportunity to reestablish sexual relations after months of forced abstinence. Dr. John Affeldt, director of the rehabilitation center at Rancho Los Amigos, discovered the sexual aspect of home visits in an unusual way. The hospital used two different chest respirators made by different companies, the Emerson Company and the Huxley Company. One day the Huxley representative asked, "How come every time the patients want to go home for the weekend, they take my Huxley off and they want an Emerson?" The staff psychologists finally uncovered the answer: "The Huxley went way down under the body, including the abdomen. The Emerson was just the chest. The patients could have sexual relations with an Emerson. They couldn't in a Huxley."[46] Patients who had reached this point in their recovery from polio were almost certainly ready to be discharged from the hospital.

| 6 |

Going Home to a Long Recovery

"**Y**OU'RE GOING HOME." Polio patients waited weeks and months to hear those welcome words. From the time they entered the isolation hospital, their goal had always been to return home to family, friends, school, and work. Few had anticipated that the disease which had begun so innocuously would lead to months of hospitalization and painful rehabilitation. But, at long last, rehabilitation was coming to an end. Rehabilitative medicine had done all it could to rebuild muscle function and to compensate for muscles permanently paralyzed. Although many polio patients had hoped that they would walk out of the hospital restored to their former physical condition and pre-polio life, they often had to settle for something quite different. Their recovery from polio was only partially completed when they were discharged from the rehabilitation facility. Many left the hospital encased in heavy steel braces, leaning on crutches, or in wheelchairs. They continued exercises at home or made frequent visits to outpatient facilities. Some would face one or more surgeries in the coming years to transplant muscles or to fuse bones in hopes of gaining greater comfort, stability, and mobility.

However much they wanted to go home, the prospect of leaving the hospital and returning to their families produced its own anxieties. The hospital had become a familiar place with a predictable routine. Days were spent among friends, all of whom were similarly disabled, and the hospital staff, in general, took good care of their medical and physical needs. But how would families react to and accommodate a crippled sibling, child, parent, or spouse? How would friends respond to their braces, crutches, and wheelchairs? Would they be able to go back to school or work and be accepted? Yes, going home was deeply desired, but it was also a step into a new and somewhat frightening world—a very different world from the one left behind when they were diagnosed with polio and entered the hospital.

When polio patients finally returned home, many of them faced a difficult period of adjustment. They were not the same persons physically, emotionally, or psychologically. Accommodations had to be made for the remaining disabilities and assistive devices. Other family members sometimes resented the extra attention paid to the polio survivor, no matter how necessary to his or her survival. In the case of adult polio survivors, the continuing disability sometimes meant that one's spouse had to become the primary income producer. Going home was only one step in the lifelong challenge of learning to live with a permanent disability.

There was no clear ending point to most cases of polio rehabilitation. Usually hospital-based rehabilitation ended when maximum muscle function had been restored and the patient had received functional training and assistive devices to compensate for any residual paralysis and disability. However, there were no precise standards by which to measure the restoration of muscle function, and many patients would continue to improve and to shed assistive devices for some years following their initial discharge. As a result of this imprecision, the decision to end restorative therapy was sometimes the result of discussions between patient and/or parent and physician, and sometimes a unilateral decision on the part of the doctor, patient or parent. Could the patient negotiate stairs with his braces? Did she have sufficient upper-body strength to propel her wheelchair? Could a respirator-dependent patient breathe on his own for up to three hours in case of a power emergency? Once the physicians were confident that the polio patient could function successfully outside the rehabilitation facility, they issued discharge orders. Not all patients and parents, however, were willing to wait for a physician's decision to release the patient. A desire to go home, or have one's child at home, and a conviction that little more was to be gained by staying in the hospital led some families to challenge the physician's authority and to negotiate an early release, or in some cases, to secure a discharge over the objections of the doctors.

Because poliomyelitis affected each patient's nerves and muscles differently, medical sources could give only general guidelines concerning the end of in-hospital therapy and the suitability of sending the patient home. For example, Dr. Philip Lewin believed that the convalescent stage, which began when muscle tenderness ended, lasted until "spontaneous improvement can no longer be observed, *i.e.,* in about one to three years." He argued that after polio patients reached "the point of maximal improvement," they should be encouraged to develop "the functional use of their muscles and braces." In describing the Kenny method of rehabilitation, Dr. John Pohl noted that after physical therapy ended in the "chronic stage, the recovery of further power in weakened muscles may go on indefinitely providing coordination and rhythm have been properly re-established." He acknowledged that "there is really no predictable end point to the recovery of function and power in muscles which are weakened but not entirely paralyzed."[1]

At the 1948 International Poliomyelitis Conference Dr. William Green summarized contemporary thinking on the convalescent phase of polio recovery. Convalescence stretched from forty-eight hours after the patient's fever ended to "about 16 months after the onset of the disease" when "no further recovery in musculature is to be expected." The length of treatment largely depended on the severity of the case, and "is as simple and short or long and detailed as necessary." While the speed of rehabilitation depended on the patient's condition, he also noted that "in general, adults are moved along more rapidly than children for socio-economic reasons." Green argued that patients should be discharged only when family members were willing and able to carry out a continuing exercise program prescribed by the doctors. For example, Green typically required parents "to come in for several days preceding the patient's discharge for instruction in the exercises and in other features of the child's regime. The parent is required to perform the exercises with the child and the patient is not discharged until they are performed satisfactorily." Green believed that during this convalescent phase "the great majority of patients who have had the disease should become normal or nearly normal."[2] Green's essay described an ideal situation. In reality, many polio patients, children and adults alike, were discharged far more cavalierly and with little instruction or training in how to proceed to become "normal or nearly normal."

Fred Davis, in his study of Baltimore polio patients, described in some detail how physicians developed a prognosis. Estimates of a patient's potential for recovery were based on periodic and careful muscle examinations made "some six weeks to three months following the onset of the disease." Relying on "years of accumulated clinical experience" rather than on "known laws of cellular deterioration and regeneration," doctors made a reasonably accurate estimate of how much muscle capacity a patient was likely to regain. This prognosis, however, was often not conveyed to either the patient or to the parents. The parents' questions "were, for the most part, hedged, evaded, rechanneled, or left unanswered." The parents' lack of full information, of course, made it easier for the physicians alone to decide when hospital rehabilitation was finished. For the physicians in Davis's study, "recovery, medically speaking, consists wholly in the patient's developing, with or without external supports, substitute or compensatory skills for overcoming as much of his functional loss as possible."[3] Given the broad and somewhat imprecise definitions of recovery and the physician's reluctance to provide patients and parents with clear and definite prognoses, it is not surprising that in numerous cases the issue of ending in-hospital rehabilitation and returning home became a matter of compromise. The physician's desire to bring about maximum recovery and the difficulty of determining when that occurred conflicted with the patients' desires to return home and get on with their lives.

Regardless of what physicians did or did not tell them, patients, including children, aided by the culture of the polio wards, quickly developed their own benchmarks of recovery. For example, the children in Fred Davis's study learned to measure the progress of their rehabilitation by the periodic muscle checks. They concluded that the second muscle check, about twelve weeks after admission, largely determined whether they would receive additional therapy or be fitted for braces. As one perceptive young girl observed, "Nobody around here walks until after they've had their second muscle check." The children in this study regarded being fitted for braces "not as a sign of severe or permanent incapacity but as proof that they were getting well and were ready to go home."[4] Although, it might take weeks of functional training with braces before doctors judged a patient ready for discharge, these experiential benchmarks provided patients with at least a rough measure of where they stood in their recovery.

Hospitals varied in the methods by which they determined that a polio patient was ready for release and the ways by which the patient learned of the decision. In some hospitals, the decision to release polio patients was a group determination involving the physician and physical and occupational therapists. John Lindell recalls that after nine months of hospitalization and therapy "a conference was held to discuss continued treatment for me, in fact, to talk about my entire future." He attended the conference with his "doctor, the therapists, [and] a couple of social workers." Relieved when the conference decided that he should be released, he soon left, along with his wheelchair, braces, and crutches. Before he could be discharged, Turnley Walker had to demonstrate his walking skills before a similar group. He remembers "stepping and swinging . . . up the hall toward the little watchful group. . . . You want the doctor's approval more than you have wanted anything else in your life." Although he was released, the doctor reminded Walker that he was "just starting. . . . You will have some return of muscle strength for at least a year. You must keep working." Not everyone, however, had his or her discharge decided in front of a committee. Louise Lake's physicians came to her room one morning and told her, "We cannot do any more for you." Soon afterward she was discharged. At the New York State Reconstruction Home, thirteen-year-old Leonard Kriegel discovered he was going home when friends brought him the news that his name was on the "Blue List" of patients to be discharged the following Thursday.[5]

The process of deciding to release respirator-dependent patients from the hospital was far more complicated. At the Northwest Respirator Center in Seattle, where Virginia Black had been treated, patients remained in the facility until "they had a home service developed to provide ongoing personal, respiratory, and medical care, as well as ongoing rehabilitation to the previous job or other rehabilitation goal." In Black's case, the customary home visit was not done, because of the distance to her Colorado home. When she was discharged, she was still completely paralyzed and could take only one or two breaths on her own. Still the doctors thought she would be better off at home. In their judgment, she had received "maximum predictable benefit." By contrast, staff at the Mary MacArthur Respiratory Center outside Boston helped Louis Sternburg and his wife, Dottie, prepare themselves and their house for his return home in his iron lung. Once the family had purchased a new home, all the necessary equipment was in place, and an attendant had been hired, Sternburg finally returned home after fourteen months in the hospital. These seriously involved patients could not go home until their families had replicated the hospital room, complete with respirator, iron lung, or rocking bed. Fortunately, in most cases the National Foundation for Infantile Paralysis paid for the iron lung, and, in some instances, paid family members to be caregivers.[6]

In contrast to these elaborate preparations, some polio survivors recall being released in a far more casual fashion. After ten months in hospitals, fifteen-year-old David Kangas decided that there was no point in staying longer in the hospital and that he "wanted to go home and just get on with my life." The physician agreed to release him, and Kangas left the next day. Ray Gullickson remembers some confusion regarding his release. He may have misunderstood the staff when they gave him permission for a brief home visit, but he told his parents to come and get him. When they arrived, the staff tried to explain that the release was only temporary, but his parents decided that "we came all this distance and if he wants to go home, then we're going to take him." Gullickson was delighted to go home, although he said that he was later ashamed to learn that he was "discharged 'under protest.'"[7] Although these patients were probably ready or nearly ready to be discharged, they or their parents took the initiative and the doctors and staff either acquiesced in releasing the child or did not prevent it.

Some parents secured the release of their child by seeking a second opinion regarding their child's progress and using it as leverage with the primary physician. For example, Chuck Andrews's father thought his son was ready to be discharged permanently following a Christmas visit home. On returning to the hospital, the boy climbed back into the respirator on his own. The physician directly in charge of the case would not release Chuck because "he didn't want to take responsibility in case something goes wrong." After consulting a specialist, Andrews's father asked for the release papers, signed them, and took his son home.[8] Even in a period when physicians operated with substantial authority and control, some parents challenged a physician's decision when they were convinced that their son or daughter would improve more rapidly under different conditions.

Although it may seem paradoxical, not all polio patients were eager to return home when the time came. Some children from poorer families found the prospect of giving up clean beds, plentiful food, attention from the staff, and the toys of the playroom difficult. Many children and adults had found friends on the polio wards where everyone was disabled, and they would miss them when they went home. Louis Sternburg wanted desperately to go home, but he also knew he would miss the respiratory center and the friends he had made there. Sternburg remembered that "saying good-bye to all of them was very hard." Similarly, Regina Woods remembers her departure from the Houston respiratory center as "bittersweet": her "treatment had been superb," and she had "made friends . . . I would probably never see again," but she was still "anxious to get home." Other patients on the eve of discharge were anxious about fitting back into the world they had left weeks and months earlier. Would they be accepted back into that world, especially with their disabilities? Leonard Kriegel, after discovering his name on the discharge list, worried about what he was going to do at home. Sharing a cigarette outside the hospital with one of his ward friends, Kriegel admitted, "Jesus, I'm scared." When Geoff Purdy's father came to bring him home from Warm Springs, he was "not a bit keen on leaving." Given the quality of care he had received, and the way in which the institution was adapted to the needs of the disabled, Ken Purdy understood his son's reluctance to leave. As Geoff told his father, "this is the best place in the whole world for a polio."[9] Nonetheless, home beckoned, and virtually all of the polio patients returned to their waiting families.

Rehabilitation hospitals differed in the extent to which they prepared polio patients for the psychological challenges of returning to their homes. Even institutions that addressed the issue could not fully prepare these newly disabled individuals for the psychological and emotional adjustments they would have to make. Living in hospitals for so long had taught Regina Woods that her "needs and wants were always to be met and that I need not share anything with others." She had become "an alien to the considerations that make a family a family." But the rehabilitation facility where Woods was sent after her physical condition had stabilized created a "family atmosphere" with shared living space to reintroduce its patients to the give and take of family life. Woods found the experience "wonderfully helpful." Warm Springs recognized the need to deal with the psychological aspects of returning home, but also acknowledged limits to their assistance. One of the psychologists at the Warm Springs Foundation told Hugh Gallagher, "You don't adjust at Warm Springs . . . That comes afterwards, when you leave. Our job is to strengthen you—physically and mentally, for the adjustment that is to come." Gallagher commented that "the patients sense this; they know within themselves that they dread this readjustment, this battle for normalcy that must come." When it was time for Lorenzo Milam to leave Warm Springs, he, like Gallagher, dreaded going home: "I am to normalize myself. I am to live at home. Several years ago, I started out to be a man, moved out of my childhood home. Then I sickened and paled and withered. Now I am going back, a child again."[10] The rehabilitation hospital might try to toughen the polio patients for the psychological challenges awaiting them outside the hospital, but it was the patients themselves who would have to meet the challenge.

At the time polio survivors were discharged, doctors, therapists, and even parents reinforced the message that it was the polio survivors themselves, not society, who would have to adjust to their disability. In the forties and fifties, American society did not provide accommodations for the disabled; the disabled were expected to find ways of managing the physical and social barriers to a full life, or to stay at home out of sight. For example, as Joyce Ann Tepley got ready to leave the hospital at Easter she "was afraid" for the first time since entering the hospital the previous July: "I was leaving the shelter of the hospital life and going back to the real world." Her father's warning that "people might stare" was "the beginning of a new self-consciousness that would haunt me for years to come." Looking back, Leonard Kriegel recognized that the rehabilitation hospital had made a "rather valiant attempt to rehabilitate" him. Still the medical and rehabilitation staff had assumed that he "should be grateful for whatever existence I could scrape together." They also assumed that whatever society "meted out to the cripple, the cripple accepted. The way of the world was not to be challenged." No one had prepared him to accept the role of an "outsider." Nor had they told him "about the fear, anguish and hatred that would swirl through my soul as I was reminded every day that I was a supplicant." [11] As Tepley and Kriegel realized, it was up to the polio survivor, and his or her family, to negotiate a place in a society which if it wasn't always hostile to the needs of the disabled, was certainly indifferent.

Almost from the moment polio survivors left the hospital and returned home they faced physical barriers that impeded their reintegration into family and society. Steep flights of stairs, narrow doorways, slippery floors, and even outhouses limited what many polio survivors could do by themselves. Some houses and apartments could be easily modified to accommodate crutches or a wheelchair, but in others the polio survivors simply had to find ways to make do. For example, Arvid Schwartz's family lived in an old farmhouse in rural Minnesota. On a predischarge visit home, his father had had to carry his twelve-year-old son to the backyard privy. Schwartz doesn't note whether the family had indoor plumbing by the time he returned home for good, but he does remember an "old winding staircase" that led to the upstairs bedrooms. His father nailed up a railing, but Schwartz still had to figure out how to get up and down the steps. He recalls that "there weren't any aids, you just had to figure out how you were going to make this work . . . at that time in the history of our country, when you were a cripple, as opposed to 'handicapped' or 'physically challenged,' you either made it or you didn't make it and it was kind of up to you to make it, with help from your family." The "physical concessions" that Charles Mee's parents made to their home were "carefully chosen." The modifications were "enough to help, [but] not enough to get me accustomed to living in any sort of specially constructed world." Parallel bars initially helped Mee climb the four steps into the house, but he stopped using them as soon as he could. His parents made no modifications in the bath, on the interior staircase, or in his bedroom. By necessity, he quickly "learned to accept the world as it was and to adjust to it" because that was "the way I had been raised." [12] Thus it was in the family that most polio survivors first learned that they, and not society, would have to make whatever accommodations were necessary for them to function.

Polio survivors were not the only ones who had to adjust upon their return home. Their families, especially parents, siblings, and spouses, also had a significant adjustment to make. Up until the time the virus had struck and they had taken their child or spouse to the hospital, he or she had been a healthy, active participant in the life of the family. Now, after weeks or months of difficult separation, the family was being reunited, but it wasn't the same family. Polio often changed relations and responsibilities within the family. Because polio patients were often discharged with significant residual paralysis, family members often had to become caregivers and therapists at least temporarily. Where the paralysis was particularly severe, as in those with permanent respiratory paralysis, the family faced the challenge of providing round-the-clock care seven days a week for an indefinite future. Even where assistance was available through the March of Dimes or other agencies, the primary burden of providing the necessary care fell upon spouses and parents. In addition, if the polio survivor had been the primary income provider (usually the husband, in these decades) and was unable to return to work, the spouse might need to secure full-time work to support the family.

Meeting the physical needs of the returning polio survivor, therefore, was often complicated by altered relationships and by unanticipated psychological dynamics. Heads of families became dependent patients; spouses sometimes had to switch roles. Adolescents who had been trying to assert their independence from their families became once again dependent children. Siblings found it difficult to reestablish old relationships when their brother or sister could do so little. While brothers and sisters might be happy to see their sibling come home, they also sometimes resented the attention parents and other family members paid to the polio survivor. Families had to work at reestablishing old relationships or forging new ones more appropriate to living with the lasting effects of polio.

Many of the polio survivors were still confined to their beds, or had only limited mobility when they were discharged from the hospital. In those cases, families had to provide the bedside care nurses and attendants had provided in the hospital and to carry or wheel their spouse or child when they needed to be moved. In addition, many polio patients were discharged with the expectation that the family would continue the exercises that had been directed by physical therapists in the hospital. For example, Richard Owen spent eight months at home lying in his bedroom on a canvas-covered frame immobilized in Toronto splints. Although a therapist came to stretch his muscles and to preserve their range of motion, his mother had to provide most of the nursing care. After their daughter returned home from the hospital, Mary Grimley Mason's parents had to put her in leg casts or braces every night for months to prevent her legs from contracting. When six-year-old Clara Yelder went home she could manage only a few steps with her braces and crutches. As a result, her parents or her brothers and sisters carried her wherever she needed to go. Her family did not have much money, and not until the community held a fundraiser when she was nine or ten and bought her a wheelchair could she get around on her own. Similarly, Paul Reitmeir's father pulled his twelve-year-old son everywhere in a red wagon until a local service club purchased a wheelchair for the boy, restoring his mobility.[13]

The burden of caregiving, however, fell heaviest on those families with a respirator-dependent member. Nursing historian Lynne Dunphy has described the task of caring for iron-lung patients in a hospital setting as a "heroic job" requiring a team of nurses and physicians. When these patients were sent home with their iron lungs, their families had to take on that heroic responsibility. Louis Sternburg acknowledged that he and his wife Dottie "never thought it would be easy," but it often proved more difficult than they had anticipated. Sternburg's return home was "only possible because Dottie, with some help from Mike [a hired aide], devoted herself to taking care of me twenty-four hours a day, as well as running the house and looking after our two small children." In taking over the role of the nurses at the respiratory center, Dottie had to learn "all the slow and complicated details of nursing a paralyzed polio patient." In several severe cases, the NFIP helped pay for the home care. For example, the March of Dimes paid for an assistant to care for Marilyn Rogers while her parents worked. The NFIP also paid for one of Roger Winter's hospital nurses to care for him at home. When that nurse became his wife, they continued to pay her to care for her husband, although they gradually cut back the amount, and after three years they phased out the payments.[14] Whether they were paid or not, and most family caregivers were not, families often had to provide significant nursing assistance as the price of having their son, daughter, or spouse back home.

Even when the polio survivor did not need round-the-clock care, families were often enlisted to assist with the prescribed exercises and therapies. Depending on the severity of the paralysis, applying the hot packs and doing the exercises could consume a considerable part of the day and often continued for months. Dick Weir's parents continued the hot packs, hot Jacuzzi tub treatments, and exercises for more than a year until he was able to walk without a walker. When six-year-old Worth Younts was sent home in 1944 his parents were given detailed written instructions on his care. They were instructed to provide a firm mattress and to ensure that their son had a daily bowel movement. The hospital also provided a daily schedule that included morning and evening baths followed by prescribed exercises. When Grace Audet left the hospital she was given a "rather strenuous exercise program" to follow at home. Her father "rigged up a library table with an overhead framework with pulleys and ropes" so that Audet could do all her exercises, which took "about three and a half hours" daily to complete. Once she returned to school, her exercise schedule was reduced to two and a half hours daily for "a couple of years." Charlene Pugleasa's father also built an exercise "machine" to help his daughter. He made leg weights using "lead fishing weights, big, huge weights and other kinds of lead weights." Her mother provided hot baths and stretching exercises. Because hydrotherapy had become a standard part of polio rehabilitation by the 1930s and 1940s, fathers sometimes constructed tubs in which to treat their children. Anita Bjorling's father, for example, "brought home a big horse tank" for her exercises. In an interesting variation Edward Barker, an electrical engineer when polio struck, designed and had constructed in his living room a 200-gallon tank heated by electricity. Unable to go to Warm Springs, it was his way of bringing Warm Springs home to Massachusetts. Of course, rather than constructing a special tub many parents simply carried their children to the family bathtub filled with hot water.[15]

Articles in the popular press and contemporary polio narratives stressed the parents' responsibility for keeping their children at their exercises. Because the exercises were often painful as well as tedious, parents often had to keep after their children to follow the exercise regime prescribed by their physicians. Some communities, such as Allentown and Bethlehem, Pennsylvania, provided out-patient exercise facilities, and polio patients were transported to this facility for daily therapy. Numerous polio survivors recall that physical therapists or other medical professionals came regularly to their homes either to supervise family-administered exercises or to do the exercises themselves. James Berry's physical therapist came to his home once a week to oversee his mother's administration of his exercises. Dick Weir remembers that his exercises were administered by a "full time nurse trained in the Sister Kenny treatment." Alexandra York, who had polio as an eight-year-old in 1955, recalled that when she was discharged from the hospital an osteopath came every morning "to work on my muscles." She further recalls her father coming home from work several times a day, laying her across the piano bench with sandbags on her forehead, arms, and legs, and forcing her to lift the weights.

The exercises were painful, and the young Alexandra cried out so often that neighbors refused to speak to her father, believing that he was hurting her more than he was helping. Ken Purdy, writing in *McCall's* about his son Geoff's polio, reminded parents that children often do better at home than in institutions provided that they "are held to strict routine." The child recovering from polio "may have to be threatened, cajoled, bribed—but he must work. If he does not, the muscles that professional skill have [*sic*] begun to bring back will fall away again." Parents persevered because they, on some level, accepted the dictum of the doctor who answered Mary Cook's question about whether her son would be crippled by saying, "He may be handicapped, but only you can make him a cripple."[16]

Doing the necessary stretching and exercises at home was not easy for either the child doing the exercises or the parents directing them. The exercises could be quite painful, especially in the early stages, and the cries of the children upset parents and sometimes neighbors. For example, Bill Van Cleve recalls that "bending those limbs was very painful" and that it was "hard" for his mother "to see a 10-year-old child crying." Both Jack Schwartz and Loreen Wells remembered resisting their mothers' efforts to make them exercise. Schwartz recalls hiding and getting a spanking when he resisted, and Wells and her mother had "terrible clashes" over the exercises. In spite of these painful memories, all of these survivors credit their parents with persisting with the exercises in spite of the physical and emotional pain involved. Jack Schwartz spoke for all of these survivors and parents when he recalled that his mother "was determined it would be through no neglect on her part that I would not learn to walk again without crutches. She succeeded."[17]

On their own or with the advice of therapists families developed a wide variety of other activities to exercise atrophied muscles and increase functioning. Several families encouraged their children to take up swimming. Ed Sass remembers being permitted to swim in a privately owned pool in Wilmette, Illinois. Stuart Goldschen's father had been a YMCA swimming instructor, and he got his son in the water as soon as possible. Other parents were instructed to have their children walk barefoot in sand to strengthen feet and legs. Still other parents rubbed their children's muscles with a variety of oils, sometimes hot, in the belief that this would help restore function. For example, Bonnie Bonham's parents "massaged and stretched my legs daily with hot olive oil." After consulting a fortune-teller, Don Kirkendall's parents rubbed him nightly with salad oil. Sharon Kimball remembers that "if somebody had a home remedy that sounded reasonable, and wouldn't interfere with anything that was already being done" her mother would try it. Her mother had heard that "rubbing cocoa butter on the muscles activated them, so she got some cocoa butter, and we tried it." Not surprisingly, "it didn't work."[18] While swimming and walking on sand certainly helped strengthen muscles, the efficacy of oil rubdowns is more questionable. However, parents' willingness to try any plausible treatment, even those recommended by fortune-tellers, is a measure of their desire to help their children recover.

Physical accommodations were not the only kinds of adjustments that families had to make when a polio patient returned home. Both the patient and the family had been changed by the experience, and both patients and families faced a period of adjustment in the weeks and months after being reunited. Siblings had to work out new relationships now that one of them could no longer run, jump, and play as they had previously. Parents had to deal with the reality of dashed dreams and of raising a child with a disability. Spouses had to rebuild a relationship that may have been permanently changed, and mothers and fathers had to find ways to be a parent from a wheelchair or rocking bed. The changed psychological dynamics of these polio-altered families could be complex and persistent.

In his family memoir, *An American Requiem*, James Carroll explored polio's psychological impact on his Irish-American family. His older brother Joe contracted the disease, but the psychological fallout affected every member of the family. Polio forced a role reversal between the brothers; James "usurped" his older brother's place by becoming "a pseudo-older brother, sibling born to lead, to try things first, to help with chores, to mind the baby, and, later, to be the outgoing one." But James could never fully enjoy his usurped role as the first-born: "Every success, since it came at Joe's expense, would feel like failure." Joe's polio also shattered their parents' happiness. Their mother "did mute penance, nailing herself to the cross of her first son's suffering. The rest of us would have to compete for the dregs of her attention." Their father withdrew from the family, devoting his time as a high-ranking military officer to "saving the Free World from Communism." From James's perspective, "the lesson of polio to all of us was that our bodies were plainly not to be trusted." His father had abandoned study for the priesthood to marry his mother, and polio's "resonance as a kind of Irish curse against a spoiled priest, his woman, and their children is what made it the radioactive mushroom cloud of our family."[19]

Fathers, in particular, seemed to have more difficulty accepting their disabled sons and daughters. Paul Reitmeir remembers that his father never really accepted his disability. Nancy Brotzman's father "didn't want any part" of his daughter with a "twisted body, head on shoulder, [and] arm turned around" so her mother always had to take her to the out-patient clinic. Dick Giddings' father "never did acknowledge that there was anything wrong" with his son. When the son was slow to complete household chores because of his polio impairments, the father described the boy to neighbors as "lazy." In other families, the word "polio" was never uttered and everyone—survivor, siblings, parents—were expected to proceed with their lives as if nothing unusual had happened.[20]

Even in families where polio was not regarded as a curse it nonetheless often altered relationships between siblings. John Swett remembered that his older brother became somewhat distant because of all the attention John received when he came home from the hospital. Although he was not fully aware of it at the time, Swett now realizes that his brother was angry at him for having polio. His brother's anger developed because John received "a little extra attention from other family and friends, plus we couldn't do the things together that we once did before I got sick." Polio also affected brother-sister pairs. Hugh Gallagher recalled that his polio affected his sister almost as much as it did Hugh. His younger sister was in her early teens when her mother almost abandoned her to spend two years in hospitals trying to keep her son alive. His sister has since told him that she also had "guilt feelings. That she feels maybe she should have been the one to have it."[21] Because a serious case of polio so thoroughly disrupted family life, it is not surprising that siblings and polio survivors found their relationships permanently altered. What is perhaps surprising is how well and how quickly most families reintegrated their sons and daughters, brothers and sisters, into the ongoing life of the family.

The daily presence of their disabled son or daughter sometimes fostered a deep sense of guilt among parents who were certain they had not done enough to protect their child from the disease. The sense of guilt, the sense that they had brought on their son's polio as retribution for their own sins, pervaded Joseph and Mary Carroll's response to their son's return from the hospital. As their younger son recalled, his mother became their "own Pietà. The spontaneous, wisecracking, affectionate young woman I first knew, as it were, simply packed up and moved out, to be replaced by the Mother of Sorrows herself, a woman privileged to be in pain." James Carroll's father fled "the sure Jansenist knowledge that his own hubris, not polluted water or 'germs,' was the true cause of his son's polio." Such attitudes were not restricted to Catholic families. Leonard Kriegel's Jewish mother blamed herself for her son's illness. "To be the mother of a cripple," Kriegel eventually came to realize, "was to be the victim of something one could not understand." His mother "had to wrestle with the suspicion that she had somehow done something to create her fate. Neither God nor his justice are blind. One received in life what one deserved."[22] These parental guilt feelings forever altered the relations between spouses as well as with their disabled child and his or her siblings.

It is not surprising that psychological adjustments to living with and caring for a severely disabled spouse or parent were complicated. When John Lindell returned home in a wheelchair after nine months in hospitals, he was particularly frustrated by his efforts to discipline his children. During his hospitalization, "many things had been allowed because there were more serious considerations at the moment." Home again, he expected to reestablish his authority and standards. But because his "discipline had been absent for so long, it was no longer recognized" and because he was in a wheelchair he "couldn't enforce it. The children soon found they could escape punishment by getting out of my reach." New relationships also had to be forged with one's spouse, especially in cases where the polio survivor had been reduced to an almost child-like dependence on others. This dependence was often initially manifest in a desire to monopolize the time and energy of the spouse. Only after he had been home for some time and had developed other friends and interests did Larry Alexander realize that he had initially been a "miser" of his wife's time. Whenever she wanted to go out at night, he would find some excuse to keep her in. Once he got involved in community affairs, he became less demanding of his wife's time and allowed her to regain a life of her own separate from his demands. Similarly, Louis Sternburg relied very heavily on his wife, Dottie, in spite of having paid assistants. He "competed with the children for her attention," and he later acknowledged that he had been selfish and possessive. It took several years and the assistance of a psychiatrist before Sternburg began to let his wife go, to let her have a life beyond the almost constant care she had provided him.[23]

While families like the Alexanders and the Sternburgs managed to work their way toward relationships that both provided care for the disabled partner and a measure of independence for the nondisabled spouse, not all families were so successful. For example, Louise Lake's husband left her once her "dancing days were over" and her "beautiful youthful days were spent." Kathryn Black has recounted how her family disintegrated after her mother contracted polio that left her paralyzed and respirator-dependent. Her parents' marriage was difficult even before polio struck, but Virginia Black's disease further upset the "balance" in her parents' marriage. Her father had relied on his wife both emotionally and physically, and after her illness he found it difficult to reverse roles and to give aid to his paralyzed wife. When his wife died, he largely abandoned Kathryn and Ken, leaving them in the care of their grandparents.[24]

Psychological studies of polio patients from the forties and fifties that examined the patient's reintegration into the family following hospitalization found mixed success. Some studies suggested that factors other than the polio or crippling lay at the root of post-polio familial conflict; after all, not all polio patients came from stable, harmonious, and supportive families. Two studies conducted in the 1940s that explored the effect of crippling on the psychological adjustment of children, including those with polio, reveal that "those with physical handicaps do not as a group seem to present any more or any different problems than any unselected group of children." Maladjustment was more likely to be "dependent upon the number and severity of the problems confronting the crippled child." In addition, "home conditions and attitudes in the family" were more likely to produce "unfavorable adjustment" than crippling alone. A study from the midfifties suggests that problems were most likely to occur "when the patient re-establishes his relations to family members and when the family is adapting itself to the new situation at home." Finally, a study published toward the end of the polio epidemics acknowledges that "the problems of readjustment on a permanent basis were formidable in the presence of far-reaching physical disability." For married patients, "there was a good deal of marital difficulty," as well as "considerable resolution of exceedingly difficult problems." The researchers concluded, however, that "about half of the patients were doing quite well from a psychological standpoint a year after discharge."[25] What is perhaps surprising is how often in these narratives the son or daughter, husband or wife, was reintegrated into the life of the family with a minimum of psychological and emotional conflict.

This process of becoming once again a fully functioning member of the family was often disrupted by the slow pace of physical recovery from polio and by the frequent necessity for continued physical therapy, new bracing, and reconstructive surgery. It could take two years or more for the body to fully recover from the initial disease and for patients to discover the full extent of any permanent paralysis. In addition, the bodies of children and adolescents were still growing, which meant that new deformities, such as scoliosis or shortened legs, could appear some years after the initial discharge from the rehabilitation hospital. Many polio survivors regularly attended out-patient clinics or spent long hours waiting to see family physicians or orthopedic surgeons. Polio survivors often feared these visits, because they so often resulted in new exercises to perform, new braces to wear, or surgeries to be endured. Going home had taken the polio patient out of the hospital, but in many cases it didn't mean the end of medical interventions in the lengthy process of recovery.

Outpatient therapy was available at some rehabilitation hospitals and Sister Kenny facilities, but others received therapy from various clinics or private practitioners. Ed Sass, for example, remembers receiving physical therapy for a year or two after his release from the hospital. He went to a clinic or hospital and was "stretched and twisted in all sorts of painful directions." Diane Baggett received her outpatient therapy at the Easter Seals Institute in Orlando, Florida, and she still remembers being "terrified of the tall whirlpools which looked like soup cans." After returning from Warm Springs, Mary Grimley Mason was treated on an outpatient basis by a physical therapist in private practice in Ardmore, Pennsylvania. Several years later after her family had moved to Montreal, she was sent to live with the therapist to continue her treatment. This arrangement ended one night when the eleven-year-old girl "went nearly out of my mind with pent-up homesickness that took the form of an acute attack of terror." [26] These outpatient sessions were generally a supplement to the home-based exercises, but they allowed physical therapists to monitor the progress of their patients and to adjust the exercises accordingly.

African American polio survivors faced other challenges in completing their recovery outside the hospital. Blacks in the South faced particular problems because there were few facilities that provided continuing rehabilitation and monitoring of African American polio survivors. One facility, as we have seen, was the Infantile Paralysis Center at the Tuskegee Institute in Alabama. Another was the Meharry Medical School in Nashville, Tennessee, which trained African American physicians. Wilma Rudolph, the future Olympic gold medal winner, lived in Clarksville, Tennessee, about fifty miles from Nashville. Because there was no place she could be treated for her polio-weakened muscles in Clarksville, twice a week for four years in the late 1940s she and her mother took the segregated Greyhound bus into Nashville for hydrotherapy and exercises. The bus stations in both Clarksville and Nashville were segregated, they rode in the back of the bus or stood if it filled with whites, and if they wanted something to eat on the trip they had to bring it with them, since the restaurants were closed to blacks. Rudolph recalls that she wore a brace during the years she was treated at Meharry, but discarded it two years after ending her treatments at age ten. She remembers that "glorious day" when her mother mailed the brace back to Meharry and Rudolph "was free at last."[27]

Even when patients did not receive regular outpatient therapy, they may have had their progress monitored in specialized polio or orthopedic clinics. Wisconsin, for example, had state-supported regional orthopedic clinics where physicians made recommendations for treatment, including bracing and surgery, and where patients could receive regular evaluations. Most rehabilitation facilities provided a similar service to former patients. Many former patients remember returning for annual checkups. Occasionally, especially when the polio clinic was part of a rehabilitation facility, a visit to the doctor could end, much to the dismay of the patient, with an immediate admission to the hospital for therapy or surgery. Kathy Vastyshak feared the regular trips to the DuPont Institute in Wilmington, Delaware, because if "they decided that you needed to stay for a procedure or whatever, you stayed right then. You didn't go home and come back. You stayed." Similarly, Gail Bias "always dreaded" her return visits to Gillette Children's Hospital in St. Paul, in part because of the possibility of additional treatment, but also because of the humiliating way she was treated. She would have to get undressed, put on a "little loin cloth, something like a diaper," and be examined by a room full of medical personnel who would "touch you, and probe you, and bend you like you were some sort of scientific specimen." She remembers these visits as "very grueling for a young child," but "you had no choice but to go down there and go through it." Of all her clinic visits, Rosemary Marx remembers only one vividly. As her mother took her clothes off and put on a hospital gown, the four-year-old Marx "started screaming and holding onto her, pleading with her not to leave me there." Having endured more than ten weeks in the hospital, the young girl feared another separation from her family.[28]

In most cases, the fear of immediate separation was groundless, but occasionally the anticipatory dread turned into an awful reality. Janice Gradin, for example, had been discharged from the Sister Kenny Institute after two months. After resting and exercising at home for two more months, she returned for a checkup. Unfortunately the home program had brought no improvement; she had, in fact, regressed, and her physicians would not let her go home. Gradin was very upset and found it difficult to accept. But accept it she did, and she spent an additional two months in the hospital before being discharged for good. It took several years of additional checkups, however, before the doctors finally medically discharged her and the specter of rehospitalization was finally removed.[29] Although regular examinations were necessary if physicians and surgeons were to monitor the long recovery from polio, these children and adolescents were relieved when they were finally medically discharged and no longer had to dread the semiannual or annual visit to the polio clinic.

In addition to examinations and treatments by physicians, many young polio patients were seen by less orthodox healers. For example, Paul Reitmeir's father was "a great believer in chiropractors" and first had his son treated by local chiropractors in Bethlehem, Pennsylvania. Then, when he was fourteen, Reitmeir spent three months in Oklahoma City with his mother and father being treated by a chiropractor, followed by ten months in a chiropractic hospital in Denver. Don Kirkendall's mother took him to two folk healers known as bonesetters. Farmers in the Dakotas, these untrained bonesetters nonetheless treated many of their neighbors by massaging muscles and aligning bones. Kirkendall returned for treatment several times, and their treatment seems to have helped him gain the muscle strength he needed to sit unaided.[30] By maintaining flexibility, by massaging and strengthening weakened muscles, these unorthodox healers replicated to some extent the more orthodox treatments available at Kenny Institutes and rehabilitation hospitals.

While most families relied on physical healers both orthodox and unorthodox, other families turned to faith healers in the hope and belief that through them God would heal their children and enable them to walk once again. In the 1950s Oral Roberts was one of the most prominent faith healers. He appeared every week on his own television program and in person throughout the country at revival meetings. Several polio survivors recall being taken to these revivals, where Roberts would attempt to heal the sick and the crippled with the power of faith. When Roberts came to Spokane, Washington, friends of Elinor Young's parents urged them to take her to the meeting to be healed: "What kind of parents are you, anyway, that you wouldn't try *anything* to help your little daughter?" They took their daughter to the meeting, and the young girl hoped for a "miracle." Although Roberts "healed," nothing happened. Young's parents assured her that it was not her fault that she wasn't healed: her "faith was just fine, and the guy was a fraud." Other polio survivors who attended Oral Roberts healings were not always reassured when their legs failed to heal in response to the evangelist's prayers. For example, Judy Garrison's grandmother suggested to the young girl that she had not been healed because she lacked faith.[31] Such comments could be devastating, since the young polio survivors had of course wanted to be healed and now had to carry a burden of religious guilt on top of the physical disability of polio.

Catholic families usually did not resort to evangelical faith healers such as Oral Roberts, but instead drew on the long Catholic tradition of appeals to particular saints or visits to shrines where healing had supposedly occurred. Some polio patients wore relics of saints in hopes of a cure. Some families took their children to noted shrines in the United States and in Canada. Although no cures occurred, the young patients usually came away impressed with the collections of discarded braces, crutches, and other devices in the sanctuaries. Occasionally a polio survivor might travel all the way to Lourdes, France, in hopes of a cure. Although miracle cures weren't recorded, some pilgrims came back with their faith strengthened, if not their bodies.[32] As recoveries stretched out, and physical therapy and exercise failed to provide a complete cure, it is not surprising that some families put their faith in God to work a miracle. But while strong faith could help one deal with polio's impairments, miracles were hard to come by.

Although it could hardly be called a rehabilitation program, several polio survivors credit farm work for their recovery. Jan Little recovered from polio on her family's farm outside Janesville, Wisconsin. The surgeons sent her home with a dismal prognosis, paralyzed from the chest down and with weakness in her arms. Little's family, however, believed that everyone needed to help out with farming. She began helping her mother in the kitchen and with ironing and eventually moved to gardening. Her father planted the garden with rows far enough apart "to let a wheelchair through without mashing the beans and peas." Using a hoe with the handle cut down, Little weeded the garden. Picking strawberries was also good therapy. As she recalled, "to get the berries, it is necessary to get down on the ground. The results were a) learning to get out of the chair onto the ground, b) crawling—or in my case, dragging my butt—on grass and c) wonderful strawberry shortcakes, pies and jams."[33] In Little's case, and no doubt others, activities of farm work mimicked the exercises of the rehabilitation gym, and surrounded by supportive family members who nonetheless expected the work to get done, polio rehabilitation went on largely independent of rehabilitation centers and clinics.

Some polio survivors developed their own exercise regimes to rebuild their bodies. Leonard Kriegel spent nearly two years in the New York State Reconstruction Home being treated for the polio that struck him at age eleven. Polio left his legs paralyzed, and he returned home to the Bronx on braces and crutches. When he was sixteen he was again bedridden and unable to walk because boils on his legs made it impossible to wear his braces. Being laid up this way forced him to reconsider what he wanted from life. He realized that most of all he wanted "vengeance—getting even" for all that polio had forced him to give up and to endure. He was, as he said, "frightened, envious, and self-pitying," but he also discovered what he wanted to do and a "plan of action, of self-creation almost, took root" in his mind. His legs were "lifeless and atrophied" and he was "still fat and flabby," but he determined to build his body as he could: "The knowledge of my arms came to me. In the arms I would mold fat into muscle. To the arms my will would attach itself. . . . In the arms was my salvation." Once the boils healed, he started his regime. "For hours at a time I exercised—pushups, situps, whatever came to mind. I knew nothing about getting into shape. I didn't want to know anything. All I wanted was to act, to feel *my* body, *my* arms, responding to the demands I made." As his arms grew stronger and he lost weight he "walked mile after mile on my braces and crutches." Kriegel did "hundreds of push-ups every day to build up my arms, shoulders and chest," and at night he would walk to a nearby playground to "do dips on the monkey bars for hours to create triceps strong enough to carry me endlessly through the days and nights of my need." Back home he would "work out to the point of collapse, lying exhausted but pleased" on the floor of his family's apartment. What drove Kriegel was not the encouragement of therapists but the deeply felt need to prove himself against American expectations of manhood.[34] In rebuilding his upper body Kriegel found the physical strength and psychological energy he needed to compensate for what polio had destroyed.

It was during this long recovery from polio that many survivors discovered whether the braces they wore would be needed permanently or whether they could be discarded following additional therapy and the return of muscle strength. While many polio patients were sent home in braces, others were fitted for braces only later when deformities caused by muscle paralysis or weakness became evident. The decision whether to brace a particular limb or the torso was not always clear-cut. In some situations bracing was an alternative to surgery, and in others a case could be made to forego both bracing and surgery, at least for the time being. Bracing was used both to support weakened muscles and limbs and to try to prevent deformities such as scoliosis from developing or worsening. While braces were often preferred to surgery, they had their own drawbacks, especially outside the rehabilitation hospital. The iron, steel, and leather braces of the postwar era were heavy, hot, and often uncomfortable. They were also very obvious and immediately marked the wearer as crippled. Although many survivors relied heavily on their braces to function, it is not surprising that, if they could, they got rid of them as soon as possible. Reducing or eliminating one's dependence on braces was a sign that recovery from polio had taken another big step forward.

Whether a polio patient was braced, and if so with what kind of brace, was often dependent upon the particular physician consulted. In addition, the patients sometimes had considerable input into the decision to brace or not. For example, Edward Le Comte recalled that in his case it seemed as if the "extent of bracing often depended on which orthopedists were on duty that particular month." Le Comte was surprised when one pair of orthopedists removed his short leg brace after a month, but he later acknowledged that "this was a case of the foot's having really become stronger." As he noted, "it was an immense satisfaction to shed something so quickly," even if "the other encumbrance [the brace on his other leg] . . . clung heavy and long."[35]

Unlike Le Comte, Irving Zola initially avoided heavy leg braces, in spite of his doctor's recommendation. Shortly after being discharged from the hospital, Zola and his parents went to a Boston polio specialist for an examination and recommendation. The physician and his colleagues "recommended full-leg bracing." Then, the doctor asked where the family lived. After his mother described a third-floor walk-up apartment, the doctor "flatly stated that since the braces were made of iron there was no way that I could navigate four flights of stairs." Instead, the doctor recommended that the sixteen-year-old Zola "be removed from home and sent to the State Residential High School for Crippled Children." He warned that failure to follow the advice would be an increased likelihood of arthritis and other problems as Zola aged. Zola and his mother conferred and because he "prized my current adolescence over my later adulthood" and because he wanted to finish at Boston Latin School, they refused the bracing and admittance to the residential high school. Zola slowly and painfully climbed the stairs every school day, sometimes taking as long as three hours to reach the apartment.[36] Choosing not to be braced had potential consequences, as Zola's physicians warned, but accepting braces had its own set of consequences, and the decision, as in Zola's case, did not always fall on the side of the braces.

Unless they were needed only briefly, bracing often meant repeated trips to the hospital or clinic to be evaluated and to alter the braces as muscles regained strength or as the bodies of the young men and women grew. The frequent need for new braces was an added expense that many families could ill afford. For example, in 1936, Larry Fournier was fitted for the first of a series of leg braces. The special shoes and the leg brace cost only forty dollars, but this was more than his family could afford. Larry was one of twelve children of a Maine mill worker who made fourteen dollars a week. In order to pay for corrective surgery (a hundred dollars) and the ten-dollar visits to the specialist, Larry's father mortgaged the family's home. This first leg brace was paid for with money from a neighborhood "sunshine basket" filled with dollar bills. Later, when Larry needed new braces to accommodate his growth, machinists in his father's mill made the braces under the doctor's supervision. Kay Brutger, like Fournier, underwent numerous surgeries and wore braces for a time. Her father had hospitalization coverage through his employer, the Great Northern Railroad, but the family had to pay for "everything else such as therapy, crutches, wheelchairs, braces, and outpatient services." Her family was "certainly not wealthy, and we stretched every dollar." While the NFIP provided braces and wheelchairs for many polio survivors in the forties and fifties, not all families were eligible for their aid.[37]

Wearing a brace meant that one stood out. Not only did braces limit activity even as they supported a weak body, they also visibly advertised one's difference from peers. Thanks in part to the NFIP's use of poster children who wore braces to raise funds, wearing leg or other braces in the postwar period usually pegged one as a polio victim. Edward Le Comte recognized that little could be done to make braces inconspicuous. He ridiculed the advice contained in a leaflet he was given with his new braces to oil and clean them regularly. Oiling "protects the brace from wear," and "prevents embarrassment" to the wearer: "It is distressing to hear a squeak with every step if the brace goes suddenly dry. This has been known to happen in the silence of a church on the way to a front pew. No one likes to be conspicuous in this way." The leaflet also recommended that the metal be "kept bright and shining," especially if worn by an active child: "Braces have a way of becoming shabby. This is distressing to the wearer and causes self-consciousness." As Le Comte sardonically observed, "it's nice to think that the little girl whose braces are showing can polish away her self-consciousness."[38]

Polio survivors often accepted their braces in spite of their weight and discomfort, because they enabled them to do things that otherwise would have been impossible. Being able to function, to move, was ultimately more important than appearances. Joyce Ann Tepley made every effort to relearn to walk without braces following polio, but after falling off playground equipment and breaking her unbraced leg, she decided to give up the goal for the sake of her own safety. Wearing braces made it easier to be involved in Girl Scouts and with friends, and she concluded, "there were other things I was more interested in doing than concentrating on walking without braces." Similarly, after several years of walking without braces, Richard Owen chose to go back to wearing a leg brace. It was at the end of his first year of medical school, he was doing a lot of standing and walking, and he decided he would be more comfortable wearing a brace. Owen noted that Sister Kenny, who had treated him during his rehabilitation, would not have approved of his decision, but "when you balance out function as opposed to what she thought was normal gait, I had to go for function."[39]

Polio survivors tried to shed their braces as quickly as possible, regardless of their usefulness, sometimes without explicit permission from their physicians. Discarding braces was another sign of recovery and return to something approaching a normal life. Most polio patients gave up their braces when their physicians decided bracing was no longer necessary. Not all doctors, however, were as cavalier as Mary Ann Hoffman's Shrine physician who, after examining her and her brace, declared, "We'll just throw this thing away. It's nothing but a mouse trap." In her case, surgery had made the brace redundant. However, many other polio survivors and their families made the decision largely on their own. Survivors generally abandoned braces when they discovered that they could function just as well without them. Diane Keyser remembers that her brace broke after she had worn it for about a year when she was in high school. The brace was sent to be repaired, but by the time it was returned, Keyser had learned to walk without it, and she went without a brace for nearly forty years. Charles Mee worked hard to achieve his goal of walking without braces. When he was finally able to keep his knee straight and to "fake walking on my left leg," Mee took off the brace and made do with crutches. For Mee, "to be out of the brace was wonderful; what was even more wonderful was not to have to wear the ugly shoes in which the brace needed to be anchored."[40]

Other polio survivors removed their braces when they thought no one in authority was watching. For example, Jim O'Meara's mother was "adamant" about his wearing his arm brace all the time, but when he played with his brothers, he would "just take the damned thing off and throw it on the ground." At school he wore it in the classroom, but at recess he removed it once again. One polio survivor undoubtedly spoke for many others when her current physiatrist asked her why she ever stopped wearing a brace, and she replied, "Because I was 13."[41] Of course, not all polio survivors could shed their braces, but those who could generally did so as soon as possible, even if, from a strictly medical point of view, they might have been better advised to keep wearing them. The temptation to appear more normal by discarding braces was simply too strong.

Not everyone, of course, could ultimately discard his or her braces. Still other polio survivors discovered that regardless of how hard they tried to walk with braces and crutches, it was easier and more functional to rely on a wheelchair for mobility. However, medical authorities were of the opinion that most polio patients could be taught to walk in some fashion. Dr. Philip Lewin argued that even "a patient with paralysis below the waist, with one good arm and one arm good enough to hold a crutch, given at least fair intelligence, can be taught to walk." Writing a few years later, Dr. Joseph Barr asserted that "practically every adult and most children with involvement of the lower extremities should be given the opportunity to attempt to walk without braces." As Barr put it, "any apparatus which the patient must habitually wear is to that extent an admission of defeat on the part of the surgeon in charge of the case." Sister Kenny's attitude is perhaps best summed up in the title of her autobiographical volume, *And They Shall Walk*.[42]

Given the emphasis that medical professionals put on the ability to walk following polio, it is not surprising that parents and patients alike saw it as a key sign of recovery. Many parents shared the attitude of one mother whose "hopes for her daughter's recovery had been realized" when she could walk with only a barely perceptible limp as well as go up and down stairs, dance, and play like any twelve-year-old. Leonard Kriegel, in looking back at his ultimately successful efforts as a teenager to stay out of the wheelchair by becoming a "crutchwalker," is stunned that he so easily accepted the widespread belief that to give up walking, no matter how hard, for life in a wheelchair was a defeat. During his two-year hospital stay, he, like most of his fellow patients, had absorbed "the belief that using a wheelchair signified some sort of spiritual surrender" and made one less of a man.[43] In spite of this medical and cultural emphasis on walking, some polio survivors concluded that while walking was nice if you had the necessary muscle strength, functional mobility was more important. For them, wheelchairs were far more effective for moving about than the cumbersome, awkward, and uncertain walking they had managed with braces and crutches.

Many of the young men and women who eventually concluded that wheelchairs offered them greater mobility with less effort discovered this only by trying repeatedly to walk with braces and crutches. Given their lack of muscle strength and control, some of them found trying to walk a harrowing experience. Paul Reitmeir remembers that for years his parents or therapists would get him out of his wheelchair and stand him up with his braces and crutches. But he never felt comfortable standing, let alone walking. Finally, after several years somebody said to him, "If you're going to give up, you know, you're go-ing to be in a wheelchair." And he recalls thinking, "I think I need to be in a wheelchair." Even though he knows he made the right choice, Reitmeir still feels guilty wondering whether he tried hard enough. Jan Little also remem-bers that in her community, "walking was proof that you had worked hard and overcome your disability. Wheelchairs were associated with old or sick people." So several times a week her mother drove her twenty miles to work with a ther-apist and Little would practice walking. Ultimately, nothing worked and Little relied on her wheelchair for mobility. In spite of his initial shame at having to use a wheelchair, Robert Lovering soon discovered to his delight that he was "mobile again." Several years later when a stranger in a department store asked him, "Isn't that wheelchair a terrible thing?" he replied, "No it is my best friend."[44]

Therapy, as we have seen, was the first strategy in polio rehabilitation. If therapy alone proved inadequate to restore function to limbs or to straighten spines, braces usually followed. The goal of most polio physicians was to re-store function without assistance, but that was not always possible. Where muscle recovery was insufficient, permanent bracing was one option for deal-ing with the remaining deformity. However, in the forties and fifties, at least, various surgical techniques had advanced sufficiently to give some surgeons confidence that almost all polio deformities could be reduced or eliminated through judicious and careful surgery. By 1948 Dr. Joseph Barr, professor of or-thopedic surgery at Harvard, was certain that "the art of the brace fitter seems to have yielded its place to the surgical art of the scalpel." But even he con-ceded that "surgery in poliomyelitis rarely succeeds in restoring normal func-tion." Timing these surgeries was crucial. Surgeons generally advised waiting for several years after the acute illness before attempting any surgical inter-ventions to prevent or treat deformities. By waiting, surgeons could be certain that maximum muscle recovery had been achieved, and, in the case of adoles-cents, that growth had slowed or ended. Dr. Philip Lewin, for example, recom-mended that surgeons try not to operate on patients younger than ten years old. He also asserted that "as a general rule, no major operations should be per-formed within a year after the acute attack." Barr also recommended that sur-geons time their operations carefully. He noted, for instance, that "tendon transplants will fail if the child's co-operation in muscle training cannot be en-listed." The result of these recommendations meant that many polio patients who had the disease as children spent their teenage years in and out of hospi-tals as surgeons tried to reconstruct what polio had destroyed. As Dorothea

Nudelman recalled, "the hospital was like summer camp for polios. Surgeries were planned. You booked a spot in advance."[45] Rather than looking forward to carefree summers, these young men and women dreaded the approach of surgery season.

Surgeons developed and described a wide variety of procedures to correct or reduce the characteristic deformities of polio. Several types recur frequently in the medical literature and in the narratives of polio survivors. Dr. Joseph Barr thought that arthrodesis, fusing the bones of a joint to achieve stability, was "most generally applicable." Other frequent surgeries that drew his attention included tendon transplantation to restore lost function and spinal fusion to correct scoliosis. Dr. Philip Lewin's book on polio describes and illustrates a wide variety of surgical procedures to correct the deformities of polio. While many of these surgeries had become somewhat standardized by the 1940s, surgeons developed numerous variations. As Barr argued, "the late stage of poliomyelitis presents such an extreme variety of problems, physical, social, and economic, that treatment must be highly individualized and adapted to the patient's needs."[46]

While the sheer variety of deformities confronting surgeons no doubt challenged their skill and ingenuity, the very necessity for surgery posed a physical, emotional, and, often, financial challenge to polio patients. However necessary medically, surgery, coming several years after the acute attack, meant once again leaving home and returning to the hospital. Surgeries were often scheduled during the summers so that loss of school time would be minimized. However, the more complicated procedures, such as spinal fusions, often required lengthy hospital stays that sometimes stretched into months. In addition, many young polio survivors had multiple surgeries to treat their many deformities, or sometimes to redo or repair surgeries that had failed the first time. Dorothea Nudelman, who had surgeries at thirteen and sixteen, recalled that the worst part "was going into the hospital feeling healthy and pretty and then experiencing pain and bodily violation in a way that was totally debilitating. It was like losing it all over again, only this time I wasn't a little kid anymore."[47] As they approached the end of their teens, some young men and women, with their parents' acquiescence, refused additional surgery, believing that no substantial improvement was likely and desiring to get on with the rest of their lives.

Not all surgery on polio survivors was done in their teens. Some who had polio when very young were first operated on when only five or six. For example, Kay Brutger contracted polio when she was nine months old. From the time she was eighteen months until she was six, she wore a leg brace to help her walk. Brutger had the first of her four surgeries when she was six. She had an operation on her "skinny and weak" right leg to correct a foot drop. She had a second surgery at eleven to stop the growth in her good leg to let the polio leg catch up. A third surgery at seventeen was intended to correct a "trick knee" and problems with a turned-in foot on her left leg. Her final surgery came eighteen years later to correct lingering problems from this third surgery. Barb Johnson, who had polio at age three, had her first surgery while in kindergarten. She had a second surgery when she was ten and then "about every other summer for the next several years." Most of these later surgeries were performed at the end of August. She would be hospitalized for two weeks and return home in time to start school. By scheduling them late in August she could enjoy most of the summer, have surgery, and still not miss school. Because she had so many surgeries, "they all sort of blend together" in her memory.[48]

Although they may have been accustomed to hospital routine, for these children and young adults the surgery itself was seldom routine. Dorothea Nudelman, for example, remembers that the ankle fusion she had at sixteen was "a rough surgery with severe unremitting pain" only partly controlled by Demerol. When the pain was still intense eight days after surgery, her doctor opened the cast to discover that the dressing had tightened with postsurgery swelling and had cut into her. When the procedure to replace the dressing was finished, she wished for her mother to "hold my head in her arms until the aching went away," but there was only more Demerol, "the cool night air, the relief from pain." Pain is a constant in these surgical memories. Sometimes the pain began before the surgery. When leg muscles had contracted, it was sometimes necessary to stretch them before surgery. This was done by putting the legs in casts, then cutting the casts at the knee, forcing the leg to straighten a bit, and then filling the hole with plaster to hold the extension. This process could be repeated for weeks before the surgery until the legs had fully extended. One polio survivor described the process as "brutal" and another remembered such constant "intense pain nobody could sleep in the same room with me at home, or stay with me during the day because all I did was cry and whimper."[49]

Perhaps the most difficult surgical experience was a spinal fusion. If polio weakened or destroyed the muscles of the torso, especially if one side was left stronger than the other, scoliosis or spinal curvature often resulted. The curve could occur at any point along the spine. The scoliosis might take the form of an S as viewed from the back, or kyphoscoliosis, which brought the head and neck forward toward the chest. In some cases, both scoliosis and kyphoscoliosis were present. If severe, the spinal curvature could compress the internal organs and impair breathing. Dr. Joseph Barr thought that "scoliosis was one of the major problems in the management of poliomyelitis." In his opinion, it could "often be prevented or controlled" if it was "detected at its beginning and treated with recumbency, vigorous corrective exercises and carefully graded activity." He believed that bracing had been used "too freely" and was not particularly successful in treating scoliosis as patients tended "to slump in such apparatus, with a slow but inexorable increase in the deformity." [50]

In spite of these admonitions regarding the ineffectiveness of bracing in preventing or treating scoliosis, many young sufferers endured years of bracing and casting in hopes of avoiding surgery. Ed Sass, for example, had polio in 1953 when he was six. A few years later he developed scoliosis. The specialist the family consulted prescribed a "Milwaukee brace" to try to correct the curvature. This brace rested on the hips and pelvis and buckled up the front. Metal bars attached to the leather pelvic girdle in front and back and ran up to the head where they attached to a chin rest to hold the head in place. In addition, Sass wore a corset to straighten his back. He wore this "ultimate traction device" almost twenty-four hours a day "for about the next five years." Following this, a new physician replaced the brace with a body cast, which Sass wore for another two and a half years. Like Sass, Chava Willig Levy's physicians tried casting and bracing to control her developing scoliosis. She was in some form of traction from the age of about five: "first body casts from chin to hips, then Milwaukee braces," which she wore almost all the time. This went on for some ten years.[51] I myself remember wearing two different braces, a molded plastic corset that laced up the front and a second one similar to the Milwaukee brace. Except for bathing and sleeping, I wore both of these all the time for several years. All of these efforts to forestall surgery came to naught, as each of us eventually had a spinal fusion between ages ten and fifteen.

Everyone who had a spinal fusion underwent some kind of process to straighten the curvature before the surgery. Many surgeons used casting to straighten the spine prior to surgery. Some patients were "hung" or "lynched" to straighten them out as much as possible. A strap around your neck and head pulled you up as you stood so that your feet were barely touching the ground or some platform and then the cast was applied. This process could take some time before all the plaster had dried sufficiently to maintain the stretched spine. Other patients remember lying on a narrow canvas strap and being stretched by straps around the head and hips before the cast was applied. Once the cast was on, various techniques were used to straighten the spine. Sometimes wedges were cut out, and the spine straightened a bit, and then the wedges would be plastered over. I remember a large screw attached to two metal plates imbedded in my cast. The surgeon would come in every day or so and turn the screw and straighten the cast until he had straightened my spine. One of the more elaborate means of straightening the spine involved a metal halo attached to the skull with four screws and to the body cast with four vertical bars. Chava Willig Levy remembers that once the cast hardened, the screws would be tightened a little more every day in order to straighten the cast and her spine. Because this "rack" didn't stretch her sufficiently, doctors drove pins through her femurs so that weights could be attached. For a month she had weights attached to her halo and to the femur pins as she lay in her bed.[52] Once casted, these young men and women spent several weeks to several months in the hospital being stretched before surgery.

The kind of anxiety and fear this process could produce is very evident in a series of letters sixteen-year-old Ruth Weinberg wrote her parents in the month before her fusion. As she lay in a cast at the New York Orthopedic Hospital, she pleaded with her parents to come and take her home. As she lay there "watching each individual patient go thru the process of being knifed," seeing them suffer on their return to the ward, and listening to "the continual moaning & groaning and oohing," her willingness to undergo the surgery rapidly disappeared. She admitted to being "a big coward" and "foolish," and acknowledged that she had disappointed her parents, but the experience was driving her "crazy" and she insisted that her parents come and get her. Her desperate parents sent five of her letters to President Roosevelt in hopes that a letter from him would give her courage. FDR wrote a brief note telling her that he hoped "she would keep up her courage." The records, unfortunately, don't reveal whether Roosevelt's letter calmed her fears.[53]

After weeks of straightening the torso, surgeons finally operated to fuse the spine. Often they operated through a hole cut in the back of the cast. In many cases, the spine was fused with bone taken either from the hip or leg bones of the patient undergoing the surgery or, sometimes, from a bone bank. Some spinal fusions included a Harrington rod or rods inserted and attached to the spine to help maintain the straightened spine. Where the curvature was particularly severe, surgeons sometimes fused the spine in two separate operations in order to achieve the desired correction.[54]

The spinal fusion was followed by several months confined to bed in a body cast as the spine healed. Because they were basically healthy once they had recovered from the immediate effects of the surgery, these young men and women were often sent home to recover. Carole Sauer spent a year lying on her back. Her father made a kind of cart so that her parents could wheel her from room to room. She recalls that "the cast was terribly uncomfortable" and she "developed sores all around the edges where it rubbed." Sauer, like most who spent months in a body cast, also remembers the itching, which she tried to relieve with "the end of a fly swatter" stuck in under the cast.[55] When I left the hospital after the surgery I was installed in a hospital bed in the back part of the living room, where I spent over six months flat on my back. Because the cast went below the waist and the top part of my legs, I couldn't bend at either the waist or the hips. Several months after the surgery, the original cast was replaced with a smaller one that allowed movement at the hips. Like Sauer, I used all kinds of devices to try to scratch the incessant itching under the cast.

Given the complicated nature of the surgery and the stresses on the spine, it is not surprising that complications sometimes developed. Ed Sass, for example, remembers being sent home in a "heavy and very uncomfortable" body cast that allowed him to walk and to attend school. One day he suddenly felt "a stabbing pain in the top of my back." When he reached under the cast he could feel a lump where the top of the Harrington rod had detached from the bone. He soon had surgery to remove the rod, and his last cast was cut off soon afterward. Sharon Kimball's cast had been lightened somewhat in the pelvic area before she left the hospital so it would be easier to use a bedpan. However, it had been lightened too much, and it soon cracked. The Kimballs lived in St. Cloud, Minnesota, and it was difficult for them to get to Minneapolis, where the surgery had been done. Consequently, "the doctor suggested that my mom just patch the cast herself, and that's what she did." Unfortunately, when the cast was later removed, the surgeon discovered that "when the cast had cracked, the fusion had slipped and hadn't healed correctly." Kimball needed a third surgery to repair the damage.[56]

There were many difficult and painful aspects of any major surgery to correct the deformities of polio, but for some young men and women the expected physical and emotional pain of surgery was compounded by being put on display for the edification of other doctors, residents, and medical students. Following his recuperation from a muscle transplant, Charles Mee discovered that the surgery, in fact, made almost no difference in his ability to walk, although Mee never admitted this to his parents, or, initially, to his doctor. His surgeon, proud of his work, repeatedly invited Mee to Milwaukee to exhibit him on stage before medical audiences. Mee "would arrive early, strip, and put on a little loincloth, like a diaper." After his physician described the surgery, the attending doctors would sometimes ask Mee one question: was he able to walk better? The first several times this occurred Mee dutifully answered yes, even though the surgery had made no difference. Finally, he realized that if he told the truth he would not be asked back. So, in response to the question from a French surgeon, Mee replied, "No, I don't think it has made any difference at all, really; maybe I'm a *little* worse." He was right; he was never asked back.[57]

Much to the dismay of some surgeons eager to operate, parents sometimes allowed their teenaged children a say in the decision whether to undergo an operation or not. When he was thirteen, surgeons recommended that Don Kirkendall's spine be fused in a straight position, which meant he would be able to walk with crutches, but could never sit down. His father turned to Don and asked his opinion, since he would have to live with the choice. Since the wheelchair already gave him mobility, Kirkendall couldn't see the advantage of walking with crutches, and saw many disadvantages in never being able to sit down. His father and mother agreed with the choice, but the surgeon was "livid with rage: 'You let a *child* decide something like this?' " His parents refused to sign the release for surgery, and the operation was never done. Similarly, Charles Mee's parents consulted him when his physician recommended additional surgery. The doctor wanted to fuse the bones in his left hip to stabilize the leg, making walking easier. However, it would mean that when Charles sat down, he "would have to slump down, sitting more on the small of my back than on my buttocks." When Mee said he wasn't sure he wanted to do this, the surgery was never discussed again.[58] In each of these cases, patients and parents were confronted with a choice that increased one function, walking, but that would have been extremely dysfunctional in terms of living one's life. Just because a surgery could be done was not always sufficient reason to do it. By the time they were in their teens, having gone through a long period of therapy and perhaps having had several surgeries already, these young men and women were anxious to get on with their lives regardless of the recommendations of their surgeons.

The accounts of severely disabled polio survivors with compromised respiratory function suggest that few made significant progress in regaining physical ability once they went home with their iron lungs or rocking beds. They generally had the longest hospitalizations of any polio survivors. Medical authorities thought that most muscle recovery in polio occurred within the first two years following the acute illness. Where muscles had only been damaged rather than destroyed, some further improvement could be expected with additional exercises, bracing, and surgery. But in the case of the most seriously paralyzed survivors, the nerves controlling their muscles had been largely destroyed, and thus no additional recovery could be expected. That did not mean, however, that they could not continue to recover something of the life they had led before polio struck. They could go home, begin to reintegrate themselves into the life of the family, continue the process of adapting to their disabilities and remaining abilities, and find meaningful ways to live their lives.

This process of recovery was different for each survivor with severe respiratory involvement. How the recovery proceeded and how far it went depended on many variables: the extent of the paralysis and incapacity, the willingness and ability of family members to take on the extensive burdens of caregiving that sometimes challenged professional medical staffs, and the ability of the survivor to deal successfully with the many psychological and emotional issues that accompanied significant disability. If each experience was in some ways unique, a successful recovery seems to have had several characteristics. First, the polio survivor could breathe on his or her own for at least some time, the longer the better, in order to facilitate care and provide a cushion of safety in a power outage. Second, the family, especially the spouse or parents, had to be willing to assume the burden of care twenty-four hours a day, seven days a week. As Kenneth Kingery's mother-in-law told him when he came home, "the entire household revolves around you now."[59] Because these survivors were so dependent and the required care so extensive, their presence in the family could easily distort relations within the family. The survivor had to be willing to let go to some extent so that spouses, parents, children, and siblings could have lives of their own. Even if life in these families could never approach cultural standards of normality, some semblance of a normal family life was necessary for all involved. Third, the survivor had to successfully deal with, if not necessarily resolve, the deep psychological and emotional issues that accompanied such extensive paralysis. Absent a successful adjustment, life could be miserable for everyone. Finally, the survivor needed to find ways to make life once again meaningful. Not all such survivors made a successful recovery; sometimes the burdens overwhelmed the physical, familial, and psychological resources brought to the task.

Before they could be released from most hospitals, polio survivors with respiratory paralysis had to be weaned from the iron lung so that they could stay outside the tank for at least part of the day. Not all facilities, however, made this a prerequisite to release. When Kathryn Black's mother was released from the center in Seattle, "she could not breathe on her own enough to survive a power outage longer than a breath or two." Nonetheless, her physicians thought she would be better off at home.[60]

A second key factor in the continuing recovery of respirator-dependent polio survivors was the willingness and ability of the family, especially spouse or parents, to take up the challenge of caring for them. Many found that their spouses, parents and families were up to the task, although that was not invariably true. Roger Winter and Arnold Beisser, for example, married women who had been their nurse or therapist and whose professional training eased somewhat the challenges and responsibilities they faced. Louis Sternburg's wife Dottie "learned all the slow and complicated details of nursing a paralyzed polio patient," although they also had some assistance from hired aides. Similarly, Norma Alexander and Fran Kingery took responsibility for their paralyzed husbands' care when the men came home from the hospital. Parents, often with the assistance of other family members, provided the necessary nursing care for Regina Woods, Alta Robinson, Marilyn Rogers, Mark O'Brien, and Martha Mason, when they brought their children home.[61]

Whatever the challenges of caring for their sons and daughters, it was far better than leaving them in institutions. Mark O'Brien's parents, for example, decided to bring their son home when they discovered that the "life expectancy of a nursing home resident was eighteen months." O'Brien, with the help of his family, not only beat the eighteen months, he went on to earn a college degree and publish his essays, poetry, and an autobiography. Not all families, of course, were as successful as these in providing the necessary care while maintaining family life. Kathryn Black has movingly reconstructed her mother's difficult and short life after being released from the respiratory center. Her grandmother took primary responsibility for the care of her adult daughter with the aid of other family members and some professional nursing assistance. Black's father, however, found it difficult to participate in the intense care his wife required. Although Black's family seems to have done all it could to care for their daughter, wife, and mother, it was not enough. Virginia Black died in her home ten months after being flown home from Seattle.[62]

Having a respirator-dependent polio survivor living at home put significant stress on all members of the family. Several male survivors recall that one of the most difficult things for them to do was to give their wives, their primary nurses, sufficient freedom to have lives of their own. Louis Sternburg, for example, admitted that although he "was dependent on Dottie, she was the focus of my anger and hostility." He refused to let her go out, even when competent care was available, and he belittled the "small domestic crises" in her daily responsibilities in caring for her husband and two children. Finally, after extensive work with a psychiatrist, Sternburg realized that "to keep Dottie, I had to let her go." So, too, Larry Alexander's wife, Norma, came to the conclusion that a key part of his recovery was regaining independence, including from her. As she put it, "The moment you let me go, the moment you stopped clinging and demanding and let me start to find interests of my own—well, that was when I started to work out my problems." Kathryn Black, in her study of polio survivors and their families, concluded that families who "coped better" with severely handicapped members were those "who tried to normalize their family life." Although it was sometimes fraught with danger and anxiety, they gave "their disabled members a place in the larger world."[63]

Recovery from polio was not only physical, it was also psychological. This was especially true for survivors with extensive respiratory paralysis. Kathryn Black quotes one physician who concluded that "it is practically never too late for the patient to realize that he is a respirator patient for life." In her study of the polio experience, she concluded that "the only way out of the maze of social expectations and personal suffering for both family and the polio survivor lay in hope." She discovered that individuals found different ways "to grasp hope, whether in stoicism, cheerfulness, fantasy, religious faith, or physical feats." For these severely disabled polio survivors, "hope could not rest on expecting a cure but on finding usefulness, physical and emotional, and then value in the life one has."[64]

Physicians and psychologists who studied the adjustment of severely paralyzed polio survivors found that certain behaviors needed to be in place if these individuals were to cope successfully with their disabilities. "Coping behavior" included "keeping distress within manageable limits; mobilizing hope; maintaining a sense of personal worth; restoring relations with significant people; enhancing prospects for recovery of respiratory and motor functions; and increasing the likelihood of working out a favorable situation after maximum physical recovery has been attained." The patients in one study of respirator-dependent polio survivors experienced a long process "through which they eventually faced and accepted the physical limitations they so much would have preferred to avoid." By dealing with their unfavorable situations in a "series of small steps," they ultimately came to recognize the "painful reality." Once that recognition was acknowledged, they increasingly adapted and made use of "whatever potentialities it offered for dependable gratifications, self-respect, and reliable relationships with significant other people."[65] Polio survivors who had the emotional, psychological, and familial resources to undertake this process eventually learned to adapt to and cope with their significant impairments. Not all survivors, however, were equally well equipped to embark on the process, and for others coping and adaptation was simply not possible.

As long as they were in the rehabilitation hospital, respirator-dependent survivors could maintain at least the hope that the continuing treatment and therapy they received would result in some physical improvement in their condition. However, when they went home with their physical condition essentially unchanged, they had to begin in earnest to deal with the unlikely prospect of significant physical improvement. Sometimes it took years before these polio survivors addressed the profound psychological issues that accompanied such severe paralysis. For example, Regina Woods had polio in 1952 when she was thirteen. The disease left her almost totally paralyzed and dependent upon respiratory assistance. Although she had seemingly made a good adjustment to her many limitations, the almost three months she spent in intensive care in 1987 to deal with a variety of physical problems plunged her into a period of depression. After returning home, she discovered that "nothing, absolutely nothing, seemed important." She felt "helpless and totally out of control" and had a "severe case of the 'I DON'T CARE's.'" Dr. David Rogers set her on a path to psychological recovery. He suggested that she begin to write about her experience. She soon discovered that nothing would change as long as she "remained under my little black cloud and that there were choices to be made about living or not living that no one . . . could make for me." Although a lot of things were out of her control, Woods finally decided "simply to acknowledge that this is the only life I have and that whatever my condition, critical or otherwise, I will live it as well as I know how."[66] Although Woods, at the urging of Dr. Rogers, engaged in a kind of writing therapy, she was not formally treated for her psychological and emotional problems.

Louis Sternburg, unlike Regina Woods, was an adult, married with two children, when polio left him totally paralyzed and dependent upon iron lungs and other respiratory aids to breathe. After several years in rehabilitation facilities, Sternburg went home reliant on a chest respirator and rocking bed. Over time, however, Sternburg found it increasingly difficult to leave the house. Finally he gave up and told his wife that he wasn't "going out anywhere, ever again." And for the next fifteen years he left his house only a few times. Eventually, he agreed to work with a psychiatrist. Sternburg acknowledges that his work with the doctor "didn't make everything magically better." His depression continued for some time, and there were repeated setbacks, but gradually he "was climbing out of the pit" and could acknowledge that his life "had some value." By acknowledging his emotions and feelings, by discussing them with a sympathetic professional, and by discovering that his life still had meaning, Sternburg learned how to tame his unruly emotions, to give his wife and children space to have their own lives, and to find ways to participate in and contribute to the life of the family.[67] As the cases of Woods and Sternburg suggest, the psychological and emotional recovery from polio took a long time. It was, in many ways, a lifelong project to recover a measure of emotional and psychological equilibrium and then to maintain it in the face of disability and dependence.

As these two accounts of the difficult challenge of finding a psychologically healthy way of dealing with severe paralysis suggest, one of the keys for these polio survivors was to find ways to make their lives meaningful in spite of their severe limitations. These respirator-dependent polio survivors had to embrace what I have called elsewhere "the covenant of grace." They needed to "achieve some level of understanding, some sense of acceptance and resignation, or some faith in God's ultimate purpose as a means of coming to terms with their remaining disability." Regina Woods, for example, found strength to continue partly in her religious faith and partly in her faith in herself. This sense of acceptance, however, was hard to achieve and difficult at times to sustain. After years of struggle to reach an understanding that would make her situation bearable, Woods concluded that "the true miracle is life itself, which becomes miraculous when, and only when, we accept it fully, problems and all, without dictating conditions." Like Woods, Louis Sternburg eventually found a measure of acceptance through his religious faith. His "growing belief" gradually restored his faith in himself, which "I thought I had lost forever when I lost movement and breathing." Part of this process of his "search for enlightenment" was a renewal of his Jewish faith. For a long time Sternburg held on to the fantasy that he would walk again. But as his faith deepened, he "finally dropped the fantasy and accepted the reality" and in the process "found an even greater strength."[68] Achieving a sense of grace, of acceptance, was not a one-time accomplishment. This coming to terms with their severe disabilities was a process that in some ways never ended, even when they had attained a measure of understanding. New physical challenges threatened this hard won faith, but once fully accepted the faith proved stronger than despair.

Not all respirator-dependent polio survivors turned so explicitly to religious faith to give meaning to their lives. Arnold Beisser, who was stricken just after finishing medical school, was not respirator-dependent, but polio left him significantly disabled and dependent upon others to meet his needs. Even with his training as a psychiatrist, it took Beisser years to fully come to terms with his own disability. As he put it, he had to be "dragged, kicking and screaming toward this new version of reality." As he developed his ideas, he acknowledged that accepting one's disability was a process, not something achieved in a flash. He argued that to accept one's disability, "there must be time, there must be fertile soil for growth, and there must be an adequate replacement" for one's prior conceptions of self and meaning. Only when these conditions are met, he argued, could "graceful acceptance occur with dignity." Beisser acknowledged that this process was "not easy," and that "grace comes from the fact that the disability has been integrated into a new way of life." "Self-acceptance is not something that occurs all at once or, for that matter, once and for all. It is a very gradual process that comes in tiny increments." When Beisser "stopped struggling [and] working to change and found means of accepting what I had already become," he discovered that he had changed. "Rather than feeling disabled," he now "felt whole again."[69]

Not everyone who confronted such severe disability was able to achieve some level of acceptance. For some, the challenge was simply too great. These men and women generally did not write narratives of their experiences. Only those who could round off their polio experience with some kind of acceptance, however tenuous, set down their stories. However, there is some evidence concerning individuals who never found satisfactory ways of dealing with their physical disabilities and attendant emotional and psychological problems. For example, Regina Woods describes how one of her friends steadily declined after going home. She had met the young woman when they were both in iron lungs recovering from polio. In the hospital they "relied on each other for support," and spent many long evenings together, since neither had many visitors. When Woods visited her friend after their release, she was surprised by her friend's "lack of responsiveness." Woods eventually learned that doctors at Vanderbilt where both had been treated said "that they had never treated a post-polio patient who had been so completely devastated emotionally by her illness." This young woman had completely planned out her life before polio struck and "could not find a way to accept the total annihilation of her dreams." The woman "gradually sealed herself away from everyone," and found "no relief until her death in 1979." Kathryn Black, in seeking to understand more about her mother's death ten months after being sent home, concluded that hope in a possible future was essential to living with a serious disability. Writing almost four decades after her mother's death, Black has no way of knowing whether her mother "could evolve to a place where she could find a measure of peace in the passive, dependent life polio left her." One of the physicians who treated her mother raised the possibility that Virginia Black had died because "she lost the will to live." A study of patients who died shortly after leaving the Northwest Respirator Center in Seattle suggests that they had physical problems similar to those who lived, but that they seemed "to lack the initiative, drive, imagination and support systems to achieve what the more successful patients had."[70] Like Kathryn Black, we can't know why some totally paralyzed survivors endured and learned to cope not only with their significant physical limitations but also with the heavy emotional and psychological burdens, while others did not. But in acknowledging the success of many, we also need to recognize that everyone brought different resources to this most difficult task, and those who succumbed to their burdens may have simply lacked sufficient resources to succeed.

| 7 |

Resuming Life after Polio

THE FIRST CHALLENGE faced by polio patients after hospitalization was often reintegration into the life of the family. The second was to leave the often-protective embrace of the family and to begin to move out into the wider world of the street, school, and work. Here, one of the biggest hurdles was to learn to deal with the stigma of being a cripple. Strangers stared at braces and crutches, asked rude questions about using a wheelchair, hurled epithets of "hunchback" and "cripple" across schoolyards, and questioned one's ability to attend school or to work.

Although some young polio survivors attended special schools for the handicapped, or were taught at home, many returned to the schools they had attended before the virus struck. They had to learn to negotiate the often inaccessible schools of the era and to find ways to become once again just another student. Particular challenges here included the ubiquitous physical education classes, athletics, and dating. For some, polio meant approaching their education with a new seriousness in order to compensate for their loss of physical ability. Older polio survivors faced the challenge of returning to work, or of finding meaningful work. The luckiest survivors had jobs to which they could return. Others faced the harder task of finding new jobs they could do with their disability, or of finding work for the first time. Not surprisingly, many of these polio survivors encountered discrimination in seeking work, in spite of the widespread public service messages urging employers to "hire the handicapped." Most of the polio survivors who were physically able to return to school and work did so successfully, but not without confronting and overcoming significant physical, psychological, social and cultural barriers.

Polio survivors returned to families with all their many strengths and weaknesses. Many survivors came from families that strongly supported the rehabilitation and reintegration of a son, daughter, or spouse. But other families' own peculiar dynamics and tensions accentuated psychological and emotional problems associated with polio. For example, Fred Davis's study of fourteen Baltimore families who had a son or daughter with polio revealed that that the "illness-generated adjustment process" was "much more difficult, prolonged, and pervasive in those families in which the child remained handicapped to some significant extent than it [was] in those families in which he did not." He also concluded that "where illness-associated problems persisted for a long period of time, there appeared to be a tendency for them to merge with older and continuing issues of tension and conflict in the family." Other studies tended to support Davis's conclusion that where there were problems in the family adjustment, some of those problems preceded polio and were exacerbated by the disease and disability.[1]

Crippling was only one factor in the adjustment of these children. Others included "broken home, poor family relationships, over-protective parents and other similar difficulties." Studies reveal that parental attitudes toward their disabled child were a major factor in the child's adjustment to his or her disability. Fred Davis argued that "the fundamental issue of identity confronting the families of the handicapped children was how to view, interpret, and respond to the many negative meanings imputed to a visible physical handicap in our society." Families in his study tended toward "normalization and disassociation" as strategies for dealing with disability. Normalization denied the disability, viewed the child as "normal" and encouraged others to treat her similarly. Families that employed disassociation "sought to insulate themselves from contacts, situations, and involvements which might force them to recognize that others, and they themselves, regarded the crippled child as somehow 'different.'" Both approaches "had inherent limitations and from time to time broke down, sometimes resoundingly." Most of the families in his study tended toward one approach, while occasionally adopting the other strategy. Ellen Whelan Coughlin's study of handicapped children classified parental attitudes as constructive or destructive. The most constructive parental attitude intellectually and emotionally accepted the child's disability and focused on how to compensate for it. On the other hand, parents with strong emotional reactions to their child's disability often projected destructive attitudes, including "overanxiety and overprotectedness" and occasionally "overstimulation of the patient to accomplish more than he was capable of." Other studies pointed to "inconsistent behavior involving careful provisions for necessary physical care, together with resentment of the burden this entails" and "outright rejection of the child."[2]

Clearly, the parents' attitudes toward their child's disability significantly influenced the child's own attitude. Families with healthier attitudes generally did a better job of integrating the polio survivor back into the family and in preparing him or her to venture forth into the uncertain world beyond the protective embrace of the family. However, children are resilient, and even many survivors from less than ideal family situations learned to function successfully in the worlds of school and work.

In spite of the potential psychological and emotional difficulties, many survivors seem to have made a relatively good adjustment upon returning home. Most families seem to have adopted some version of what Fred Davis described as "normalization," that is, treating the child as close to normally as possible, and expecting them to take up their family responsibilities as they could. Parents were often warned against being overprotective and of the dangers of coddling their disabled children, and many parents seem to have taken the advice seriously. For example, Dorothea Nudelman remembers that her mother insisted that she do things for herself if she had her braces on, even if it took twice as long. Her mother was simply following the "doctor's orders" to "make her [daughter] independent as soon as possible." Many survivors remember being expected to pitch in with chores as they were able, especially if they lived on farms. Stanley Lipshultz recalls that he was exempt from most of the outdoor chores, but he also "washed more than my fair share of dishes and did other chores that did not require a lot of walking." He experienced "what amounted to the tough love of the 50s." Gail Bias believes that she "was never treated any differently by my parents or other members of my family." She never felt excluded, and like her siblings was expected to do chores. While she didn't bale hay, she did drive the tractor and perform practically all the other chores, or at least she tried. She does acknowledge, however, that she felt some pressure to prove herself by keeping up.[3]

Sometimes, however, polio and the survivor's presence in the family created an emotionally tense environment. Charles Mee remembers that his efforts to do things by himself often produced conflict. For example, when his mother asked "if she could help me reach a book or turn on the television, or get out of a car or put on a shoe, I would say patiently, 'No, thanks,' or sometimes I would snap at her that I could do it myself." He felt, as he said, that "I needed to defend myself against my mother's instinct to help; and my mother and I survived the strain of that negotiation only because we were so close." Many of the polio survivors studied by Richard Bruno and Nancy Frick

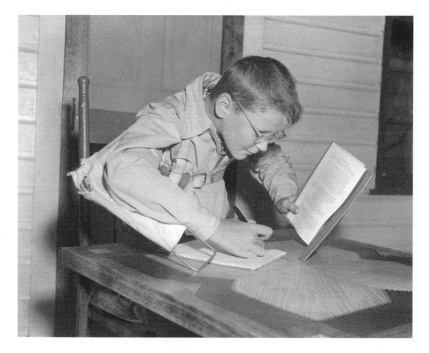

FIG. 18. Larry McKenzie, 12, the 1951 March of Dimes poster boy, studying on his family's farm. 1950.

also recall unhealthy family responses to polio, reporting being "physically trapped by their parents' refusal to make accommodations for their physical limitations." Some parents tried to "'forget' about polio by requiring children to equal or exceed the level of physical performance they exhibited before their illness." Other parents expected their sons and daughters to "outperform their peers academically." Still other parents sought to isolate their crippled children and sometimes the entire family in an effort to avoid the "'shame and estrangement' at having been 'singled out' by polio."[4] Not surprisingly, family dynamics in response to polio ran the gamut, from healthy reintegration into family life to toxic emotions that added a psychological burden to the physical recovery.

In many families, siblings found ways in which to incorporate their crippled brothers and sisters into neighborhood play. For instance, Don Kirkendall remembers that his older brothers would tie him in a buggy to take him hunting. Even with "useless legs and only one good arm" he could still "get a bead

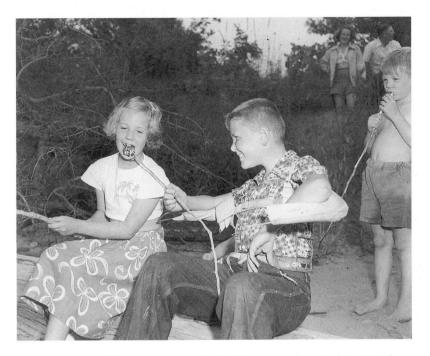

FIG. 19. Larry McKenzie, 12, the 1951 March of Dimes poster boy, sharing a toasted marshmallow with a friend. 1950.

on a gopher." Later, after he got his own wheelchair, he could be "part of the gang and take part in their games, brace, chair, and all." Kay Brutger "did most of the things the other kids did." She "jumped rope, played basketball, even ice skated." With her brace and built-up shoe she "wasn't particularly good at all the things" she tried, but she "was able to do most anything the other children did, as long as it didn't involve running or climbing trees." She recalls that "the kids never made fun of me and generally included me in what they were doing."[5] Very often siblings and neighborhood kids were more interested in figuring out what you could do and how you could participate than in excluding you. Since so many childhood games and activities were improvised anyway, it wasn't hard to find ways to include somebody wearing a brace or using a wheelchair.

The children who faced the most daunting task in reintegrating into family life were those who returned home in iron lungs or reliant on other respiratory devices. They were far less mobile and the gravity of their condition also imposed a barrier to trying to resume their pre-polio childhood. For example, Marilyn Rogers was eleven when she returned home in an iron lung. Installed in the converted dining room, she recalls having to get reacquainted with her younger brother, whom she hadn't seen since entering the hospital. Although her old neighborhood friends visited, something had changed. They no longer "had anything in common." Polio had aged Rogers quickly, and her return home ended her childhood; the new friends she made were usually adults. When his parents brought him home from the rehabilitation hospital, Mark O'Brien was able to spend several hours a day outside a chest respirator, although he still slept in it. He recalls that while he "couldn't fully participate" in the games that his older brother and friends played, he "enjoyed them and the companionship of the boys, who, though puzzled about how to include me, welcomed me with a simple warmth that I seldom sensed in adults." Regina Woods remembers that when she returned home her days were divided between schoolwork and listening to the radio. Like Rogers, she made new friends, but was distressed when some old friends drifted away. She could only conclude that they "simply could not deal with the radical changes that had taken control of my life and made me into a person much different from the one they had known."[6] Although these three survivors all wanted to resume their childhood or adolescence, the severity of their impairment and their need for continued respiratory assistance proved a major obstacle.

Mothers and fathers, husbands and wives who returned home in iron lungs or on rocking beds faced a different set of challenges. Resuming life meant taking up once again the role of parent and spouse and, for the men, especially, returning to one's job or finding a new way to support one's family. This was difficult when your paralysis made you as dependent as an infant. Contemporary studies of such severely paralyzed polio survivors suggest that several conditions needed to be in place if the individual was going to make a good transition from the respiratory center to home. For some, continued physical progress after discharge from the hospital helped morale, but not all survivors continued to regain strength and ability. Several other factors seemed to be necessary to make a good adjustment at home. These included being able to depend on prior familial or professional relationships, having an important and needed role in the family, finding a role in the community, achieving a level of economic security, learning to accept assistance, persistence in "working toward restoration of physical functions, interpersonal relationships, and a satisfactory socio-economic position," appropriate medical and psychological care, efforts to improve appearance, developing interests that did not require physical prowess, setting achievable intermediate goals, "pride in strength," "stoicism," and achieving "sexual gratification" for both partners. The challenges facing survivors with extensive paralysis were formidable. However, among patients in these studies "there was a remarkable degree of resolution in some cases and impressive evidence of resourcefulness."[7]

Kenneth Kingery, an air force officer stricken on his last day in the service, wasn't sure he would be "at all good in the role of disabled deadbeat." He discovered that "with no job, no career, no achievement whatever, the constant taking without ever giving began to gnaw at my innards." He realized that he "had to work at *something* in order to merit my wife's respect and affection." After he talked to the Veterans Administration about additional education to become a freelance writer, Kingery finally saw some hope of regaining the man's role of a worker supporting his family. As he put it, "I believe a man must have the dignity of a job to feel that he's needed by mankind; an income to prove that he's doing his job well."[8]

Like Kenneth Kingery, Roger Winter, who used a chest respirator, wanted to support himself and his new bride when he returned from the hospital and they set up housekeeping. His wife, Theresa, had been his nurse in the rehabilitation hospital, and initially the National Foundation for Infantile Paralysis paid her to be his full-time attendant. Winter believed strongly that a family could not continue to be supported by charity if it "is to hold heads high." With the help of vocational rehabilitation the Winters began a magazine subscription business out of their home. It earned them $500 in 1955 and over $5,000 in 1961. Winter did the typing for the business using a mouth stick, and his wife handled the telephone. The other challenge for Winter was learning to be a father. They tried to make the situation for their daughter Lori "as normal as possible," although Winter admits that his medical equipment made for some unusual toys. His daughter also took on new responsibilities as soon as she could, such as putting paper in his typewriter, getting things, and helping to feed her father.[9] Only when Winter found a way to support his family did he feel that he had really taken on the roles of husband and father.

When Louis Sternburg returned to a new home that would accommodate all his medical equipment, he and his wife Dottie had to figure out ways to meet his time-consuming and demanding medical needs, care for their two young children, and find a way to earn an income. At home Louis found that he "was the center of everyone's attention . . . instead of being one of the inmates controlled by the hospital rules." But in time life settled into a routine, and he began to worry about money. What helped Louis most to achieve some sense of progress in this new life was going back to work. Louis knew that he "had to help support my wife and children, if I was going to get back any of the self-esteem that had been knocked out of me by this demonic illness." [10]

Kathryn Black's mother was still dependent on the rocking bed or chest respirator when she left the respiratory center for her newly rented house near her own mother's home in Boulder, Colorado. What Black remembers from the summer of 1955 when her mother came home was not so much "the strangeness of our family life, with Mother paralyzed in the dining room and Dad nowhere in sight," but the fact that her mother "was *there* again, talking to me and listening to me." During the nine months that she lived at home, Black's mother was a real presence in her life, although her grandmother took over most of the responsibility of raising her and her brother. After her mother died, Black's surviving family members, "grandparents, father, brother" and herself, "spun free of each other, into separate realms, unable to cope with our own grief, unable to help each other." In succeeding years as Black and her brother grew up under their grandparents' care, neither their mother nor polio was mentioned.[11] In this case, the severity of Virginia's paralysis, the fragility of her health, and the family dynamics prevented her from fully taking on the role of mother and wife upon her return home.

Children who lived with a paralyzed and respirator-dependent parent often faced a difficult childhood. With one parent immobile and dependent, and the other preoccupied with the many details and pressures involved in the care of their paralyzed spouse, children often had to fend for themselves. Dottie Sternburg recalls worrying about what kind of home she and her paralyzed husband could provide for their young children. She remembers thinking, "I didn't want any of us to be ashamed of the way we lived or isolated by fear of what other people thought. I wanted our home to be approachable to everyone, not just pointed out as the house where the man on the rocking bed lived. I wanted the children to love Lou as a normal father, even though he wasn't, and to go to him not out of duty but out of desire." Their children, David and Susie, had somewhat different reactions to their childhood and adolescence. David, the older, felt that his father's illness and paralysis "was a terrible loss for my father and mother, but for me, as a child, it was mostly gains." Only two when his father contracted polio, David was very close to his father and never hesitated to bring his friends over. His friends usually came back because his father was "fun and good company and they liked to be with him." As he grew older, his caring for his father increased, although his mother usually insisted on doing things if she was available. Susie, who was eighteen

months younger than her brother, found the family's situation more difficult. She didn't talk much about her father at school, and she didn't bring
many friends home when she was young. She acknowledges that her parents
wanted to bring them up as normal children and to encourage their independence. However, unlike her brother, in her teens Susie "stopped accepting
the situation and thinking it was normal. It became the focus of my rebellion."
At fourteen, she "couldn't stand" either of her parents, and they "couldn't
stand" her. After her teen rebellion faded, she grew close to her father again,
and she became a confidante of her mother. Like David, she has come to realize that her parents' goal was "to bring us up as normal children, and they've
succeeded." [12]

In seeking to understand why her family disintegrated under the impact of
Virginia Black's paralysis, Kathryn Black concluded that "those who coped better . . . were the ones who tried to normalize their family life." The more successful families "approached obstacles cheerfully." They, along with the paralyzed member, went "to restaurants, stores, concerts, and church, and even on
vacations, with the help of portable respirators, wheelchairs, slings, and lifts."
These families didn't isolate themselves; instead, they gave "their disabled
members a place in the larger world." What emerges from the narratives
and from Black's quest for answers is a complex picture of family dynamics in-
tersecting with the course of polio and its lasting legacy of paralysis. Some
marriages and some families had the psychological, emotional, and financial
resources to survive the paralysis of one of the parents. Others did not. In addition, the course of polio recovery varied widely. Virginia Black survived for
about twenty-two months following the acute disease. One study revealed
that, like Virginia Black, about 10 percent of the patients discharged from the
Seattle respiratory center died within two years. The patients who died "didn't
necessarily have different physical problems . . . from those 'who succeeded,'
but rather seemed 'to lack the initiative, drive, imagination and support systems to achieve what the more successful patients had.'" [13]

One of the challenges for all polio survivors, although it was perhaps more
acute for those with severe paralysis, was making a decision to reenter the
larger world outside the safety of hospital and home. Regardless of the severity of their disability, polio survivors feared the stares of curious adults and
children, the pitying eyes of strangers, the intrusive questions, and the stigmatizing label of "cripple." Responses ranged from curiosity to hostility, but
all stigmatized the survivors as cripples. Fred Davis in a study of "deviance disavowal" argued that handicapped individuals needed to learn how to manage

"strained interaction" if they were to successfully negotiate "everyday social situations." Because negative attitudes about individuals with disabilities were widespread in society, every encounter outside one's intimate circle risked rejection. As Davis put it, "the visibly handicapped person must with each new acquaintance explore the *possibilities* of a relationship." However, because individuals with disabilities did not "comprise a distinct minority group or subculture," there was more ambiguity in the encounter with an able-bodied individual than was the case in other cases of "intergroup stereotyping" such as between black and white in the segregated South. Davis's study suggests that the polio survivor's fears of being stigmatized as they moved outside the hospital and home were real, but they also had opportunities to move the strained relationship to a more normal one.[14]

Most polio survivors took their first moves into public without the kind of supportive community that the rehabilitation ward had provided. Once they returned home, polio survivors had little contact with others who had survived the disease. Ward friendships were hard to maintain because the individuals who shared nearby beds in the rehabilitation hospital might have come from another town, another county, or even another state. And even if a long-distance friendship was maintained, the support and encouragement it provided lacked the immediacy that was so important during rehabilitation. In spite of the large number of survivors from the epidemics of the forties and fifties, there was typically only one in a neighborhood, school, or workplace. Even where there was more than a single polio survivor, they didn't necessarily become supportive friends. For example, I went all through Catholic grade school with another boy who had had polio, but I don't recall ever talking about our respective experiences or being especially supportive of one another. I suspect that was due in part to having internalized the social and cultural message that we needed to become as normal as possible. As Tobin Siebers observed, "one cripple is invisible compared to two cripples," with the result that many polio survivors chose for decades to be "strangers to each other."[15] In getting on with our lives, polio survivors wanted very badly to fit in. Keeping company with individuals who were disabled by polio or other causes only set us apart even more. And so we entered public life alone, largely bereft of the comradeship that had lightened the pain of rehabilitation.

Going out in public for the first time was a big step psychologically and emotionally and one every polio survivor needed to take if he or she was to have a social life, or go to school or work. For example, Jan Little remembers that in her community "being in a wheelchair carried a fair amount of shame."

After her parents took her to a local concert, one of their neighbors chastised them for "taking a child like' that out in public." Arnold Beisser remembers that it was a "major step" to go out in public after having been isolated for years in a hospital. When he first went to a restaurant in a wheelchair with his friends, "it seemed as though all eyes were on me, as if daring the pariah to invade the domain of those who belonged." On one of Hugh Gallagher's initial forays into the outside world a young girl "crossed herself as we passed." Gallagher was shocked, especially when "she said a prayer that she wouldn't be like me." Even at home in his rocking bed Louis Sternburg discovered that he had to put visitors "at ease to reassure them that this wasn't a horror show." Some old friends never came to visit and of those who did he could "see fear in their faces. They're worried, tense, and pale. They stutter a bit and grope for words, so I have to carry the conversation." Eventually, his anxiety about the reliability of his portable breathing equipment and the effort and even pain of going out caused him to withdraw, and over the next fifteen years he went out only twice.[16] Most polio survivors didn't withdraw, however, and they found ways to respond to stares, inappropriate comments, and discrimination.

For younger polio survivors, going to school often produced considerable anxiety about their treatment by classmates and teachers. Although some survivors were educated in special schools for the handicapped or at home, many were mainstreamed into the public schools. Here they faced a number of challenges. Many worried about falling behind their grade because of their long hospitalization and convalescence at home. Although most rehabilitation hospitals tried to enable patients to keep up with their education, the schooling the children received was not always comparable with their regular school. For those with significant lower-body paralysis or weakness, the physical construction of most midcentury schools posed a potential barrier to returning. Most schools were multistory buildings, often with a steep flight of stairs up to the front door, and few had elevators. Schools often permitted students reliant on braces and wheelchairs to return, but the students generally had to figure out how to negotiate the stairs. Finally, there were the psychological and emotional concerns about being accepted by one's peers, about performing adequately, and about finding a secure place in the social environment. While many classmates and teachers were helpful and understanding, fellow students could be also cruel and insensitive in their comments. Many of those who returned to school found that they did better academically than they had before polio struck. Excelling in class work was a common way to compensate for the loss of one's physical abilities. Still, polio survivors found ways to participate in activities, such as physical education, athletics, and band, that required some physical prowess. In spite of the anxiety it produced, returning to school and joining in activities with old and new friends was a significant step in one's recovery from polio.

School-age polio survivors often feared being held back in school because of the classes they had missed while in the hospital and recovering at home. Polio was enough of a burden without being held back, especially in smaller communities and schools where everyone knew what grade you were supposed to be in. Consequently, as soon as they had recovered sufficiently to focus on their schoolwork most young survivors attempted to keep up with their schoolmates. In some cases parents hired private tutors to teach their children until they could return to school. In other cases the school district made arrangements for teachers to come into the home to teach those not yet ready to return to school. For example, Dorothea Nudelman had received some instruction in the hospital and regular instruction for a year at home, but she had still missed two years of regular schooling. When she returned to school, the district wanted to hold her back a year, but her parents argued for keeping her with her friends who were entering seventh grade. As Nudelman recalls, "I was devastated by the idea of being 'left back.'" Because the sixth grade was full, she entered seventh grade on a trial basis. Eager to succeed, she worked hard and at the end of the year won an award for the highest grades in class. Irving Zola was tutored by a retired schoolteacher during his absence from the Boston Latin School, the most rigorous high school in Boston. Nonetheless, Zola was afraid that he might not be able to enter his senior year. For him, as for other polio survivors, "the words 'being kept back,' 'repeating a year,' 'falling behind' were terms for personal failure." When it came time to return to Boston Latin, his tutor argued that Zola be put on probation for the first part of his senior year and if he passed that he be given credit for the year he missed. After the school agreed to the proposal, Zola went back to school and became an honor student.[17] Motivated by a strong will to succeed and by a desire to avoid the additional stigma of failure, young polio survivors generally discovered that they could keep up with their classmates when they returned to the class, in spite of the time and assignments missed.

Some polio survivors, especially those with significant paralysis and dependent on some form of respiratory assistance, never returned to school. They received all of their schooling at home. Marilyn Rogers had some teaching during her two and a half years at the Sister Kenny Institute, but her school district had no resources for homebound students, so she skipped the fourth through the seventh grades. After the district started a home program for un-wed mothers and extended it to students with disabilities, Rogers received four hours of instruction a week, but only in some subjects. Mark O'Brien's schooling was equally erratic. For much of his elementary schooling, a teacher employed by the town visited disabled children two or three times a week. In fifth and sixth grades, the school district experimented with home instruction with speakerphone two hours a day. In junior and senior high school O'Brien was taught by teachers who came to his home after the regular school day. O'Brien believes that he "got a pretty good education because I was working one-on-one with the teachers and I was very eager to please them." He eventu-ally passed the test for the general equivalency diploma.[18]

Polio survivors who could return to school faced a number of obstacles. Schools in the forties and fifties were generally not prepared to accommodate students with physical disabilities, and some chose not to readmit polio sur-vivors. Other school districts segregated students with disabilities in their own building, often mixing physical, mental, and cognitive disabilities in the same room. Jan Little, who lived in southern Wisconsin, was tutored at home for grade school. When it came time for high school, the superintendent of schools refused to admit her. He told Little's mother that "since the high school was a multi-story building, the classes would have to be rearranged, and that wasn't convenient." He also conveyed the impression that it was a waste of time to educate crippled children. His final argument was that it would be depressing for the other students to have to look at her every day. Two years later, after listening to repeated family protests and after construct-ing a largely one-floor high school, the school board finally admitted Little when the family promised not to ask for any special favors. Even so, her home-room teacher apologized to her class for their having to be in the room with her. In addition, Little had to get through the six- to seven-hour school day without using the bathroom, since the doors to the girl's bathroom were too narrow for her wheelchair.[19]

Clara Yelder was even less fortunate. After she returned from the Tuskegee Institute polio facility, her parents wanted to enroll her in the local Alabama schools. Her father was told that she could not attend, and that the district refused to take responsibility for her education. She stayed home with her mother and read her brothers' and sisters' books and their homework. Later, one of her sister's teachers, "out of the kindness of her heart, decided she would come out at least once a week and go over homework" with her. Occa-sionally Yelder took night classes, and eventually, at the age of twenty-nine, she completed her general equivalency diploma.[20] It is hard to know to what extent the fact that Yelder was African American made it easier for the superintendent to exclude her, but clearly the district was unwilling to educate this polio survivor.

Some polio survivors received their education in a variety of venues. For example, Kathy Vastyshak had just started first grade when polio struck. After returning from the hospital she had teachers at home for her first three grades. Starting with fourth grade, she was assigned to a school very near her home. The fourth-grade teacher "just assumed it was his responsibility to come and get" Vastyshak, so he picked her up at home and took her to class. If she tired early, he would take her home at lunch. This lasted for only one year; after that she "went to specialized classes for orthopedically handicapped kids." For junior and senior high school Vastyshak transferred to regular schools. Both were new buildings and were accessible for her wheelchair, although she needed help getting up a step into the high school. In high school she took the business course and encountered a teacher who had had polio. Vastyshak could type with only one hand, and since the teacher didn't know of a method for this, she developed one herself and taught it to Vastyshak. Like Vastyshak, Paul Reitmeir had a varied experience with schools. He had attended a Catholic elementary school for two years before he had polio. After he recovered, the parish priest refused to readmit him, telling Reitmeir's parents, "Well why should we educate him, he's not going to amount to anything." His parents then turned to the public schools, which provided a teacher to come to their home once or twice a week. This was followed by classes in a special school that brought all the disabled students together in one room. Later, while undergoing chiropractic treatment in a Denver hospital, Reitmeir was taught by a teacher provided by the Denver school system. When he returned home to Bethlehem, Pennsylvania, the high school was inaccessible. Two of the high school teachers, one in English and history and one in business, came to his home once a week to provide instruction. Thus, he was able to graduate with his class, even though he had never really been in class with them.[21]

Most youngsters were welcomed back by their classmates, and in some cases found themselves treated as heroes for overcoming polio. Sometimes, however, the first challenge was simply getting to school and learning how to get around the building. For example, Kay Brutger had to take a taxi to school, since there was "no such thing as a handicapped accessible school bus." Those who could use a school bus wanted very much to be treated like all the other students rather than as someone who was disabled. Ray Gullickson, for instance, was embarrassed on his first trip back to school when the driver drove the bus all the way into the farmyard to pick him up. That made him "feel very 'crippled,' so every day after that, I walked the three-fourths of a mile to the bus stop." For other students, the obstacles appeared when they arrived at school. Boston Latin, after pressure from his family, allowed Irving Zola to use the private elevator and the teachers permitted him to arrive late and leave early. His friends, as Zola recalls, "took turns carrying my books and occasionally even me." David Kangas needed help to negotiate his inaccessible high school. In order to get from floor to floor, "a crew of several students would have to grab my chair and lift me up the steps." Although he didn't like being dependent on others, he also knew that "it was the only way I was going to get up to those other classes and continue" his schooling. He also admits that "the guys who helped me were quite willing to do it." [22] A strong will to succeed and ingenuity enabled these young men and women to devise ways to get to school and to class with the help of parents, bus drivers, administrators, teachers, and, especially, friends.

Polio survivors often worried about the reception they would receive from the classmates when they returned. Many were welcomed back, others were embarrassed to be held up as role models of heroism, and some encountered curious questions and teasing. Most of these polio survivors were the only ones in their classes or schools with a disability and they stood out. Richard Owen recalls his return as a "strange event" for his classmates because at the time "it was unusual for a child with a physical disability as severe as mine to be integrated in a regular classroom." Even though he knew most of his classmates, it was odd to return "on two crutches and lugging a fifteen-pound brace." Similarly, Gail Bias returned to the one-room school where everyone knew her, but "it was very difficult to be the only child in the school with a disability." When polio survivors returned, teachers sometimes celebrated them as heroic role models, which didn't always endear them to their classmates. For example, Dorothea Nudelman recalls that when she returned to her Catholic school, the nun described her as "the sterling example of the seventh grade," which only "separated" her even more from her classmates. In addition it attributed to her "special spiritual strengths" she didn't have. When Edmund Sass returned to school wearing a very obvious Milwaukee brace to correct his developing scoliosis, the brace became "the major topic of conversation around the school" for several weeks. Sass recalls that "it was almost like the other children were delighted to have this new curiosity in their midst." Sass, however, wasn't so sure he liked the attention and notoriety.[23]

As the novelty of their return wore off, many polio survivors remember being teased by their classmates. Jennifer Williams recalls that the neighborhood children who knew her didn't give her a hard time when she returned to school, but that others whom she didn't know would tease her and "say things like, 'Hey gimpy, you walk like a duck.'" She learned that if she didn't respond, the teasing generally stopped. When Gail Bias returned to her one-room school, others made fun of her, although "after a while they accepted me pretty well." She thinks they became accustomed to her and her limitations. However, when she went into town for high school, she again had to deal with being teased both about being a "country kid" and about her built-up shoe and limp. Tobin Siebers's nickname throughout elementary school was "Chester," for Marshal Dillon's sidekick who walked with a limp on the television show *Gunsmoke*.[24]

Polio survivors quickly learned ways of dealing with the teasing that almost all experienced. A common response was to ignore it, no matter how much it hurt, in the hope that it would end, as it usually did. Lacking a response, most taunters sought out more likely targets for their scorn. Other survivors discovered that their friends often came to their assistance. As Jennifer Williams recalled, she "had a lot of kids who liked me, and they would go over to the ones who'd taunt me and say, 'Leave her alone. She's nice.' That helped a lot." Sometimes the very things that made you different also helped gain a measure of reprisal. Vivian Johnson Reagin recalls that boys liked to "pop" the girls on their backsides by bringing two or three fingers down quickly "like a whip." Bending over a water fountain one day she was "popped," which was immediately followed by "jumping and shouting." The boy had popped her on her steel brace and was convinced that he had broken his fingers. She remembers that "his fingers were not broken, but I was never popped again." When Edmund Sass got tired of explaining his Milwaukee brace, he told kids who asked about it, "Well, my dad's a carpenter, and one day he got careless with the electric saw and cut my head off. The brace holds it on." The looks he got "were amazing." What was "even more amazing is how many kids believed that's why I wore the brace."[25] Almost all youngsters are teased and taunted at one time or another, but having a visible disability often singled polio survivors out for special treatment. Even when they achieved a measure of revenge, it still hurt and added to the challenge of returning to school.

One of the concerns facing survivors with mobility impairments who returned to multistory schools was what to do in case of a fire drill, or more important, in case of a fire. Schools had different ways of handling the problem. Sometimes the school required the student to demonstrate that she could get out of the building on her own in case of a fire. In one case this meant being able to negotiate four flights of stairs. Often, schools allowed such students to stay in their classrooms during fire drills. This, of course, didn't address the problem in the event of a real fire instead of a drill. Other schools assigned older boys to help students with disabilities evacuate the building, including carrying them if necessary. For example, Joyce Tepley remembers that when she was in sixth grade on an upper floor, "the school arranged for a muscular eighth grade boy to carry me down the stairs during fire drill." She was "embarrassed, more so out of my budding sexual feelings, but secretly liked the special attention." [26] However it was handled, these procedures once again set the polio survivors apart from their peers.

Once they returned to school, polio survivors wanted to participate fully in its activities. The activities that provided the greatest challenge, of course, were those involving physical skill, such as physical education and sports. An inability to participate, or a relative lack of skill in these activities, stigmatized boys and girls in a school culture that valued physical ability. Not everyone wanted to participate in sports, but many polio survivors found the required physical education classes to be one of the most difficult and painful parts of their school experience. Some schools solved the problem by making alternative arrangements for students who couldn't take regular physical education classes. For example, Grace Audet began in a "modified" PE class, but she was able to switch to a modern dance class where she "did pretty well," even if she wasn't able to do everything. In junior high Jennifer Williams was excused from physical education, but after California passed a law requiring every student to take it, she "was shoved into a room for what they called adaptive P.E. It was like a study hall." Ed Sass's "asymmetrical body made me embarrassed and self-conscious" while swimming and showering in the locker room, and there were some things in class he "just couldn't do." For example, when Sass couldn't do some of the expected exercises he would listen to what other students were reporting for their scores and "then just report one that was respectable, but a little below average." The teacher "was nice enough not to confront" him. This teacher also helped when the class played basketball in the gym. Sass's team always wore their shirts and the other team was the "skins." Sass is sure the teacher "knew that playing basketball in the gym without my t-shirt would have been embarrassing." Tobin Siebers remembers that gym was the only time he could take his brace off, because his shoes would have ruined the floor. One morning exercising in his tennis shoes he "cracked my bad ankle against the floor." In explaining how this happened, the gym teacher told the principal, "They want so to be like other children and don't like to be left out."[27] Like no other class, physical education pointed up the difference between polio survivors and the other students.

One of the traumatic moments for polio survivors in both formal physical education classes and in informal school yard and sandlot games was the picking of sides, usually by the two best athletes. If they could run, polio survivors were usually the slowest players on the field and almost invariably were chosen last when teams were picked. In Millie Malone's school there was a "very nice boy who used to make sure I was not picked last on the teams that were chosen for sports." She was "usually next to last, but he always made sure I was not the very last." As she notes, "it is sad when one is always last." Bob Sellars wasn't allowed to take physical education, but the boys he hung out with after school played a lot of sports. He recalls that "they always counted me as half a man." He "always hated standing there as the sides were chosen. Wanting to be one of the first players to be picked, but always being the last." Sometimes they "would flip a coin" to decide which side he played on, or they would declare, "we have peg leg, you have to spot us 5 points."[28] I learned early that if you brought the bat and ball to the neighborhood games you were automatically one of the team captains who got to pick the other team members. That way you were first instead of last.

Sports and physical education classes may have given polio survivors the most difficulty in school, but they were not the only activities they tried to participate in. They were game for almost all the activities the school offered. In rural southern Wisconsin, for instance, Jan Little was active in 4-H. As she observed, "I was just another 4-H kid—swinging between being a good kid and a pain in the ass. It was pretty incidental that I ran around the fairgrounds and got in trouble using a wheelchair instead of my legs." In high school, Little participated in forensics and debate, which didn't require standing and walking. "Roger and Bill, my debate team partners, managed to carry me up and down stairways in schools all over southeastern Wisconsin and only drop me a little way one time." The coach in Arvid Schwartz's small Minnesota high school asked him to be the student manager for the sports teams. Schwartz now belonged: "I became part of the group. I rode the players' bus, I was friends with the players and the cheerleaders." Mary Ann Hoffman was active in school activities. She "was in student council, . . . editor of the school yearbook, . . . [and] sold tickets at the games."[29]

Faced with their physical limitations, many young polio survivors focused their attention on their classes and excelled in their schoolwork. Jim Doherty, who grew up in a rough Chicago neighborhood, believes that polio made a substantive improvement in his life. Barred from physical activity, and needing braces and crutches or a wheelchair to get around, Doherty was sent to the Chicago high school for students with disabilities. Here he "soon felt the beginnings of a new life and a wider and totally different perspective" from his pre-polio outlook. He mingled with kids "whose interests were not solely confined to sports and postmortems on the last rumble." In high school he "discovered a host of other interests (apart from girls, of course) such as politics, music, theatrical stagings, strategies to end (we thought) certain unpopular school administration policies, and other mind-centered pursuits." These new interests and his studies eventually led him out of his tough environment to college and a professional career.[30] Polio survivors often compensated for their lack of physical ability by throwing themselves into the many other activities mid-century high schools offered and, especially, by becoming good and even excellent students, substituting mind work for physical work.

Understanding and supportive teachers eased the polio survivor's return to school and helped her fit in with her classmates. Unfortunately, some teachers contributed to the torment these boys and girls felt in school. Good teachers included the fourth-grade teacher who picked up Kathy Vastyshak and took her to school and the typing teacher who devised a one-handed typing method for her. Others included the coaches who urged Arvid Schwartz to become team manager or ensured that Edmund Sass always played on the team that wore their t-shirts. There was also the high school physics teacher who encouraged Jan Little to work in his lab and in the visual aids department. On the other hand, there were many teachers who did not know how to work with students with disabilities, had no desire to learn, and openly displayed their displeasure. For example, Jennifer Williams's second-grade teacher "just couldn't relate to a child with a handicap." This teacher was always hard on the young girl and refused to believe she was any different. As Williams remembers, "she would always say things like, 'They're doing it, so you have to do it too. You know we can't play favorites.'" And Wanda Peterson's sixth-grade teacher would talk about her in front of the class. The teacher would declare, without naming Peterson, "Some people in this room think they are so great because they aren't supposed to run in P.E." The teacher also made her move her desk away from everyone else's. Soon, the girls in her class began to imitate the teacher in their treatment of Peterson. Interestingly, the teacher never stopped the harassment, but "finally the boys in the class . . . put a stop to it. They told the girls off in no uncertain terms."[31] The attitudes and actions of teachers could make all the difference in the class. Those who were supportive helped polio survivors to fit in as best they could and to excel where they were able. The worst helped make school a living hell.

Other than sports and PE, dating probably caused the most anxiety among polio survivors. Dating, and whom you dated, was a measure of one's social acceptance. Since polio survivors were often perceived as cripples, as damaged goods, it was difficult for these young men and women to find classmates willing to date them. In part, their lack of dates was due to the perceptions of their classmates who couldn't see beyond the physical limitations, but in part the problem was internal. The survivors had internalized some of those same attitudes and couldn't conceive why someone would want to date them. In addition, the risk of being turned down was too great; it was easier to stay home on Friday night. Some polio survivors went through their entire high school years without a date, while a few did manage to date occasionally. Arvid Schwartz remembers that the "only thing that really bothered" him about high school was that he didn't date. He "figured that no one would want to go out with me, so I didn't have a girlfriend." Gail Bias didn't want to dance "because I was self-conscious of my limp." She didn't want people staring at her on the dance floor, and she hated having people "gawk and laugh" at her. As she put it, "I think all teenagers are self-conscious, but when you have some physical disability, it really magnifies that self-consciousness." When James Berry asked one girl to dance, she replied, "Oh, are you able to dance?" He remembers being "so insulted" that he "just turned away." When his invitations were repeatedly spurned he "entertained the notion that these rejections were coming because I had polio," and he "began drowning my sorrows in alcohol."[32]

Some polio survivors, however, were more successful at the high school dating game. Mary Ann Hoffman remembers having both good and bad experiences with dances. She had been excited about the freshman dance, but "no one asked me to dance all night." She "was just crushed" and remembers thinking, "Is this the way things are going to be for the rest of my life?" However, after transferring to a new high school she "even started to get asked to dances, and not just school dances, but community dances too." Irving Zola's friends at Boston Latin arranged his first date after he returned to the school. Zola was relieved when the young woman accepted, and shuddered "to think what would have happened if the girl had refused the date and later my advances." Charles Mee shared the anxieties, but he managed to date a cheerleader. He had learned to drive a car and he and "Suzy Harvey . . . began dating. She was a cheerleader, which is to say, she was not only pretty and energetic and popular, she was also the mainstream." His cheerleader took him "into the mainstream with her."[33]

Whether one was successful in dating or not, almost all polio survivors felt betrayed by their bodies. In a culture that put a premium on looking good and fitting in, paralyzed limbs, twisted torsos, braces, crutches, and wheelchairs set polio survivors apart. Although a high percentage eventually married, the high school years were especially difficult because of adolescent high expectations and the casual cruelty of so many of one's classmates.

Since jobs requiring substantial physical activity were not an option for many polio survivors, many of them went to college after graduation. Colleges, however, were no more accessible than elementary and high schools. In some cases, polio meant that young men and women who might not have gone to college because of their social or economic backgrounds decided to pursue their education. State departments of vocational rehabilitation often provided the funding for college. For example, Jim Doherty acknowledges that without polio he probably would not have gone to college. His "parents didn't have the money for it and in the neighborhood where we lived it was generally not 'the thing to do.'" His college costs were paid by the Illinois Department of Rehabilitation, but he quickly found out that in college he "had to change into a serious student capable of developing and applying good study habits, or I was sure to wash out fast." Bill Van Cleve's education at Rutgers was paid for by the New Jersey State Rehabilitation Program. The experience changed his life, as he was the first in his family besides his father to attend college.[34]

Not all state vocational rehabilitation programs were so supportive. Jan Little, for example, had to battle with the Wisconsin Division of Vocational Rehabilitation to win their support for college. Her high school counselor told her that "no college or university would accept a person in a wheelchair as a full-time, residential student," and the state psychologist recommended that she "consider typing envelopes at home." Thanks to the swim coach she learned of a program for students with disabilities at the University of Illinois and she entered the university in the fall of 1957.[35]

Even polio survivors dependent on iron lungs insisted on going to college. Ed Roberts, however, found that he had to challenge the California Department of Rehabilitation when he decided to transfer from San Mateo Community College, where he lived at home, to the University of California at Berkeley, where he would live on campus. The Department of Rehabilitation initially refused to fund his college education on the grounds that "spending money on Roberts would be wasted since it was 'infeasible' that he could ever work." The state eventually gave in as the result of extensive negative media publicity, but Roberts still faced obstacles in being accepted at Berkeley. One dean told him, "We've tried cripples before and it didn't work." Finally, when the head of student health services offered to allow Roberts and his iron lung to move into the university's student hospital, Roberts was permitted to attend. Although this state financial support was invaluable, the rehabilitation counselors had their own preconceptions about what polio survivors could or could not do. In the fifties and sixties they generally held to the medical model, which defines disability as a "deficit located within individuals that requires rehabilitation to correct the physiological defect."[36] Since college would not correct the significant physical limitations of severely impaired polio survivors, these professional counselors often had trouble conceiving why these men and women were so desirous of a college education. Prisoners of their own assumptions, these professionals sometimes added to the obstacles polio survivors faced in attempting to further their education.

The difficulties didn't end, of course, when polio survivors arrived on campus. Almost no campus was accessible in the fifties and sixties, and students with disabilities were expected to make their own arrangements to gain access to buildings and classes. The more severe one's impairment, the more difficult it was to negotiate the campus. For example, Richard Owen had gotten rid of his long leg brace and used only a cane for support when he went to Indiana University. However, he still had to plan in advance how he would get around, since Indiana was "a huge campus with a lot of ups and downs and hills and lovely wooded trails between buildings." When David Kangas went to the University of Minnesota in 1955 he found that an accessible apartment was nearly impossible to find and that the campus and dorms were not accessible by wheelchair. Nonetheless, he eventually found an accessible off-campus apartment. He drove from his apartment to the university in his hand-controlled car, but since there were no parking spaces reserved for the handicapped, he "had to find these sort of secret places where I could park without the University patrol coming along and ticketing me." When confronted with steps he would "have to get a bunch of volunteers or just recruit people as they were rushing from class to class." It was more difficult than in high school, where his friends had been a reliable lifting crew. At the university other students sometimes helped and at other times left him sitting, unable to reach his class. "It took me five years to graduate because I had to drop so many classes," Kangas says. "I just couldn't get to some classes enough because accessibility was such a problem."[37]

When Jan Little entered the University of Illinois in the fall of 1957 she went to one of the few colleges in the nation that had a program for students with disabilities. However, since she had missed so much schooling, she wasn't prepared for college, either academically or socially. Little also wasn't physically prepared for independent living. After her parents dropped her off, she realized that she was not used to getting in and out of bed by herself, nor did she have a "legitimate plan of attack for using the bathtub." By watching others, she figured out how to get out of bed, use the bath, and transfer to a car. Although classes were more difficult than she anticipated, she survived these as well. Once she got over the initial hurdles, Little threw herself into college life. She became both a freshman advisor and a cheerleader for the wheelchair basketball team. The director of the program, Tim Nugent, had predicted that she wouldn't be able to take care of herself, but Little was determined to prove him wrong and did.[38]

When Berkeley finally admitted Ed Roberts in the midsixties, neither he nor the university realized the profound changes that would result. Living in the campus hospital wasn't ideal, but it was a start. Roberts had attendants, paid with state funds, to push his wheelchair, to assist him with dressing and eating, and to help him figure out how to get into buildings that at first seemed inaccessible. He could stay out of the iron lung long enough to attend classes and participate in other activities, including partying and drinking. Ultimately he got a powered wheelchair, which gave him both more mobility and more privacy, since he could then go where he wanted by himself. As news of Roberts's experiment spread, other students with significant physical disabilities applied to Berkeley, and by 1967 there were twelve living in the campus infirmary. They adopted the name "Rolling Quads" and began to push the university to eliminate the barriers they faced. They took their cues from the contemporary civil rights movement and began to develop the notion of civil rights for individuals with disabilities. The Rolling Quads also pushed the university to develop accessible housing in something other than an infirmary and pressured the city to install curb cuts. By 1970 with the aid of federal funding the university established the Physically Disabled Students Program to help students find places to live, hire attendants, negotiate the university and the city, and be as independent as possible.[39]

Roberts and his colleagues, however, went beyond simply making the university more accessible to students with physical disabilities. They began to rethink how they, the university community, the larger society, and health professionals ought to conceive of disability. Roberts and his cohorts rejected the medical model of disability that measured the success of rehabilitation by how much function one regained through medical interventions including physical therapy and surgery. Instead, Roberts "redefined independence as the control a disabled person had over his life. Independence was measured not by the tasks one could perform without assistance but by the quality of one's life with help." The newly christened "independent living movement" assumed that the person with the disability knew better what she needed and wanted for daily life than did some doctor or health professional. "And what disabled people wanted most of all was to be fully integrated in their communities, from school to work." The success of this student movement at Berkeley widened the horizons of men and women with disabilities who were not in college, and in 1972 Roberts and his friends helped establish the first Center for Independent Living. "It would be run by disabled people; approach their problems as social issues; work with a broad range of disabilities; and make integration into the community its chief goal. Independence was measured by an individual's ability to make his own decisions and the availability of the assistance necessary—from attendants to accessible housing—to have such control."[40] What began as a simple effort to go to college ended as a civil rights movement to free people with disabilities from cultural assumptions, from medical control, and from social and legal restrictions on their ability to live independently and to make their own decisions about how they would lead their lives.

One of the polio survivors to benefit directly from the work of Ed Roberts and his colleagues was Mark O'Brien. O'Brien had been paralyzed at six and in his midtwenties still slept in his iron lung. After his father learned of the program at Berkeley he began trying to get his son admitted to the university. After several years of additional rehabilitation and intense lobbying by Walter O'Brien, Mark was finally admitted to Berkeley in 1978 at the age of thirty. His iron lung was moved into a dorm by crane and "attendants pushed him to class in a reclining wheelchair and treated him as he had never been treated before—as an adult." O'Brien recalled that he had to make a major adjustment in his thinking at Berkeley: "I had to accept the idea that I was in charge, which was very difficult for me in the beginning. I had to be my own social worker, dealing with four or five different agencies. I had to learn not to be intimidated by the bureaucracies and to insist, insist, insist and make myself a real pain in the ass." Eventually he got a customized electric gurney, operated by the only parts of his body below the neck that he could move: his left foot and knee. Like Roberts's power chair, this gave O'Brien freedom to move around the university and the city. O'Brien graduated from Berkeley after five years with a 3.4 GPA and a B.A. in English.[41] What Ed Roberts and his colleagues had established in the sixties and early seventies made it easier and more likely for those who, like Mark O'Brien, came after.

Going to school and college, getting an education, was an important step toward independent living, but it was only a first step. Most polio survivors assumed that they would return to the jobs they had left or that on finishing their education they would enter the world of work. Perhaps the survivors who had it the easiest were those who could return to the jobs they held when polio struck. Some companies held jobs for their ill employees to which they could return when they were physically able. Others, however, and especially the more severely paralyzed, found it harder to return to work or to find new, well-paying jobs. And as polio survivors graduated from high school and college they too sought work in a society that might urge employers to "hire the handicapped," but that in fact threw all kinds of obstacles in the way of these men and women seeking to support themselves and their families.

A study by Charles Lowman and Morton Seidenfeld published in 1947 gives some indication of the difficulties polio survivors faced in seeking work. The study looked at the psychosocial effects of polio on 203 male and 234 female randomly selected patients at the Orthopedic Hospital in Los Angeles. The authors admitted that "visible physical limitation" adversely affected employability: "The capacity for the job and the ability of the individual to render efficient service in a normal environment, are often overlooked or ignored. Individuals with minor alterations in capacity but with obvious deformities are discriminated against by prospective employers." At the time the survey was taken, 44 percent of the men and 18 percent of the women were employed, although the authors note that they did not include in their figures the 30 percent of women who were married and "did not seek employment outside their household." The percentage of men working varied significantly by the severity of their disability. The authors concluded that "the individual with a good educational background is considerably better off in securing employment." Later studies demonstrate that a much higher percentage of polio survivors eventually found work. For example, Margaret Campbell's 1997 study of 120 polio survivors revealed that only 3 percent of the sample never worked.[42] This suggests that over time almost all polio survivors who wanted to work and who could work found jobs. However, the individual stories of polio survivors reveal that the effort to find meaningful and remunerative employment was often difficult, especially for those whose impairments were more severe.

Some older polio survivors were fortunate in that their employers held their jobs for them while they recovered, and the extent of their impairment did not preclude returning to their former position. Jim Marugg, for instance, was a sports writer with the *Los Angeles Star-News* when he contracted polio in 1952. Although he spent time in an iron lung, his respiratory muscles recovered and he was soon able to breathe independently. His legs, however, remained permanently paralyzed. As his recovery and rehabilitation proceeded, Marugg assessed his impairments and his possibilities. He noted, correctly, that "polio rarely affects the intelligence" and his "higher responses—sight, hearing, touch, taste, smell"—were unimpaired. Because his hands had not been affected by polio, he could still be a sports writer. The fact that the paper had kept his job and supported him during his recovery was a major source of encouragement during the long months of rehabilitation. Like Marugg, Bea Wright returned to her job. She was a single mother of three boys who worked for the Wayne County, Michigan, chapter of the National Foundation for Infantile Paralysis when polio struck. As soon as she was able, she began working from her hospital bed, with the nurses relaying messages from the office. Once she had recovered, she took a position with the national office of the NFIP in New York that had been held for her while she regained her strength. Both Edward Le Comte and William Foote Whyte were college professors when they came down with polio. Le Comte contracted polio in France, where he was on leave from his position at Columbia University. After a long recovery, he returned to his classes at Columbia. William Whyte was in Cambridge to sign a contract at Harvard when he developed polio in 1943. After polio struck he was unable to take the Harvard position, but in the spring of 1944 he was offered a position at the University of Chicago, and in June, after he finished his rehabilitation at Warm Springs, he moved there with his family.[43] Although both men used canes for assistance, neither of them found them to be an impediment to their teaching.

Other polio survivors found that they had to change jobs as a result of their impairments. For example, John Lindell had been a soil scientist with the Soil Conservation Service in Nebraska before polio. This position required considerable fieldwork checking the types of soils under cultivation. He had hoped to return to his old job, but it became clear that his paralyzed legs made that impossible. He gradually recognized that, as he put it, "any work I would do in the future would have to be of a sedentary type. For me there would be no walking across fields, digging in soil, and recording my findings on maps." Eventually a friend at church offered Lindell a job keeping the accounts for his business. Just as he was settling into the position, the controlling partner in the business visited the firm. After the partner left, Lindell was fired. The controlling partner had made it clear that "no disabled persons were to be allowed to work in his business." Disappointed, Lindell attended the National Business Institute (instead of the University of Nebraska, which was not accessible), eventually earned his CPA, and secured employment with an insurance firm.[44] This kind of odyssey was not unusual for polio survivors who had to contend with the prejudices of employers in their efforts to support themselves and their families.

Polio survivors who were children when they had the disease confronted some of the same problems in finding jobs when they finished their schooling. Don Kirkendall even found it difficult to get work in Portland, Oregon, during World War II when there was a shortage of workers. He worked at a number of part-time jobs, including stints as a musician, as a radio show host, and for the ration board, but nothing lasted very long. In one three-week stretch when seeking another position, he was turned down for twenty-nine different jobs. Finally, an official in an employment agency told him, "It is the wheelchair, Donald. Nobody seems to want to take the risk of hiring a man in a wheelchair, no matter how well he can do the job." Ultimately Kirkendall concluded that the only way he would have a job would be to start a business of his own. After Jim Doherty graduated from the University of Illinois he applied to the Chicago Board of Education for a teaching position. He was rejected "on the grounds that my physical disability would prevent me from shepherding students out of the school to safety in the event of a fire." Doherty held a number of jobs before he accepted long-term positions with the State of Georgia and later with the Social Security Administration.[45] Persistence enabled these young men to find employers who paid more attention to their abilities than to their disabilities, although in the case of Don Kirkendall that employer turned out to be himself.

The careers of Arvid Schwartz and David Kangas illustrate some of the other ways in which polio survivors negotiated the world of work. After high school Schwartz attended the Minnesota School of Business, and when he graduated he took a job with an insurance firm. After two short-term accounting jobs, he took a position at an insurance company in 1961, stayed for twenty-five years, during which he completed his college degree, and rose within the firm to become treasurer and financial vice president. After leaving the company he became involved in a successful land development company in the Twin Cities. Later, after buying a farm, he discovered that he still loved farming and decided to take it up full time.[46] It is clear that Schwartz's changes in jobs were the result of his own changing interests rather than related directly to his disability. Like Schwartz, David Kangas had a varied career. After graduating from the University of Minnesota, Kangas and his wife, whom he had met at the university, moved to California to avoid the harsh Minnesota winters. In both California and later in Minnesota he took civil service exams and eventually worked for state and county government agencies. Kangas recalls that "back in the 1960s, if you were disabled, just getting any type of job was a mammoth undertaking. If you could even get an interview, you were lucky. There was no affirmative action at all, and it quickly became apparent to me that in private industry, opportunities were virtually nonexistent." Finally, he realized that "with civil service, if you took the exam and got first, second, or third highest score, they would at least have to give you an interview."[47]

Arnold Beisser's encounters in the 1950s with medical administrators in his efforts to secure a residency and finish his medical training demonstrate that health professionals could be just as prejudicial as any other profession toward individuals with disabilities. Beisser had completed his medical degree when polio struck, but he had not yet completed a residency in a specialty. Polio had left him substantially paralyzed. When he considered the possibilities for a residency, he finally decided that "psychiatry had the fewest physical demands and seemed the most logical." Beisser "applied to countless programs for residency training in psychiatry. Most programs did not even answer after learning of my physical condition." Beisser discovered that the physicians who were program directors were not "immune to awkwardness in dealing with a disabled person." Finally, the director of a new residency program at a state hospital decided to give Beisser a chance. Within six months, Beisser had convinced the director that he was going to survive and that he "might even turn out to be a pretty good resident." His salary was doubled and the hospital offered Beisser and his new wife a house on the hospital grounds. Beisser eventually completed the three-year residency and the two additional years of supervised practice as well as passing the certification examination to become a board-certified psychiatrist.[48]

Even polio survivors needing continual respiratory assistance sought meaningful paid work. Although they needed to work out of their homes in many cases, they still wanted to contribute financially to their own care and to support their families. Male survivors, in particular, saw work for wages as crucial to their sense of masculinity. A man ought to be able to support himself and his family, and that self-conception didn't end with near total paralysis. In addition to whatever income they could earn, working boosted their self-esteem and sense of worth. Not until they had work could they begin to feel that they were once again contributing members of society and of their families, that they had regained an important part of their manhood.[49]

Polio left Roger Winter and Louis Sternburg needing almost continual respiratory assistance, and they established businesses at home with the cooperation of their wives. The NFIP initially paid Winter's wife, Theresa, to care for him when he left the hospital. However, that would not last forever, and the young couple began a business selling magazine subscriptions by phone from their home. In addition, they began selling greeting cards, and Winter did typing for Goodwill Industries and administrative work for a fund-raising firm to earn additional income. Before getting polio Louis Sternburg had a business selling clothing labels. Once he had returned home permanently he began to think of how he could get back to work. As he put it, "It was vitally important to get myself involved again. We needed the money. Our families were generous, but I wasn't going to live off them. I had to support my wife and children, if I was going to get back any of the self-esteem that had been knocked out of me by this demonic illness." They established a business with his wife at the head, since he "couldn't keep records or do any bookkeeping or correspondence." He got on the phone to his old customers. Gradually he reestablished his customer base and the business became successful. In addition to the welcome income, the phone calls he made every day took his "mind away from introspection and self-pity," made him "feel useful and productive," and bolstered his "shattered self-esteem." Ultimately, while continuing to maintain his label business, Sternburg earned both a Masters degree and a Ph.D. from Brandeis University in psychology.[50] Like many other polio survivors, when Winter and Sternburg focused on their abilities, they found ways of making a successful living and in so doing restoring the self-worth and sense of masculinity shattered when polio struck.

Adult women who contracted polio had somewhat different goals from adult men. Those who were married at the time polio struck hoped to be able to return home and resume their roles as wife, mother, and homemaker. They had to find ways to do all the tasks involved in maintaining a household and raising children, or to find ways of getting assistance to do what they could no longer do. The more severely paralyzed they were the more they had to battle the perceptions of family and health professionals that they were too disabled to resume their roles within the family. In cases where their husbands left them these women also had to figure out how to support the family financially. When Sylvia Gray contracted polio in 1951 she already had two young children and a third on the way. After four months in the hospital she returned home and gradually learned to take care of the house and children from her wheelchair. After 610 days in the hospital, Harriet Griswold discovered that reestablishing relations with and authority over her three-year-old son and eight-year-old daughter would be challenging. The son, especially, quickly realized that if he ran away his mother could not chase him. A second challenge was to arrange her household so that she could do as much as possible for herself. She also had to deal with the housekeeper, who expected her to be an invalid. Griswold, however, could still "order food and plan meals even if I couldn't take stock of what was in the refrigerator." [51] These women found that being an effective mother and homemaker was not simply a matter of being able to do physically all that these roles entailed. Being a part of their family's lives, even if in a largely supervisory role, was more important than what they could no longer do physically.

Some of these women, however, found that in addition to figuring out how to resume their expected tasks they also had to learn to be single mothers when their husbands left. When Louise Lake left the hospital using a wheelchair, she and her daughter lived in a relative's apartment while she learned how to take care of herself and how to do the many things she would need to be able to manage her own house. After several months she and her daughter moved to a new apartment that friends helped decorate and outfit to her needs and abilities. For example, "a new ironing board was made, with proper height for the wheelchair and clearance underneath." She soon started "to cook and wait on others, and soon people were depending on me." However, some four and a half years after polio struck, her husband decided he wanted to end their marriage. Lake concluded that "there was nothing to do but serve the dual role of parenthood." She soon got a job in a department store to support herself and her daughter.[52]

Polio left Jane Boyle Needham paralyzed from the neck down and reliant on respiratory assistance to breathe. When she contracted polio in 1949 she and her husband had three children, aged two, three, and four. The physicians involved in her care were convinced that she could never go home and recommended custodial care. Although Needham's husband had been supportive during the early stages of her recovery from polio, as her months in the hospital stretched into years, he eventually decided that he wanted a divorce and custody of their children. Needham, however, was determined to care for her children. Everyone, from medical professionals on down, thought that it was impossible for a woman in an iron lung to run a house and care for her children. Nonetheless, Needham was determined to try. It wasn't easy, but she left the hospital, moved into a home of her own, and regained custody of her children. Although she still received considerable financial assistance from the county, she cost them less in her own home than in the hospital, and at the time she wrote her narrative, she felt well cared-for by her teenage daughters.[53] Although she faced more obstacles than many, Needham simply wanted to resume her life as a mother and homemaker in her own home. The role of mother and homemaker was much more than the physical activities, which could be done by almost anyone, whereas no one could really replace the mother in the family.

Returning to school or working, or taking up once again the duties of running a household, marked only the beginning of learning to live with polio. Because their disabilities were permanent, polio survivors continually faced physical obstacles and the possibility of prejudice and discrimination as they sought to get on with their lives. Most of them, however, would find ways to meet these challenges in the coming decades.

Living with Polio

FOR MOST AMERICANS, the memory of polio quickly faded in the decades following the success of the Salk and Sabin polio vaccines. Polio, if it was remembered at all, was recalled as a once-dreaded disease vanquished by medical science. In the 1960s even the March of Dimes turned its attention away from polio to focus on birth defects. Polio survivors, however, found it harder to forget the disease, for they had to live every day with the physical and psychological consequences of their encounter with the virus. Even as the number of polio cases dropped dramatically, polio survivors struggled to finish their schooling, to find and keep suitable employment, to marry and raise children, and to enjoy rich, rewarding lives. Many did so burdened with significant physical impairments and with lingering psychological issues unresolved during their recovery. Polio survivors also faced tremendous pressure from their families and society to integrate themselves into the mainstream of American society long before there was an Americans with Disabilities Act designed to facilitate the participation of people with disabilities in all facets of American life. If accommodations were made in those decades, it was because polio survivors found ways to overcome the obstacles to their full participation.

The cultural context of midcentury America in which polio survivors sought to resume their interrupted lives encouraged them to "put polio behind them," to get on with their lives as though they had no disability. Polio survivors, as we have seen, were encouraged to focus their energies on their physical rehabilitation and to repress or deny their feelings and emotions about their experience. They took pride in pushing themselves, in ignoring pain and discomfort, in forging ahead in spite of their disabilities. In many ways, denying the severity of their impairment, proceeding as though all obstacles could be overcome, and refusing to accept limitations were useful strategies. Polio survivors in large numbers finished their education, went on to successful careers in many fields, married and raised children, and participated in the social and cultural lives of their communities. But while these strategies were successful in many ways, there was sometimes a hidden cost in terms of both physical and psychological well being.

In addition to problems that can plausibly be connected to their physical disabilities or to the psychological consequences of living with polio, polio survivors experienced all the other joys and challenges facing Americans in the second half of the twentieth century. Not all marriages were strong and harmonious and families were not always happy and supportive. Children did not always turn out as one hoped. Jobs were not always stimulating and rewarding. And there were medical problems, such as heart disease and cancer, that were unlikely to have been related to having had polio. Clearly, the fact of having had polio could exacerbate problems in a marriage or on a job, but polio was not always the cause of the difficulties these men and women faced in their careers and in raising their families.

Polio was a disease that could and often did alter the plans young men and women had made for schooling, jobs or careers, and military service. Although some polio survivors with minimal damage had careers in the military, polio kept many survivors out of the armed forces. During World War II, especially, many young men wanted to serve their country, and some polio survivors were disappointed when military recruiters or local draft boards rejected them. Jack Dominik would have liked to have served during World War II, especially in the air corps. He recalls going to the draft board with some high school friends, "and this doctor told us to drop our pants. He just looked at me and wrote 'obvious' on the form, and that was that." Bill Van Cleve also wanted to join the military, and he went with high school friends to a navy recruiting physical. Van Cleve had convinced himself that "my country needed me enough that they would ignore this slightly smaller leg." When the navy rejected him, he remembered, "I was just crushed. I almost felt like I had been drummed out of the male corps or something." Polio also kept survivors out of the conflicts in Korea and Vietnam. Arnold Beisser was a naval reserve officer reporting for active duty during the Korean conflict when polio struck. As he writes, "there was an unexpected change of plans in my childhood agenda, and there began a future life for which I was totally unprepared."[1] My draft number during the Vietnam War was low enough that I was at risk of being drafted, and I was relieved when my draft board reclassified me as 4F. Especially during World War II, when many young men were eager to join the fight against Germany and Japan, polio survivors regretted being kept on the sidelines.

If polio often closed off the option of military service, it sometimes created opportunities for advanced education. Polio did not generally affect the intellectual faculties of its victims, and even though hospitalization and rehabilitation could interfere with schooling, most survivors returned to school and performed at appropriate grade levels. Polio survivors soon recognized that given their physical impairments they could not consider jobs requiring physical strength, significant physical exertion, or the ability to stand for long periods or to walk long distances. Thus taking education seriously acquired a new urgency following a serious case of polio. Richard Owen recalled that before polio struck when he was twelve, he was "constantly in trouble" and "fought to and from school." In addition to fighting, he also "loved to play football and baseball and things like that." He remembers that prior to polio he "had only read about three books in my whole life." After he returned to school following a year of rehabilitation, he focused on his studies. He could no longer compete athletically, but he could in the classroom. Owen is convinced that if he hadn't had polio he probably wouldn't have become a physician. Dale Jacobson acknowledges that polio made him realize that he "needed to pursue a career in which my physical limitations would not handicap me." That insight turned out to be an advantage for he ultimately pursued a career in dentistry that was more suited to his interests and abilities. Finally, Mary Ann Hoffman grew up on a farm in rural North Dakota, and although she was satisfied with farm life, polio pushed her to explore a wider world. Following graduation from her small high school she entered the University of North Dakota to study occupational therapy and she later lived and worked in Iowa, Arizona, and Wisconsin.[2]

State departments of vocational rehabilitation provided many polio survivors with the means to attend college. Jim Doherty lived in a neighborhood where making money took precedence over spending money on college. In his case, however, since the Illinois Department of Rehabilitation provided money for college, it was the obvious thing for him to do. Doherty realized that "then as now, not too many employers were hiring folks with disabilities, and especially those who had no educational credentials beyond the high school level." Bill Van Cleve never intended to go to college, and expected that he would get a blue-collar job. However, thanks to the state support, Van Cleve attended Rutgers University intending to become a teacher. He recalls that New Jersey paid him more than the federal government paid returning veterans under the GI Bill. As we saw in chapter 7, state vocational rehabilitation departments, however, were not always so supportive of the college plans of polio survivors. Jan

Little in Wisconsin and Ed Roberts in California had to battle for the support they needed and deserved. In a nice irony, California governor Jerry Brown eventually appointed Roberts to be director of the very department that had earlier declared it "infeasible" that he would ever work. Although state departments of vocational rehabilitation were supposed to assist individuals with disabilities get the training they needed to be productive citizens, polio survivors sometimes found that their first challenge was surmounting the agency's assumptions about proper training for individuals who used wheelchairs or who were as severely physically impaired as Ed Roberts.[3]

Polio survivors generally needed jobs that emphasized the mind over brute physical strength. But a college degree or specialized training did not guarantee employment or a career. In spite of frequent "hire the handicapped" programs, many employers were reluctant to hire men and women with disabilities regardless of their abilities. Although a high percentage of polio survivors worked for wages or as homemakers, it was sometimes difficult to find and keep employment because of the attitudes of employers.[4]

Some polio survivors encountered discrimination when they sought employment. Judy Heumann trained to be a teacher. After she graduated from college, the New York City schools denied her a license to teach. She had passed the oral and written exams but failed the medical exam. "The testing physician questioned whether she could get to the bathroom by herself or help children out of the building in an emergency." Heumann sued the board of education for discrimination and took her case to the newspapers, "which were happy to tell the story of a qualified teacher up against a coldhearted bureaucracy." Realizing they would likely lose, the board of education settled out of court and granted Heumann her teaching certificate. However, no school would hire her until the principal of the elementary school she had attended in Brooklyn offered her a job. Heumann, after becoming an advocate for individuals with disabilities, served in the Clinton administration as assistant secretary of education. Like Heumann, Cass Irvin, who relied on a wheelchair for mobility, tried to find a teaching job after graduating from Kentucky Southern College in the sixties. In the era before disability awareness and laws she quickly discovered that no school in her community would hire a teacher in a wheelchair. Irvin later realized, however, that even had she been hired as a teacher, the salaries were so low that she "could never earn enough money to pay the expenses of living with a disability." Robert Gurney confronted at least two different forms of discrimination. He had been hired on his first job while his boss was away serving as a colonel in the army. When his employer returned from the war, Gurney discovered that the man "couldn't tolerate seeing an imperfect person." So, even though the job did not require physical strength, Gurney was soon fired. Gurney eventually worked at another firm for twenty-four years, but even there "every time there was a promotion at work, somebody else always got it." When he asked why he had been passed over for the promotion, his employers would refer to his disability, saying, "Oh, you can't walk very good."[5] In the sixties and seventies institutional procedures and individual prejudices sometimes frustrated polio survivors who had sought an education in order to work and support themselves.

Paul Longmore, who is a professor of history at San Francisco State University, encountered another kind of hurdle in seeking a career in academe. Undergraduate and graduate professors discouraged him from pursuing his goal on the grounds that no college would hire him with his disability. Longmore, however, persisted. The California Department of Rehabilitation initially refused to support him in graduate school. Longmore continued his education with some private assistance and with what little he could save monthly from his Supplemental Security Income (SSI) checks. When he applied for fellowships he was rejected because, as they told him, "nobody is ever going to hire you as a teacher." After struggling for six years, Longmore finally received some assistance in 1977 when section 504 of the Rehabilitation Act of 1973 took effect. Because the university received federal funds, it was now obligated to provide him with assistance. In addition, the California Department of Rehabilitation began to provide some tuition money and, more important, funds for transcribing services. Finally, Longmore could do the work he wanted. As he looked to the future, another problem loomed. Because he received SSI, Longmore was eligible for health insurance through Medicaid and for in-home support services, which he needed to live independently. However, SSI regulations prohibited recipients from earning more than $300 a month for nine months. These regulations had been drafted when it was assumed that individuals with severe disabilities would not work and would always be dependent on government assistance. Longmore knew he could earn more than $300 a month, but he also knew he couldn't earn enough to pay for the assistance he needed to live on his own. He faced the very real prospect of having to turn down a job because he couldn't afford to lose the government assistance that made it possible for him to get the job in the first place. In 1988 Congress changed the regulations, allowing people to get a job and still maintain eligibility for a time. Finally, Longmore could search seriously for a teaching position. Since securing a position, Longmore has had a distinguished career as a biographer of George Washington, as a historian of disabilities, and as an advocate for individuals with disabilities.[6]

Other polio survivors remember fewer polio-related problems in their careers. Many of the thirty-five survivors whose oral histories were published in Edmund Sass's *Polio's Legacy* reported experiencing little or no discrimination during their careers. For example, Kay Brutger worked at factory jobs for most of her life, as well as in a bank and with a local government agency. After finishing graduate school, Edmund Sass worked as a school psychologist, and since 1977 he has taught at the College of St. Benedict in Minnesota. Len Jordan trained to be a printer with the assistance of the state of Minnesota and worked as a linotype operator, then had a career in graphic sales and ownership. After many years as a mother and homemaker, Mary Ann Hoffman took a job as coordinator of the Center for Independent Living in Menomonie, Wisconsin, where she trains peer advisors for others with disabilities. She has also become involved in the handicapped rights movement. Finally, Pat Zahler went to college, graduated, and was a social worker for fourteen years before taking five years off when her children were young. She has since returned to working in an elementary school and doesn't believe that polio has held her back.[7]

The very ordinariness and variety of the careers of polio survivors is significant. They were ordinary people living ordinary lives. If they succeeded in some measure they did not necessarily become role models for other polio survivors. Still, polio survivors in general expected that they would be able to fulfill their goals and to succeed in their careers, in finding a spouse, and in raising their children. In part, at least, their expectations were rooted in the story of President Franklin D. Roosevelt, perhaps the best-known polio survivor. From the 1930s onward, Roosevelt was held up as the role model for polio survivors. As Amy Fairchild has observed, "Roosevelt himself, journalists, and the National Foundation for Infantile Paralysis all helped create and promote a core polio narrative featuring FDR's triumph over disease and disability, which became a national myth." Many polio narratives testify to the power of Roosevelt's example in motivating individuals to confront and overcome obstacles. For example, Dorothea Nudelman recalls being inspired by a biography of FDR she received as a birthday present. As a young man in the rehabilitation hospital, Leonard Kriegel's daily battle was inspired and motivated by Roosevelt's example. Kriegel believed that "the promise of his victory was that I would win, too" and that FDR "was a great and mighty god. There was nothing he couldn't do." In addition, many of the polio survivors who wrote to

Roosevelt while he was president testified to his importance as a role model. However, Roosevelt was, at best, an imperfect role model for polio survivors. Lacking Roosevelt's financial resources and the assistance he commanded as president, few polio survivors could emulate what Hugh Gallagher has called Roosevelt's "splendid deception" of establishing and maintaining the illusion that he had completely recovered from the polio that had paralyzed his legs.[8]

While Roosevelt's story and the success stories of other polio survivors such as Olympic gold medalist Wilma Rudolph could inspire polio survivors, these heroic tales could also demoralize men and women whose impairments precluded running Olympic races or whose lack of wealth and social position closed off opportunities FDR enjoyed. Eventually, some polio survivors began to criticize the Roosevelt story and to critique its usefulness to them and to other individuals with disabilities. Using Roosevelt or other prominent and successful polio survivors as role models was a double-edged sword. Polio survivors Hugh Gallagher and Irving Zola ultimately realized that when individuals with disabilities commit too heavily to measuring their own success by the standards of role models they could set themselves up for disappointment and failure. Hugh Gallagher ultimately found that he was unable to emulate FDR's method of denial. While working on his study of Roosevelt and while experiencing the fatigue and weakness associated with post-polio syndrome, Gallagher concluded that Roosevelt "was Super Crip; I opted for human." Irving Zola, a medical sociologist who studied the experience of disability, argues that "in almost all the success stories that get to the public there is a dual message. The first one is very important—that just because we have polio, cancer, or multiple sclerosis, or have limited use of our eyes, ears, mouth, or limbs, our lives are *not* over. We can still learn, be happy, be lovers, spouses, parents, and even achieve great deeds." However, Zola came to "abhor" the second message. This was the belief that "if a Franklin Roosevelt and a Wilma Rudolph could *overcome* their handicaps so could and should all the disabled. And if we fail, it is our problem, our personality defect, our weakness."[9] The challenge was to balance inspiration with a realistic appraisal of what one could plausibly achieve given one's impairments.

A good job was one measure of success for midcentury Americans; marriage was another. "During the postwar period, marriage was seen as an essential ingredient for a full and happy life. Fewer than one American in ten believed that an unmarried person could be happy." The postwar American dream envisioned "successful breadwinners supporting attractive homemakers in affluent suburban homes." And these successful breadwinners and attractive homemakers desired healthy, happy children to complete the family. As Elaine Tyler May observed, "children provided tangible results of a successful marriage and family life; they gave evidence of responsibility, patriotism, and achievement." Most polio survivors, whether they married in the postwar era or were born during the baby boom years, joined the parade to the altar. Several surveys in the 1980s and 1990s revealed that nearly 90 percent of polio survivors eventually married.[10] In spite of the worries of many young polio survivors that their disabilities would keep them from dating, finding love, and eventually marrying, the statistical evidence and the testimony of the narratives suggests that most polio survivors who wanted to marry eventually did.

It is impossible to know how many of the polio survivors who avoided marriage did so because they were gay or lesbian. Only one polio narrative, Lorenzo Milam's *The Cripple Liberation Front Marching Band Blues*, is also a coming-out story. Milam seems to have been attracted to men from at least his late teens, but even he married and fathered a daughter. He admits that he married at least in part to "cure" him of "this boodle called Man-Love." When the cure didn't work, a divorce soon followed. Single again, Milam eventually took himself to Europe in 1960 in search of sex, love, and companionship.[11] Milam is surely representative of a larger group of gay or lesbian polio survivors, but it is not surprising that I have found only one such narrative, since homosexuality was even more deeply stigmatizing in these decades than disability.

Teenaged polio survivors, as we saw in chapter 7, had many anxieties about dating and finding someone to love them. Their disabilities set them apart and sometimes kept them from participating in athletics, going to dances, and joining in the other activities where boys met girls. In some cases, even where the physical impairment was slight, a fear of rejection kept polio survivors out of the dating game. However, as polio survivors grew out of adolescence they often found it easier to meet individuals for whom the physical impairment was no barrier to intimacy. Many polio narratives mention marriage and family as a matter of course and without elaboration. For example, Mary Ann Hoffman remembers that she met her husband while she worked in Des Moines, Iowa, and he was an intern in psychology: "After we were married, we moved to Tucson, Arizona, where he finished his doctorate. We had four children, so I got my wish of being a mother and a homemaker." Many survivors simply report "I am married and have a terrific wife and three wonderful children." Or "I led a very normal home and family life. I was married, had four children, and now have seven grandchildren. My wife died of cancer in 1985, and after being alone for 10 years, I am now planning to remarry." Women, as well as men, report their marriages very matter-of-factly. June Radosovich and her husband have "been married for 39 years and he's an angel to me. He always has been." And Millie Teders feels "fortunate" to be "able to live quite a normal life after all my early trauma. I'm married, and I have four children and eleven grandchildren."[12] Where polio had set them apart, their marriages and families affirmed polio survivors' place in American culture and society.

Still, when one was disabled, the process of taking those first steps toward dating, and the big step of getting engaged, were fraught with more than the usual anxiety. Arvid Schwartz's experience points to the challenges facing polio survivors. Schwartz met his future wife, Judy, while they were both working in St. Paul. Initially, Schwartz didn't "consider it 'dating,'" but they "were together more and more" and he soon began thinking, "Wow, I've finally got a girlfriend." They were engaged in 1960, married the following year, and eventually had four children. Schwartz articulated the thoughts that must have been in the minds of many polio survivors when he remembered that "back in those days, I guess I thought that 'crippled' people didn't usually get married. Though I knew I would be a good husband and father, I had to convince one other person of that." He was afraid that because his handicap "would require her to do some extra things," Judy would turn him down when he proposed. They discussed the "complications" that his disability caused, but decided they could deal with them. Schwarz still recalls the joy he felt when she said yes.[13]

In a few cases, polio survivors married individuals who had helped care for them in the days and months following their illness. Polio care involved close interaction between patient and nurse or therapist, and sometimes the ward relationships blossomed into something more intimate. Roger Winter had been dating a young woman while in college. Their relationship endured the early months of his recovery and rehabilitation, but she eventually ended it when it became clear that Winter was permanently paralyzed. Winter first met Theresa Drenth when she became his nurse at the rehabilitation hospital. They seemed to form a special bond from the beginning, but it took almost a year before their mutual fascination began to develop into a serious relationship. They conducted a "rather public" romance in the hospital. Theresa spent her off-duty time there with Winter, and "to get a little privacy we would go out for a 'walk' around the hospital, or up on the roof." They were married in October 1954, a little over two years after polio left Winter paralyzed from the neck down. They had a daughter three years later.[14]

Like Roger Winter, Arnold Beisser eventually married one of his caretakers, Rita, who had been one of his physical therapists. From the time she first appeared on the ward, Beisser had noticed her because she "stood out" among the physical therapists: "Slender and graceful, she perfectly filled out her starched white uniform." But she also "took her responsibilities very seriously and simply and purposefully went about her business." Despite the joking about sex, or lack of sex, on this all-male ward, Beisser recalls that at the time he "was both surprised and mistrustful of any evidence of interest in me by young women." He was wracked by "many self-doubts, and was so embarrassed about my body" that he feared "disclosing" his feelings. His relationships with women had become "rather superficial and impersonal." Although he found Rita attractive, he didn't have the nerve to let her know, even when she was friendly. In spite of their growing affection for one another, Beisser found he had to get over his feeling that polio had made him unattractive. Rita, however, saw his considerable physical problems as "minor inconveniences." While he was pessimistic about their relationship and about his ability to find work as a doctor, Rita was certain that things could work out. When Beisser was hired as a resident in psychiatry at a state hospital and was able to move out of the hospital, everything proved difficult, including finding acceptable attendants. The only relief, he remembers, came "on the weekends, when Rita came to visit. Everything suddenly turned easy then." They were soon "married by a judge one weekend, me in my reclining wheelchair, alternately lying flat and sitting up, feeling like the creature from outer space, and Rita in her usual radiant naturalness." For all his initial misgivings, Beisser gives Rita credit for making it possible for him "to live almost as if I were not paralyzed at all."[15]

Individuals who were already married when polio struck faced an entirely different set of problems from those whose illness had come earlier. The disease and the long period of convalescence that followed often tested the bonds of love and marriage. Sometimes those bonds were strengthened and the marriage survived; in other cases, the marriage could not stand the additional strain of dealing with a permanent disability, and it dissolved. Perhaps the most extended and most personal account of how polio affected a marriage is that of Louis and Dottie Sternburg, who had been married for several years when Lou was almost totally paralyzed by the disease. Their jointly written account of how they dealt with Lou's severe respirator-dependent paralysis, raised two children, found ways to support the family, and worked through the inevitable strains on their marriage suggests some of the ways in which polio and its attendant paralysis could affect a marriage.[16]

Louis Sternburg's polio in July 1955 forced a substantial reorientation in his marriage to Dottie. Until polio struck, he had been "in charge," but now everything depended on her. Dottie's first reaction was "disbelief. This couldn't be happening to us. This was the first crisis in our marriage. Up to then, everything had been beautiful." She was determined to preserve what she valued: "I had a wonderful husband whom I admired and adored. . . . I was damned if this virus was going to take my husband away from me. . . . If he died, I saw myself as a depressing young widow, with two small children and very little money." Dottie remembers being overwhelmed by all that needed doing to care for her three-year-old son David and fifteen-month-old daughter Susan, as well as for her husband. As she put it, "I did it because there was nothing else I could do." Dottie "plunged in and did first things first. Whoever seemed to need me the most got the attention. The house came last." Dottie was determined to maintain as much of a normal family life as possible. She "spent a lot of time thinking about the way I wanted our family to be seen by other people—our friends, the neighbors, the world we lived in." She recognized that she and Lou "would never live a normal life again," but she also wanted their children to "live like other children." [17]

The Sternburg's marriage had all the needs of most marriages. Lou Sternburg was able to revive his business selling labels for clothing, and thus provide for his family. The other thing that helped relieve his pain and boost his self-esteem was sex. Although privacy was lacking, since his bed was in the middle of the first floor of their home, the Sternburgs "managed to find again the satisfying sex life that had been one of my main reasons for wanting so desperately to get home." Lou viewed making love as a "reaffirmation of manhood, of life itself," and the best way for the two of them to express their love. [18]

In spite of their evident love for one another and Dottie's commitment to caring for Lou, assisting in their business, running the home, and taking charge of their growing children, the marriage had its tensions. As they portray it, much of the strain came from Lou's possessiveness regarding Dottie and his fears that his breathing equipment might fail. For nearly fifteen years he rarely left the house, and during most of that time he expected Dottie to be there when he wanted and needed her.

For this marriage to survive and for Dottie to continue to be Lou's main support and chief attendant, she needed to carve out time away from her family and he needed to let her go. Gradually, with the help of psychiatrist Ed Payne, Louis allowed his other attendants to do more, and "Dottie went out, at first for a short while in the daytime and then, when we both got up the courage, out to dinner in the evening." Since she had done no socializing on her own following their marriage, it took some time for her to feel comfortable going out alone. Because she was "lively and amusing," she soon had many invitations and "she forgot her shyness and began to enjoy herself." Ten years after Lou contracted polio, Dottie took her first vacation, a week-long visit to Florida with a friend. During this first separation, Lou was too fearful to stay at home with attendants, so he returned to the Mary MacArthur Respiratory Center while his wife was away. Dottie soon began to take longer and more frequent trips. She quickly saw the benefits of change: "Lou appreciates me more and I miss his companionship when I'm away and am reminded of what it means to me." Several years later Dottie needed surgery and spent a week in the hospital while Lou had to function without her and to rely on his attendants. Even after she returned home her physician restricted her physical activities for two months so that the attendants had to continue their primary role in Lou's care. She was in her midforties, and she realized she needed to change her "superwoman habits." As Dottie put it, Lou came to realize that "instead of loving him less, I would love him more if I had more freedom. This was my new beginning." [19] Although the circumstances of Lou's paralysis made this marriage unusual, it was also marked by many of the features of any marriage: love between the partners, good sexual relations, a willingness to trust the other and to let him or her find and enjoy a measure of independence. Polio complicated and circumscribed their lives, but it also provided a vehicle for them to eventually come to a deeper understanding and appreciation of one another.

Like Lou Sternburg, Kenneth Kingery was paralyzed from the neck down and required respiratory assistance. Kingery was thirty-three in 1952 when polio struck on his last day in the U.S. Air Force. Kingery had a wife, Fran, and three young children aged nine, five, and two, and was looking forward to civilian life. As with Dottie Sternburg, Fran Kingery became Ken's major emotional support and his sometime nurse during his long rehabilitation and after he returned home able to move only few muscles in his hand. After he passed through the acute phase of polio, Kingery shed "bitter tears" over all the "grief" he had caused his wife by getting sick. Now she would have "to lead two lives—one of fragments, tension, and austerity at the hospital; one of a lonely widow at home." He loved his wife more than ever: "It dawned on me that my feelings went far beyond being just used to, or devoted to, or loyal to my wife; I was crazy about her. How I longed to share our bed together again—to run my fingers through her soft smooth hair—to hold her cool young body in my arms." [20] While his physical recovery proceeded slowly, the Kingerys worked toward a new relationship that embraced those parts of their relationship that had sustained the marriage this far, but that also incorporated the changes brought by his paralysis and dependence.

For Kingery, as for Sternburg, physical intimacy was an important part of his relationship with his wife. On his first reunion with his family at the hospital while using a portable chest respirator, Kingery was able to spend a few minutes alone with his wife, who held his arm around her. As he recalled, "I nearly swooned with the sensation of silk and softness against my hand. Faint, exquisite stirrings . . . told me unmistakably I was still the man of the family." Later, on the evening of his first day back in their home, Kingery again felt physically attracted to his wife. Lying flat on his rocking bed, he "wanted desperately" to be with her: "Even though I couldn't hold her in my own arms, I wanted her to hold me—to press her full length against me—and to match the passion of my kisses. Was this asking too much? Can a girl come to a man who cannot come to her?" Unable to take his wife in his arms, "the magic moment was over, the spell was broken. Every-night conversation resumed." [21]

Kingery's utter dependence on his wife posed a major challenge to their relationship. Fran was determined to do everything for her husband. She "took on the odious chore of doing personal things" he would ordinarily have done himself. This, as Kingery put it, "took some getting used to." To be dependent in the hospital was one thing, but in his own home he was "supposed to be the man of the house. . . . Head of the family. Tower of protecting strength." Kingery's dependence on his wife changed their relationship. He had "no authority, no initiative, no confidence at all," and he had to ask Fran for everything. He wondered if their "once-mellow love had been taken from us by that sinister virus called polio." When he questioned his wife about her feelings, she replied that things were "just not the same now," and she admitted that perhaps she had changed as a result. Kingery concluded that the situation had become "all too clear: paralysis meant loss of initiative, meant loss of sex appeal, meant loss of the normal life I'd lived for." Still, he could understand her point of view. She had all the "tension" and "tedium" of caring for a "total invalid." With "a husband's help subtracted, and a lot of effort added" perhaps there wasn't "any room for romance." [22]

One night, following a relapse of respiratory problems necessitating a return to the iron lung, Kingery came to a new understanding regarding the love of husband and wife. As a worried Fran stood next to his iron lung while he struggled to clear his congested lungs, Kingery recognized the love in her "worried gaze. Here lay love far deeper than the passion of youth—love that dwarfed mere sex by its gentle giving, its total understanding. Here was the greatest power. Love was the key." He concluded, "life would always be worth living if there were a special someone to share my life—a mate to share the love I had to give." Kingery survived this crisis, and he gradually adjusted to the reality that he could no longer "hope for a quick, or even gradual recovery." As he became less demanding, and began "independently answering letters or reading for hours at a time, with little to bother her," Fran "smiled more easily, relaxed more often." And gradually, "a narrow rivulet of the broad, mellow old affection began flowing back" into their relationship. Even Fran noticed that they "never seem to get tired of each other." Kingery acknowledged that "we might never achieve the same sort of bliss we'd known before the polio virus wrecked a happy marriage, but I would continue to pray. Perhaps the desired things weren't the most important. At least now, again, we were sharing each other's thoughts, re-discovering old depths of love and affection between us."[23] Here, as with the Sternburgs, polio had significantly altered the marital relationship in ways that neither anticipated. The Kingery's marriage proved resilient until his death in 1964 shortly before his autobiography was published.

It did not happen often, but occasionally both husband and wife were stricken with polio. In these cases, the couple faced significant challenges in meeting all the demands upon them. For example, both Charles and Ann McLaughlin caught polio in July 1955, apparently from their nine-month-old son who had "a mild case with no aftereffects." Both of them, however, were much more severely impaired by the disease. Ann had bulbar polio, which affected her ability to swallow and speak; Charles had spinal polio that paralyzed his legs. During the long months when both were in the hospital, Charles's mother and a nurse cared for their son, John. Once Ann had recovered sufficiently to use a wheelchair, she spent considerable time in Charles's room. Ann was able to leave the hospital before her husband, and "the first weeks living outside the hospital, playing with Johnny, taking him for walks in the morning, napping, and going to the hospital to eat my picnic supper with Charlie were full of excitement." She also found a first-floor apartment that could be made accessible for both. In May 1956, some ten months after polio struck, all of them moved to the new apartment, along with the babysitter nurse who had taken care of Johnny. Both McLaughlins went on to successful careers as college professors. Looking back from the perspective of forty years, Ann McLaughlin remembers how they sometimes speculated "about how much easier it would have been if only one of us had developed polio, for there have been times when our combined disabilities have limited us severely."

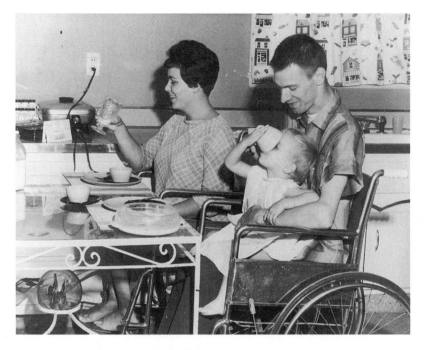

FIG. 20. Nancy and Lloyd Burkhardt at home with daughter Mindy. Both parents used wheelchairs. 1961.

However, the experience "bound us together as well and increased our understanding for each other." She concludes "there is nothing heroic about a person who had polio, nor about a couple that contracts it simultaneously. Polio," she notes, "creates limitations and a lot of tedious tasks." [24]

Unlike the McLaughlins, Bonnie and George Bonham had had polio as children many years before they married. When they announced their engagement, they received mixed reactions from family and friends. Most were supportive, but others questioned how they "would ever get along." There would undoubtedly be complications, but, as Bonnie wrote, "with our love to bind us we could certainly take care of each other." When they had a son and then three years later a daughter, family and friends again wondered how they would manage. One of the first challenges was how they would carry the children. George used crutches to walk, while Bonnie walked unassisted, but could not carry anything heavy, because it took everything she had to balance herself. They ultimately settled on using a portable crib to move the children

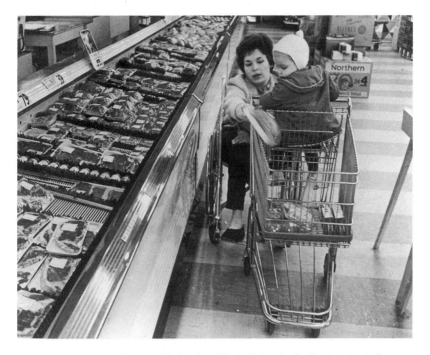

FIG. 21. Nancy Burkhardt, with daughter Mindy, doing the family shopping in her wheelchair. 1961.

around, and when George began using a wheelchair following a hip-breaking fall, he often carried the children on his lap.[25]

The Bonhams found that despite their desire to be independent, they also became adept at accepting assistance. George worked as a dental technician from a laboratory in their home, and Bonnie was his assistant. As they raised their two children they discovered that "his strong arms compensated for my weak ones." She could push the stroller, and he could lift it in and out of the trunk. While they had worked out how to feed, change, dress, and play with their babies, they did not feel safe bathing them. Fortunately, a grandmotherly neighbor volunteered to give the children their daily bath. Bonnie and George also learned to trust their young children not to wander away from their parents on outings. For Bonnie, what made it all work was "a net to support us if we falter—a net woven with love."[26]

In the case of failed marriages among polio survivors it is not always possible to tell whether the spouse became unwilling or unable to continue in a

relationship so significantly changed, or whether the disease simply exacerbated preexisting tensions and problems. In some narratives, however, the
spouse with polio believed that the disease had broken up the family. Louise
Lake, for instance, had polio in 1945 while living in St. Louis while her husband was in the military. However, he seems to have played no role in her recovery, for although she mentions her young daughter and other family and
friends, she almost never mentions her apparently absent husband. Then,
some four and a half years after the onset of Lake's polio, her husband sought
a divorce.[27] Lake went on to a successful career and to raise her daughter by
herself. Since she was determined not to dwell on her "heartaches," it is impossible to tell what role polio played in the breakup, but Lake certainly believed it was the crucial element.

Jane Needham's husband, Jim, supported her through the acute illness and
recovery. She had married this "startlingly handsome" military officer in 1943.
When she embraced her new husband after their wedding, she was convinced
they would live "happily forever and ever." But polio intervened, and "forever"
lasted "six years, two months, and twenty-seven days." In the years that followed their marriage the Needhams had three children, two girls and a boy.
Needham acquired polio while on a family vacation at Lake Tahoe in July 1949.
Polio left her totally paralyzed and respirator-dependent. Jim was supportive
during the acute phase and by her side as she began her long recuperation.
Needham had hoped Jim would fight for her to be released, even though she
still needed an iron lung: "Jim could say he needed me, that the children
needed me. Surely a wife and mother in an iron lung was better than no wife
and mother at all." Jim, however, had other ideas. Without consulting his
wife, he had placed the three children in foster care. His business had soured,
he was having trouble making payments on their house, and he thought the
foster mother, who was a family friend, could better care for the children.
Soon, Jane moved to the County Hospital because her condition required custodial care, and her family could no longer pay to keep her at Children's Hospital in San Francisco.[28]

Following the move to the County Hospital, Jane saw her children more frequently, but they often came with family friends rather than with their father.
She recalled that "the breach between us widened. Jim came rarely and when
he did we quarreled, mostly about the children." Gradually, Jane realized that
Jim had ceased to love her, and she sensed that he wanted his freedom. She
soon learned of her husband's girlfriend. Jim finally told her that he wanted a
divorce and custody of their three children. Needham tried to understand his

point of view. He was "a young and virile male" and "life is for the living." Still, she believed that if the situation had been reversed, had Jim been in an iron lung, she "could not have pulled out." Jane then concentrated on getting out of the County Hospital into a home of her own and gaining custody of her children. Jim's girlfriend put Needham in "a very strong bargaining position. He wanted her, I wanted the children. Very well, we'd trade. A divorce for their custody." Friends found her a house, and the doctors were eventually persuaded that she could live outside the hospital. Finally, after more than five years in hospitals, Needham moved into her new house with her children. Three days later in a court session held in her living room, she was granted a divorce and custody of Ann, Susan, and Craig. Needham admitted that she and Jim had "differed on the big things *and* the little things" even before polio entered their lives.[29] Perhaps the marriage would have been stormy in any case, but polio clearly came between Jane and Jim.

Not all of the marriages of polio survivors that ended in divorce had polio as the cause of the dissolution. The divorce rate in the last half of the twentieth century was high, and the marriages of polio survivors ended for many different reasons. Polio in one or both spouses did not by itself guarantee either marital success or failure. For example, Don Kirkendall's first marriage, to a waitress in a favorite restaurant, lasted two and a half months. His second marriage, to a woman who ran a restaurant, lasted nine months. After his second marriage, especially, Kirkendall asked himself whether his failures in marriage were due to the fact that he "moved on wheels." He decided he could not use his paralyzed legs as an excuse, but he still wondered why his marriages had failed. He met his third wife, Mary Ann, when he hired her to help with his business. Soon a business relationship turned into a social one. Mary Ann was divorced with two children, and when Kirkendall proposed, she said yes. Before long they added a child of their own, and unlike his first two marriages, this one lasted.[30]

In her narrative, Mary Grimley Mason, whose legs were affected by polio, describes both her marriage to Herb Mason and its long breakup. After they were introduced by friends in Chicago, their relationship strengthened in Cambridge, Massachusetts, where both attended graduate school. Mason recalled that as "we became closer, I became less and less conscious of my disability. It did not seem to play a part in our relationship." Herb was aware of her disability, because he opened doors and carried heavy packages, but they did not talk about it. Mason wonders whether that was a mistake, but it helped her feel like everyone else, and that was what she wanted at the time. They were married in September 1954. By marrying Herb, Mason had "achieved one agenda that had driven my life unconsciously." She "had done what my sisters and many of my friends and most 'normal women' did." She had "found an eligible, handsome man and married in my twenties" and prepared to live "out the story of a traditional woman of the 1950s."[31]

As part of that tradition, the Masons had three children. Early in her marriage Mason tried to deny her disability and she asked for no special accommodations other than a hand-controlled car. She "insisted on acting as an able-bodied wife in a traditional marriage," and Herb acquiesced. Later, as her strength waned, probably from post-polio syndrome, the balance of their marriage changed. Their marriage also changed in the 1970s as Herb's career took priority over family life, and Mason "felt the strain of a loss of sharing and intimacy that had been so much a part of our relationship." In the mid-1970s Herb began the first of a series of affairs, many of them with his students. After his first affair ended, Herb made an effort to keep the family together, but the marriage became more and more difficult for Mason, until 1979, when "Herb walked out peremptorily and permanently."[32] Although Mason does not directly address the question of what role her disability had in the dissolution of her marriage, she implies that it was an unspoken factor from the very beginning and that her post-polio syndrome contributed to the widening rift between Herb and her. Still there were other factors in this marriage—Herb's devout Catholicism, his immersion in his work to the neglect of his family, and, of course, his affairs—that certainly contributed their part in the disintegration of this marriage. Mason's marriage followed the arc of so many marriages of the fifties—marriage, children, divorce—so it is hard to know precisely what role her disability played.

Although most polio survivors who wanted romantic relationships and marriage were successful, some 10 percent of them never married. There are no doubt many reasons for their failure to marry. Whether their disability was what kept them from marrying is difficult to ascertain. As we have seen above, even very severe disabilities did not necessarily bar one from developing romantic attachments and eventually marrying. Polio survivors who did not marry could react quite differently to their lack of success in forming intimate romantic relationships. Both Regina Woods and Mark O'Brien were almost totally paralyzed and dependent on respirator assistance from the time of their illness when she was thirteen and he was six. Woods, in her memoir, makes no direct mention of a desire for romantic relationships or disappointment in her failure to marry. She writes that she never had a "grand design" for her life or dreams of what might have been had she not had polio. When she had polio, she "had not even visualized a life in which I appeared as an adult." She regards herself as "fortunate not to have had dreams that died along with my nerve cells." Woods writes that after polio "the big dreams simply did not come to mind." She was content to be "an eternal kid," living and enjoying life day to day, without lamenting dreams lost.[33]

Mark O'Brien, however, is much more open about his feelings. In an essay reflecting on the experience, O'Brien explores his complicated feelings about sex, love, disability, and his frustrating failure to form lasting romantic attachments in spite of having numerous close female friends. Although he had normal sexual feelings, when they occurred he felt "accused and guilty." Sex had been a taboo subject in his Irish Catholic family; it simply wasn't discussed. Into his thirties he remained embarrassed by his sexuality, especially when he became aroused during baths. Still, O'Brien "wanted to be loved . . . wanted to be held, caressed and valued," but his "self-hatred and fear were too intense." He had previously fallen in love with several people, male and female, and had waited in vain for them to initiate a date or to seduce him. In the mid-1980s he began discussing with his therapist the possibility of seeing a sex surrogate. After a long period of anxiety about what his parents would think, what God would think, what his friends would think, O'Brien called the surrogate. Cheryl was not repelled when she saw his twisted and shrunken body, and over the course of three meetings she initiated O'Brien into sexual play and intercourse.[34]

Working with Cheryl, however, didn't substantially change O'Brien's life. He was still isolated, in part because polio forced him to spend most of his time in the iron lung and in part because of his personality, which he described as "low-key, withdrawn, and cerebral." He wonders whether seeing Cheryl was worth it in terms of "hopes raised and never fulfilled." He wonders, too, if he had had intensive psychotherapy earlier in his life whether he would have been able to participate in "the more familiar pattern of flirting, dating, and making out which seems so common among people who have been disabled during or after adolescence." He has no desire to engage a prostitute, in part because that arrangement is too much like the "impersonal, professional service" he already gets from nurses and attendants. He concludes the essay by asking just what it is that he wants from a romantic relationship. Is it "someone who likes me and loves me and who will promise to protect me from all the self-hating parts of myself?" Or is it "an all-purpose lover-mommy-attendant to care for all my physical and emotional needs?" Or perhaps it is "a shapely savior" to rescue him from the "horror" imposed on him and by him. He ends where he began. He acknowledges wonderful female friendships, but laments that none of these women have expressed any romantic interest in him. His project of pursuing women appears "doomed." And his "desire to love and be loved sexually is equaled by my isolation and my fear of breaking out of it."[35]

O'Brien is hardly a typical polio survivor in terms of the severity of his disability, his failure to form lasting romantic and sexual relationships, or his willingness to write explicitly of his attempts to become a sexually active adult. However, several of O'Brien's observations apply not only to his rather extreme position but to the experience of polio survivors more generally. In order to be seen as potential romantic and sexual partners, polio survivors first had to see themselves in such terms. Their physical impairments and their psychological and emotional responses to the illness, recuperation, and their crippled bodies sometimes formed barriers to romantic love and sexual intimacy. Whether polio left you with paralyzed legs, a withered arm or leg, or a twisted torso, bodies marked by polio did not conform to the beauty standards of late twentieth-century America. Polio, because it often impaired mobility, sometimes encouraged passivity in the men and women who survived. Limited mobility often meant that polio survivors found it difficult to do the many things that counted as dating among young men and women. In addition, there was the always-present fear of rejection—rejection because your body did not conform to some ideal or because you could not do the things friends and lovers customarily do. Clearly, given the high marriage rate among polio survivors, most of them overcame these psychological and emotional barriers to intimacy and found lovers and spouses. But O'Brien forcefully reminds us of disability's power to complicate and frustrate the polio survivors' search for fulfilling and romantic sexual intimacy.

Children of parents with polio were also affected by the disease. They were aware from an early age that their mothers or fathers were in some sense different. Perhaps they limped or wore a brace, or used a wheelchair for mobility, or even lived on a rocking bed or in an iron lung. Children, however, have a tremendous capacity to accept the given as the norm, and regardless of any disability, to respond as children do to parental love and support. With the exceptions of Kathryn Black and Louis Sternburg, children in these narratives generally appear through the voice of the memoirist rather than in their own voices. Polio survivors recall that their children accepted their disabilities as natural and that having parents with disabilities taught these children to accept other individuals with disabilities. Robert Gurney, for example, doesn't believe that his disability affected his relationship with his wife and children. As an example, he recounts his young daughter's reply when her teacher said "Your dad is Bob Gurney. He's the one who is handicapped." His daughter replied, "No he's not. He's my daddy!" Richard Owen, who became a physician, speculated on the impact his polio and disability had on his three children. He noted that his daughter "married one of the spinal-cord-injured fellows on my wheelchair basketball team, and they have been terribly happy." Owen believes that watching him and his wife deal with his disability helped his daughter be "very sensitive to accessibility and mobility needs." His oldest son is a psychiatrist, and Owen thinks that his own friendships with disabled people helped his son in medical school. Finally, his youngest son is the ball boy on the wheelchair basketball team, and being around people with a variety of disabilities has "made him very accepting of a variety of people."[36]

Louis Sternburg's narrative is primarily in his voice, but his wife, Dottie, and his two children, David and Susan, speak in their own voices in several sections of the book. David's and Susan's observations suggest that even when children accept a parent's disability there are difficulties and challenges to negotiate. Only two when his father contracted polio, David doesn't have any memories of his father before that. As a result, having a father who lived on a rocking bed "was normal." Over the years David and his father "formed a much closer bond than most sons and fathers." David tried to include his father as much as possible, such as accepting Louis's sideline advice on throwing and batting a ball. David doesn't remember resenting his mother's focus on taking care of her husband, which sometimes meant that the children's needs and desires took second place. From an early age, David was willing to help his father and to relieve his mother. Still, he doesn't agree with the people who have felt sorry for him. Instead, he believes he had an "amazing man" for a father. Susie's memories of her childhood are somewhat different from those of her older brother. When she was small she "wasn't aware that there was any difference between us and everybody else." Susie, however, was more reluctant to bring friends home, especially after one friend was "so scared by the bed that she ran out of the room and down the street." Like her brother, Susie doesn't resent the time her mother spends on her father. "It had always been like that." Even at an early age she recognized that the family was "working together as a team to overcome what had happened" to her father. Like David, she acknowledges that her parents tried to raise them as "normal children" and they encouraged her to "be independent."[37]

As they grew older and entered adolescence, both David and Susan found that their relationships with their parents became more complicated, and in the case of Susan especially, more difficult. As Sternburg writes, "we had wanted our children to grow up as normally as possible, and now we had a normal teenage household, where the only thing the parents could be sure of was that everything they did was wrong." David recalls that he never rebelled, because, as he put it, "I was still too worried about pleasing my parents, my mother because she could make your life hell if you didn't, and my father because he needed it." As he got older, his caring for his father steadily increased to the point where he was handling such things as bedpans. At one point David moved to California to work, but he eventually returned to Boston because he observed problems developing in his parents' relationship. The years had taken a toll, and he believed his presence could help defuse the tension. As he got older David became the one his father talks to in his "down moments." While David sees his childhood in a positive light, as an adult beginning to establish himself in his career he views the help he provides as more of a sacrifice. David knows that if his mother is ill, or unable to care for her husband, she would count on him to drop everything and help out, at least temporarily.[38]

Susie's adolescence was more troubled than David's, and she acknowledges that her father's and the family's situation was at the root of her rebellion. By the time she was a teenager she had "stopped accepting the situation and thinking it was normal." Still, she "grew up, and they grew up, and we've all changed." Since she broke away from her family she "can look back and love them as the people they are, without feeling obligations or guilt."[39]

All four Sternburgs described their situation as trying to live a normal life under rather extraordinary circumstances. What they meant by "normal" was more than establishing a façade of suburban, fifties normality, which was impossible given the family's situation. "Normal" in this context meant that Lou would be a full participant in the life of the family, earning an income, participating in decision-making, teaching his son to play ball, and continuing to be the head of the household. Dottie had always expected to be an at-home mother taking care of her children and her husband. After polio struck, her responsibilities as her husband's chief caregiver were a vastly expanded version of that role. In addition, as her son suggested, she had to take on some of the burdens of "the man of the house."[40] When David and Susie speak of having a "normal childhood" they mean that they had two parents who loved them and provided for them, that they were encouraged to bring friends home and to get involved in a whole range of activities inside and outside of school, and that they felt free to develop independence and even go through a typical teenaged rebellion. Being normal in this case didn't mean denying or minimizing Lou's disability, but rather accepting it as a fact that needed attention and then getting on with all the busyness of life that any family experiences. That said, the passages in David's and Susie's voices reveal some of the tension, anxiety, and strain of growing up with a severely disabled parent.

Kathryn Black's book about her mother's polio and the impact that it had on her family powerfully explores how the disease could destroy a family. Like Louis Sternburg, Virginia Black was completely paralyzed and dependent on a respirator or a rocking bed to breathe. But whereas the Sternburgs survived as a functioning family, Virginia's polio began the slow dissolution of her family. Even more than thirty years later, Kathryn Black can "hardly bear to contemplate the heartbreak" she suffered as a four-year-old when her mother disappeared. She remembers feeling guilty, as if she "had done something to send her away." She felt "naked, vulnerable, and afraid" without her mother's protection. During that first summer with her mother "submerged in hospital life," Kathryn and Kenny, "confused and lonely, limped through the summer in the care of our grandparents."[41]

In looking into the early years of her parents' life together, Black discovered a "passionate marriage with emotions running high," but also a marriage that was "rocky" from the outset, which her father attributed to "too much poverty and too different personalities." During the long months that Virginia Black was in the Northwest Respirator Center in Seattle, her two young children in Boulder wrote her occasional letters. In June 1955, a year after contracting polio, Virginia Black was discharged from the respiratory center and the air force flew her home to Denver. After greeting the plane that brought her mother to Denver, Kathryn and Kenny saw their mother in an iron lung once during the week she was in the hospital. Once acclimated to the altitude, Virginia Black was moved to a rented house near her parents and installed on her rocking bed.[42]

When she reconstructed the summer of 1955 from memory, Kathryn Black recalls that "those summer months seemed tranquil" because her mother was back. She wasn't "impressed by the strangeness of our family life, with Mother paralyzed in the dining room and Dad nowhere in sight." What did impress her was that her mother was "*there* again, talking to me and listening to me." She doesn't remember questioning "the circumstances. It was enough that Mother had come back, however pale and small and unmoving she was in a giant bed that did move." Black's father eventually returned from Seattle, but as we saw earlier, never really reestablished his place at the head of the family. Kathryn was vaguely aware of how "powerful emotion eddied around us: grief, sadness, fear." On an April morning in 1956 while Kathryn and Ken were at school, Virginia Black died. Following the funeral, Black's father disappeared and she and her brother moved to their grandparents' home nearby. They became, "in deed, if not in fact," orphans. Kathryn and Ken were raised by their grandparents with their mother as a kind of unmentioned shadow. Kathryn remembers that in "the first years, in the dark, alone," she permitted herself to miss her mother. Gradually, Kathryn and her brother "fashioned a façade." For example, they called their grandmother "Mom." She remembers that her life appeared normal to anyone unaware of what had happened. Gradually she "became so accustomed to never speaking of Mother that I lost sight of the oddness of being reared by grandparents." She rarely spoke of her situation to anyone inside or outside the family. "And so," she painfully recalled, "I became an adult who had no name for my mother."[43]

In writing her book Black gained some perspective on her own difficult encounter with the disease. She acknowledges that the "silences of my father and grandparents compounded the loss of our mother for my brother and me," but her discoveries also helped her "begin to stop blaming them and to feel compassion for the losses they, too, suffered." Each member of her family knew his or her "own pain beyond measure." It was "pointless to try to decide whether the agony of a child who loses her mother is worse than the devastation of a mother who loses her child."[44] Black's story and the stories of those other spouses and children who lived with polio forcefully remind us that polio not only changed the lives of those who had the illness, it also affected the lives of all the family and friends who came in contact with the disease.

While dedicated families often cared for severely disabled polio survivors, as time passed polio survivors sometimes had to take on the role of caregiver. Martha Mason provides a striking account of what can happen when an aging parent can no longer care for a severely disabled child. Martha and her brother Gaston both had polio in 1948 when she was ten and he was thirteen. Gaston died shortly after being admitted to the hospital, and Martha was left totally paralyzed and dependent on an iron lung except for brief periods of free breathing. Following rehabilitation, the doctor's prognosis was that Martha would not live long, and her parents decided to bring her home in her iron lung and to provide her care for however long she lived. Mason lived well beyond the physician's gloomy prognosis, eventually earning a college degree from Wake Forest, where she graduated first in her class and was elected to Phi Beta Kappa. Her parents provided excellent care, but eventually their health became an issue. Her father had a severe heart attack in 1961 that limited his ability to help in her care. Until his death in 1977, Mason's mother had to care for both her daughter and her husband. Her mother managed with the aid of paid attendants until a series of strokes in 1993. Mason then had to begin to manage her mother's care as well her own, and from an iron lung. It was not always easy, especially when her mother began experiencing episodes of dementia or attendants were discovered smoking marijuana or stealing from the grocery money. But eventually reliable aides were hired and Mason supervised her mother's care until she died in 1998. Since then, she has had only her own care to organize.[45]

Almost from the beginning of their rehabilitation polio survivors were encouraged by health professionals, families, and the National Foundation for Infantile Paralysis to believe that they could surmount the disease and resume a normal life. Most polio survivors wanted nothing more than to complete their educations, get good jobs, marry and have children, and generally participate in American life and culture as though they had never had the disease. This "polio tradition," as the anthropologists Jessica Scheer and Mark Luborsky have argued, is "a condensation of some core American values learned during the rehabilitation and recovery phase and reinforced in the broad context of American values." Many polio survivors used the "work ethic to minimize physical limitations" and as "one passage to normalization." They perceived themselves not as handicapped, but as "simply unable to perform certain functions." In addition, many polio survivors were encouraged "to forget their polio and put the past behind them." Scheer and Luborsky note that these behaviors had "survival value, especially during the first years of being disabled," but that they could also become psychologically and physically costly during a lifetime of living with polio.[46]

Lauro Halstead and Carol Gill reinforce Scheer and Luborsky's arguments from the dual perspective of health professionals who have treated individuals with post-polio syndrome and as polio survivors themselves. Lauro Halstead directs the Post-Polio Program at the National Rehabilitation Hospital in Washington, D.C. He writes that "virtually every polio survivor" he has met has told a story of how "individual will power" enabled him or her to achieve "a full and productive life." This achievement was often "made possible by denying our disability and the reality of what was lost and the life that might have been." Halstead acknowledges that "we knew we weren't physically normal, but, if we thought about it at all, we considered ourselves inconvenienced, not disabled." Carol Gill, a clinical psychologist who has treated polio survivors, has written that despite the fact that "three of my limbs were paretic, my scoliosis was severe, and I practically lived in heavy leg braces, no one in my family ever uttered a word suggesting I had a disability. Polio was a 'sickness' and I was 'getting well.'" She was brought up to believe that "nothing lay beyond my abilities if I worked hard enough. I learned to see myself not as disabled but as a regular child challenged and inconvenienced by some obstacles to surmount." Later, as a clinical psychologist working with post-polio clients, she realized "how common it was for polio survivors to view themselves as different from others with disabilities." Gill argues that polio survivors from very early in their recovery saw "hope in our family's, the health professionals', and teachers' eyes that we would never be like the pitiful dependent outcasts who were truly crippled. We learned what we had to do to be valid human beings, namely, overcome our weaknesses and refuse to be disabled."[47] For polio survivors, the attitude that Gill describes was functional as they moved from the rehabilitation facility to home and from home to school, work, marriage, and parenthood. Many polio survivors expected to be able to do all that their able-bodied family and friends did, and by pushing themselves, and sometimes society, a high percentage succeeded.

By seeing themselves as "challenged and inconvenienced" rather than as crippled or disabled, polio survivors expected to resume a normal life following their recovery. "Normal" in this context meant doing what their able-bodied family and friends did in terms of education, career, and marriage. Polio survivors wanted nothing so much as to fit into American culture and society as full participants in spite of whatever physical impairments they might have. Lennard Davis has recently argued that the notion of "normality" as applied to bodies and people is a nineteenth-century invention that poses significant problems for people with disabilities. Unlike the earlier concept of the "ideal," which by definition no one can attain, the "normal" forces individuals to conform to cultural and social standards or risk marginalization and ostracism. As Davis writes, "We live in a world of norms. . . . There is probably no area of contemporary life in which some idea of a norm, mean, or average has not been calculated." Davis argues that "the concept of the norm, unlike that of an ideal, implies that the majority of the population must or should somehow be part of the norm." Thus, in any "society where the concept of the norm is operative, . . . people with disabilities will be thought of as deviants."[48]

By and large, however, polio survivors were neither marginalized nor ostracized, although the costs of their success were sometimes high both physically and emotionally. Although the repression and denial undoubtedly helped polio survivors succeed in so many areas of a normal life for so many years, just as the body wore out after decades of struggle, these defenses could not always be maintained, especially when the new muscle weaknesses, pain, fatigue, and increased impairment of post-polio syndrome appeared decades after they thought they had beaten polio. Post-polio syndrome thus forced a new and unwelcome reckoning with both the physical and the psychological consequences of living with polio.

| 9 |

An Old Foe Returns: Post-Polio Syndrome

A S THEY ENTERED MIDDLE AGE, most polio survivors of the midcentury epidemic years believed that they had put polio behind them. They had worked hard to achieve physical recovery, they still believed that with suffi-cient willpower and hard work they could accomplish anything they wanted, and they had finished their educations, entered careers, married, and had fam-ilies. Polio survivors were convinced that they had beaten polio and they had little more to fear from the disease or its aftereffects. It was with some sur-prise, then, that twenty to thirty years after the initial onset of the disease, po-lio survivors began to experience increased muscle weakness and pain, debili-tating fatigue, more frequent falls, and an inability to do things they had once done. Doctors initially had few explanations to offer for these unexpected de-velopments: perhaps age was catching up with them, perhaps it was somehow related to polio, perhaps it was all in their heads. Neither polio survivors nor physicians initially realized that these were all symptoms of what would soon come to be called post-polio syndrome (PPS). The disease they thought they had conquered had at least one more surprise for polio survivors.

Many polio survivors found the symptoms of post-polio syndrome particu-larly difficult to deal with. For survivors who had pushed their bodies and themselves to recover from and compensate for paralysis, the new weakness, fatigue, and pain often conjured up frightening images from their past. Men and women who had considered themselves "inconvenienced" by their impair-ments now faced the prospect of being newly disabled. As the symptoms of post-polio increased, polio survivors often faced the challenge of returning to using assistive devices they had so gladly discarded decades previously. Those who had gotten out of braces, or given up using canes or crutches, discovered that they needed them once again. Individuals who had risen out of their wheelchairs to walk found they needed the wheelchair once again to travel any distance, and then, perhaps, all the time. And those who had used manual wheelchairs for decades found their arms would no longer propel them, forcing them to make the sometimes difficult transition to electric wheelchairs or scooters.

While the physical changes were difficult enough to accept, many polio survivors experienced at the same time a profound sense of failure and defeat. The hard lessons learned in the rehabilitation hospitals, the cultural expectations of post-World War II America, and the injunctions of parents, physicians, therapists, and teachers to succeed at all costs meant that it was difficult for polio survivors to slow down, to conserve energy and muscle strength, to seek assistance, and to rely on assistive technology for support. For some polio survivors this new disability has given rise to full-blown psychological depression. Whether mild or severe, the emotional and psychological responses to the physical symptoms of post-polio syndrome seem rooted in the repression and denial of the disease and disability that allowed polio survivors to function so successfully in the world of the able-bodied. But what had once been functional was functional no more, and many survivors not only had to contend with new physical limitations they also had to develop a new emotional and psychological response to the disease that had shaped their lives for so long.

While the onset of post-polio symptoms in a large population of polio survivors caught both survivors and the medical profession by surprise, the fact that individuals who had had polio could experience late effects had been noted in the medical literature as early as the 1870s. Dr. David Wiechers's search of the medical literature discovered what was "probably the first explanation for the late effects of polio," offered by the great French neurologist Jean Martin Charcot in 1875. Several other reports in the French medical literature of similar cases followed this initial description. The first reports in the German literature appeared in 1879 and in English in 1899. By the end of the nineteenth century some twenty medical reports had drawn a connection between an initial case of poliomyelitis and the subsequent development of new symptoms of fatigue, weakness, and pain. These early reports of post-polio-like conditions were based on relatively few cases, in part because in the late nineteenth century polio had only begun to take on the epidemic form that would dominate the first half of the twentieth century.[1]

Medical reports of the late effects of polio appeared occasionally in the early twentieth century. Although they described similar symptoms among the individuals in their studies, the physicians gave these symptoms different names reflecting their theories of causation. In addition, it was not always clear that polio, rather than some other paralytic disease, had given rise to the new symptoms. Furthermore, a lack of long-term follow-up meant that ultimate outcomes were not recorded. By the 1960s and 1970s, reports of the late effects of polio began to appear with more frequency. By the early to mid-1970s, Wiechers found an emerging "agreement about an association between the late onset of progressive muscle weakness and a previous attack of poliomyelitis." In addition, it appeared that "this late-onset weakness generally occurred 30 to 40 years post-poliomyelitis," although cases were seen as early as five to ten years after the acute disease and as late as seventy to seventy-five years. Medical studies of the phenomenon increased in the late 1970s and the term "post-polio syndrome" began to be used to describe "those conditions that are the direct effects of progressive muscle weakness or the indirect result of the late effects of polio."[2]

Given the increasing number of polio victims in the twentieth century and the significant expansion of polio research undertaken in the United States and Europe, it is surprising that so few studies of the late effects of polio were undertaken before the 1970s and 1980s. The early epidemics, and especially the 1916 epidemic in New York City and the northeastern states which produced over 27,000 diagnosed cases of polio, resulted in many survivors who were probably experiencing significant problems by the 1930s and 1940s.[3] I suspect that there were several reasons for the paucity of studies before the 1970s. First, scientific and medical attention was rightly focused on the significant challenges of finding the cause of this newly epidemic disease and discovering how to prevent it.[4] Isolated reports of late effects attributed to the disease had a much lower priority in polio research when the acute disease still posed a major threat and was not fully understood. Second, given the increasing number of polio survivors who needed extensive rehabilitation immediately following the acute disease, doctors, nurses, and therapists again rightly focused their attention on developing methods of physical therapy to restore muscle strength and function, and devising surgical techniques and assistive devices to compensate for what the virus had destroyed. Again, I suspect that the significantly smaller number of older survivors reporting new difficulties simply didn't appear to be a problem when set against the thousands of new cases that needed attention every year. While the polio epidemics raged, the late effects experienced by polio survivors were obscured.

There are three reasons why the late effects of polio emerged in the late 1970s as a growing problem for polio survivors and for the medical profession. First, with the waning of the epidemics in the 1960s as a result of the success of the Salk and Sabin vaccines, there were few new polio cases every year. As late as 1960, there were still more than 2,500 paralytic cases a year, whereas by the late seventies and early eighties there were generally fewer than 10 a year. The increasing number of polio survivors reporting new symptoms no longer had to compete for attention with thousands of new acute polio cases per year. Second, the sheer number of polio survivors from the severe epidemics of the mid-twentieth century ensured that when the problems of the late effects of polio emerged they would affect a significant number of people. Exact figures on the number of polio survivors are almost impossible to obtain. Data provided by the *Morbidity and Mortality Weekly Report* listed 457,088 paralytic and nonparalytic polio cases in the United States between 1937 and 1997. This number, however, very likely understates the total number of cases in that period because reporting requirements were not uniform nationwide and not all cases were reported.[5] A 1987 survey by the National Center for Health Statistics estimated that there were 1.63 million polio survivors in the United States. About 641,000 of these individuals had paralytic polio and were at the highest risk for developing post-polio symptoms. Another 833,000 had nonparalytic polio and were at somewhat less risk. In the late nineties an estimated 120,000 to 240,000 polio survivors were experiencing the symptoms of post-polio. These figures, too, are probably understated, and some authorities suggest that as this population ages increased numbers will experience at least some of the late effects of polio.[6] Whatever the actual number of polio survivors who have developed or will develop post-polio syndrome, these individuals represent a significant medical problem that has drawn increasing attention from science and medicine.[7]

The third reason for the growing awareness of PPS among the public and among medical professionals was the advocacy and activism of polio survivors who were initially unable to get from physicians either an explanation of what was happening to them or any alleviation of their symptoms. A 1979 article by Larry Schneider in *Rehabilitation Gazette* "drew attention both to the deleterious effects of aging on polios and to the lack of doctors who knew anything about the disease." Schneider's article inspired polio survivors who were experiencing their own disturbing symptoms. The *Rehabilitation Gazette* under the leadership of Gini Laurie sponsored a 1981 conference in Chicago to address the question "Whatever Happened to the Polio Patient?" The conference attracted over 200 attendees, many of them polio survivors reliant on wheelchairs and respirators. A second conference held in St. Louis in 1983 marked the creation of the Gazette International Networking Institute (GINI) to coordinate "information and networking on the late effects" of polio. GINI has continued to hold post-polio conferences (eight through 2000), to advocate, lobby for, and support additional research into the causes of PPS and the development of effective therapies and to provide a clearinghouse for information regarding PPS.[8]

Research over the last two decades has led to a growing understanding of PPS, although a diagnosis is still, in Julie Silver's words, largely "a diagnosis of exclusion." As a syndrome, PPS is a "collection of symptoms that characteristically occur together." There is no single test for PPS and a diagnosis of PPS is given only if the patient meets "specific criteria established by the medical community, and only after all other reasonable (and testable) conditions have been eliminated as possibilities." The symptoms indicative of PPS, according to Silver, are: "new weakness, unaccustomed fatigue, muscular pain, new swallowing problems, new respiratory problems, cold intolerance, and new muscle atrophy." New muscle weakness is the "most important criterion" in this list. Silver lists four criteria for a diagnosis of PPS: "1. An individual must have a known history of polio. . . . 2. The individual must have had some improvement in strength following the initial paralysis. 3. There must have been a period of stability (at least one or two decades) in which the individual had no new symptoms. 4. The individual must present with new symptoms that are consistent with PPS and not attributable to some other disease." Unfortunately, these criteria remain frustratingly imprecise for both polio survivors and physicians. The lack of a definitive test for PPS causes polio survivors no end of trouble and leads to frequent misdiagnosis.[9]

Physicians have developed a set of recommendations to alleviate PPS symptoms and to prevent any worsening. Each polio survivor presents a unique set of problems under the umbrella of post-polio syndrome and, consequently, the recommendations for alleviating the problems will differ from case to case. However, some general recommendations have emerged. In patients exhibiting muscle weakness, reports Halstead, "every effort should be made to provide more rest and support for those muscles." Where individuals have been pushing themselves and their muscles excessively, "a change in lifestyle with *more rest* and *less stress* is absolutely essential." Polio survivors, however, should not abandon exercise entirely, as "there is considerable evidence that almost everyone can benefit from some form of exercise." The key is to develop a program with knowledgeable physicians and therapists that is helpful and supportive rather than destructive. Managing fatigue, like managing weakness, usually requires steps to conserve energy and often lifestyle changes that reduce strain and stress on the body. According to Halstead, "the successful management of both new weakness and fatigue is essentially accomplished through a succession of small changes rather than by one dramatic intervention." Over time, Halstead notes, these small changes can accumulate and "eventually provide significant relief." [10]

Although the emergence of new symptoms is often overwhelming for polio survivors, there is good news from the research and clinical experience of the last two decades. Halstead advises that "with persistence and common sense, most of the symptoms of PPS can be improved with a combination of lifestyle changes, 'bracing and pacing,' and medications." [11] However, as we will see, this news is often a bitter pill for polio survivors struggling to deal with unexpected and unwanted new symptoms that painfully recall the losses incurred when polio struck decades before.

The onset of post-polio syndrome was often insidious. Polio survivors who had become adept at coping with their disability began to notice that they tired more easily, that they couldn't walk as far as they once had, that their muscles seemed weaker, or perhaps a leg collapsed, that their breathing was more labored. Accustomed to some daily fluctuation in their energy and strength, and relying on the lessons learned so long ago, many pushed ahead in spite of the new fatigue or weakness. Doing more, not giving in to one's body—following the injunction "use it or lose it"—had always worked previously. Most did not want to explore the possibility that these emerging problems were related to their polio in some fashion. Polio was something they had put behind them years previously and they had no desire to revisit that painful time. Many had also developed a healthy aversion to doctors and hospitals and chose initially not to seek medical advice on this puzzling development. If they sought medical advice in the late seventies and early eighties, they often found physicians equally baffled, younger doctors who had never treated a polio patient, and physiatrists who recommended physical therapy to strengthen weakened muscles.

The emergence of the symptoms of post-polio often began innocently enough. Tobin Siebers first noticed the "toll" that "overexertion and bravado" had taken on his polio-affected muscles when his children were small. At one time he "could carry a suitcase for a mile, if I had to, through sheer determination." However, when his children arrived, he discovered he "could not carry a two-year old for three blocks, no matter how hard I tried." Carrying his children up steps was simply impossible, and Siebers "began to notice that other people were picking up my children and carrying them around." William Whyte first noticed weakness when he was in the garden. He had no trouble

getting down on the ground to help with the weeding, but it became so difficult to get up that he soon gave up helping his wife with the gardening.[12]

Dorothea Nudelman, who had polio in 1949, discovered post-polio syndrome while reading a magazine in her optometrist's waiting room in 1980.
"The article focused on polio survivors in middle age who were experiencing
some alarming new symptoms." When the doctor called, she was "happy to
put the story aside, grateful that I wasn't among that chosen group." Six years
later Nudelman and her husband Mike built a new home and moved into it.
She did much of the packing, and her "fatigue was insurmountable." Once
they moved into the new and larger house, Nudelman expected that her exhaustion would subside. However, it took longer and longer to reach distant
parts of the house. Neither her internist nor her orthopedist when consulted
thought her problems might be connected to post-polio. They speculated "that
middle age and difficult physical challenges made everyone more tired, and
recommended moderate exercise." Although she continued to read and learn
all she could about late effects of the disease, one day she "put post-polio out
of my mind. It was too depressing to think about." A year later on vacation
Nudelman found that she "was doing practically nothing, getting plenty of
rest, but still stumbling over myself and still tiring out fast." She found it
difficult to negotiate the four steps into the cabin and her husband had to install a handrail so she could manage. She could no longer deny that something
serious was happening.[13]

When Leonard Kriegel was a young adolescent in the New York State Reconstruction Home learning to walk with crutches and long leg braces, he
learned to fall safely so as not to hurt himself when the inevitable happened.
"Falling," he writes, "rid a man of excess baggage; it taught him how each of
us is dependent on balance." But equally important to Kriegel was learning
how to raise himself to a standing position once again. As he put it, "As long
as I could pick myself up and stand on my own two feet, brace-bound and
crutch-propped as I was, the fall testified to my ability to live in the here and
now, to stake my claim as an American who had turned incapacity into capacity." But he always knew the day would come when he could no longer pick
himself up. One rainy night in 1983, some thirty-nine years after polio, while
walking with friends to dinner in Manhattan, his left crutch slipped and he
fell to the sidewalk as he had so many times before. But when he turned over
and tried to use one crutch to boost himself to his feet, he discovered that he
couldn't. It wasn't a matter of strength. Rather "it had to do with a subtle, mys-
terious change in my own sense of rhythm and balance." His body, as he later

observed, "had decided—*and decided on its own autonomously*—that the moment had come for me to face the question of endings." His friends finally had to help him up. Later that night, Kriegel pondered the implications of the evening: "I would . . . never again get to my feet on my own. A part of my life had ended."[14] Kriegel sees the event as rounding out his life. It also almost certainly meant that Kriegel had begun to experience the symptoms of post-polio.

Because the onset of post-polio syndrome was gradual, polio survivors often denied that the new problems were permanent or that they represented a new stage in their relationship with impairment and disability. In denying or ignoring the growing evidence of new problems, polio survivors often resorted to the tactics that had worked for so many years. However, to their dismay, the tried and true methods learned decades earlier now no longer worked. The problems only increased. For example, by the 1980s Linda Priest had become a wheelchair athlete competing in basketball, track, and road racing, in addition to swimming. However, while competing actively she began to develop problems with her shoulders and wrists. She was also much more fatigued than previously and didn't recover from 10K races as quickly. She also noticed that "other 'jocks' with polio seemed to be experiencing the same problems." Priest first heard about post-polio syndrome at the National Wheelchair Games in 1980 or 1981. She remembers that she "would not even listen to the conversation." She recalls thinking then that "it was true, but it took a long time" for her to admit it to herself. She had come from an athletic family, had grown up watching from the sidelines as family and friends competed, and "finally, after all those years I had been able to experience the joy of competition." She didn't want to give all that up: "It just couldn't be true. It had to be a lie. They told us that we were not going to get worse, that one of the good things about polio was that our condition was stable. What kind of sick joke was this to change their minds!" Still, no matter how hard she tried, Priest could not ignore the pain in her shoulder, the fatigue and the gradual decline in her strength. Priest finally went to a post-polio clinic at Warm Springs. To her dismay, after four days of tests the physician recommended that she "consider major lifestyle changes including stopping all house work and going into a motorized wheelchair." She was "in shock." She was still playing wheelchair basketball and trying to regain her strength so she could resume road racing. "A motorized wheelchair, that was a fate worse than death."[15]

It took Linda Priest several years to begin to come to terms with what she had been told at Warm Springs. She began to read about post-polio syndrome and she did give up wheelchair sports. However, she "did NOT quit doing housework," she "did NOT go into a motorized wheelchair," and she continued to care for her young children. Because her marriage was ending, she soon took on even more responsibility for raising her children. She also did not go back to Warm Springs. As she put it, "being the typical post-polio, I decided that I could handle this on my own." As she continued to research post-polio on her own, her reading in both popular and medical journals gave her a new awareness of how widespread the problem had become. She came across references to GINI and its efforts to establish a network of support for polio survivors. Eventually, through contacts made with GINI's assistance, Priest and several other polio survivors in Atlanta, Georgia, established the Atlanta Post-Polio Association. And, fifteen years after it was initially prescribed, Priest finally began using a motorized wheelchair.[16]

Nancy Baldwin Carter's post-polio symptoms emerged over a number of years, but she steadfastly resisted the implication that these new problems required any major change in her life or in her way of dealing with polio's legacies. For her, the "changes began in my thirties. At first it was merely a matter of fatigue." She began adjusting her schedule so she didn't travel on days she had to lead a seminar or workshop, but the fatigue continued and she "could not get away from the pain that tore through my body." Carter found herself spending "more and more time in bed, eliminating activities that stole strength from my work." Eventually, she was forced to give up her career as an adult education program administrator. "Somehow I knew this had to do with polio," she recalls, but she was not yet ready to explore that insight, so the new problems "baffled" her. She took a more sedentary job keeping the books in her father's law firm, but found it dull. However, she thought this was "the price I had to pay to accommodate my irritatingly uncooperative physical condition." Carter hoped this would be a lasting accommodation to her body's new demands. As she puts it, "I thought I could tap dance for time, do a little diversionary waltz clog to earn a bit of cash while buying some peace for my body." And it worked for a time, but "almost imperceptibly fatigue returned." Now "exhaustion blended into weakness that somehow produced pain," and she found it increasingly difficult to drive, to stand for more than a few minutes, to vacuum or to make the bed. It was only at this point that Carter sought medical help.[17]

Many polio survivors had become experts at burying their painful memories of polio. Post-polio threatened the self-image constructed by so many polio survivors. Stanley Lipshultz, for instance, had learned very early the "mainstreaming rules," and for years he had followed them "to the letter." He became, as he said, "the consummate *passer*" and he "functioned just fine for the longest time." "Passing," however, "came with a price. . . . Being 'normal' took an enormous amount of energy, both physical as well as emotional." After years of trying to be normal, Lipshultz's first intimations of a change in his body "occurred rather innocently." He "noticed a new weakness in my 'affected' limb," and "I seemed to be tired all the time, especially after walking a few blocks." He finally went to a northern Virginia hospital to see whether a new brace would help. After several tests he was diagnosed with "aging athletes' syndrome." He was also told to see a psychiatrist. His response was to do nothing. Several years later he read a magazine piece by Dr. Lauro Halstead describing the problems experienced by aging polio survivors. As he puts it, "The good news is you are not crazy. The bad news is you have post-polio syndrome. Some message!"[18]

Like Lipshultz, the writer Wilfred Sheed "had taken the arts of concealment to such dizzy heights" that he was "genuinely surprised" when others asked if he needed help. In retrospect, Sheed admits, "I was probably always a lot more handicapped than I let on, either to myself or others. My knacks were all geared to the same end, a massive cover-up, a down-right Watergate of the nerves and muscles, in order to pass inspection." However, when he began in his fifties to experience the symptoms of post-polio, "it weakened the whole physical apparatus just enough to call my bluff on all fronts at once." As he writes, "no one could have been more surprised than I to realize quite how much I'd been faking it for all these years."[19]

As these stories suggest, the symptoms of post-polio threatened the polio survivors' conceptions of themselves as perhaps inconvenienced by their impairments but not disabled. Carol Gill, herself a polio survivor, discovered in her work as a clinical psychologist that for many polio survivors, "seeking the company or support of disabled peers would mean admitting on a deep emotional level that they *had* a disability." This admission would lead to an unraveling of "all of the other tenets of the polio 'nondisabled' identity, such as the belief that all things can be accomplished by trying harder, or the taboo against saying 'I can't.'" For example, Nancy Baldwin Carter couldn't conceive of herself as disabled even though fatigue and weakness forced her to give up the job she loved and to stop doing many daily activities. As she put it, "With everything that was in me, I did not want to be disabled. The word itself was repugnant to me. It meant defeat, hopelessness, the end. I refused to be disabled. I may have been using a wheelchair, unable to complete household tasks, struggling with breathing and swallowing, but by God, *I was not disabled.*"[20]

The physicians whom suffering polio survivors consulted didn't always know much about polio or post-polio and sometimes suggested that the symptoms had simply been imagined. When she was in her late thirties Janice Johnson Gradin began to experience "terrible pain" in her joints and muscles. She went to a doctor who performed a number of tests and prescribed pills and physical therapy. "Nothing helped." Another physician, as she said, "even suggested that my problems were all in my head. He said, 'Are you sure you don't just *think* you have all these problems? You don't look sick, and the tests don't show any problems.'" In the mid-1980s Jennifer Williams "seemed to be getting weaker and more fatigued every day." She went to a doctor who, on seeing her medical history, sent her to a neurologist. The neurologist did an EMG test using electrodes inserted in the muscles and concluded that there was indeed evidence of old polio but no evidence of new polio. When Williams asked him about post-polio syndrome, he responded "Well, what's that?" The neurologist "had never seen anyone with polio, let alone anyone with post-polio," and he couldn't tell Williams anything she didn't already know from her reading. Notwithstanding his lack of knowledge, the physician sent Williams to a physical therapist who "put her on a very difficult regime of exercises" as if she were recovering from an injury. The therapist told her, "Do it until you can't do it anymore. Do it until it hurts." As Nancy Baldwin Carter's problems increased in severity she finally "sought professional help." As she recalled, "I saw an unbelievable seven physicians, each one diagnosing his own specialty— the rheumatologist said I had arthritis, while the orthopedist was sure that poor posture was the culprit." Eventually, a doctor at Warm Springs diagnosed post-polio syndrome and provided her with a set of recommendations to be carried out under the direction of her local physician. But when she took the diagnosis and recommendations to her doctor he "scoffed" at them. Her local physician "called the entire PPS theory ridiculous. He said that he, himself, had contracted polio as a young man and that he was fine." Ultimately, he gave Carter the name of a psychiatrist whom he thought could help her.[21]

These instances could easily be multiplied many times over, especially from polio survivors who began to experience post-polio in the late seventies and early eighties. Even today, after two decades of medical research into the problems and widespread publicity about the late effects of polio, some physicians, particularly those with no experience treating polio, reject the concept of post-polio syndrome.²² The challenge for polio survivors, who knew the problems were not in their heads, was to find doctors who would listen to their concerns, take them seriously, and seek to find out more about the late effects of polio before pronouncing an uninformed diagnosis or prescribing unneeded and often harmful exercises. In some cases assistance was found in familiar places, such as the Sister Kenny Institute in Minneapolis or at Warm Springs, Georgia, where the long-term problems associated with living after polio had never been completely forgotten. In other cases, survivors found open-minded and sympathetic physicians with whom they could form a team to devise a successful strategy for dealing with the persistent physical problems and the emotional and psychological issues that accompanied them.

Most polio survivors who have experienced new weakness, fatigue, and pain have eventually found doctors who recognized the condition and whose recommendations helped rather than hurt. For example, Ray Gullickson's family doctor had originally prescribed a tranquilizer for his depression, but nothing for the weakness and pain he was experiencing. Later, after running tests, a neurologist told Gullickson that he was in "excellent health," except for "post-polio syndrome." Gullickson's initial response was disbelief. When his own physician referred him to the Sister Kenny Institute in Minneapolis the doctors there confirmed the diagnosis of post-polio syndrome and told him that it "would be harmful to fight it because that could damage my other muscles." Only after getting this confirming diagnosis did Gullickson concede that "positive thinking isn't going to do the job this time." Sharon Kimball saw her family physician when she began experiencing joint and muscle pain, but he suggested that she needed to consult someone more knowledgeable. However, she admits that it took him about five years to persuade her to get another medical opinion. She finally accepted a referral to the Sister Kenny Institute even though she was "afraid they were going to tell me I had to withdraw from life."²³ Getting good medical advice about the late effects of polio required two things. First, polio survivors had to recognize that the new weakness, pain, and fatigue represented another stage in the process of living with polio and that dealing with these issues required knowledgeable medical assistance. Second, they had to find physicians who acknowledged and recognized post-polio syndrome and who knew how to treat it.

Even though most polio survivors probably suspected that their disturbing symptoms were somehow related to their polio, acknowledging that new reality has proven difficult. A diagnosis of post-polio syndrome conjured up all the unpleasant memories of polio, hospitalization, rehabilitation, the struggle to deal with braces and wheelchairs, and the stigmatization of being crippled. For example, Sharon Kimball has found it particularly difficult to adapt to the new realities of post-polio. She writes, "The hardest thing for me now is to realize that all of the thought processes that helped me overcome my handicap, the attitudes of 'If it's painful, I'll work through it; if it's hard, I'll work harder. If there's a task to be done, I'll do it; I don't need any help,' no longer apply." Because so much of her life has been "serving and living up to people's expectations," she finds it difficult to live within these new limitations. Kimball concedes that "the basic problem" is, as she puts it, "that I still really have trouble seeing myself as handicapped." After making an appointment with the Sister Kenny Institute to have her new problems evaluated, Janice Gradin found that "thinking about dealing with polio over again was more than I could handle." She recalls that she "just fell apart," and "cried a lot." After being diagnosed with post-polio at the Sister Kenny Institute, Gradin "needed first to accept that I had it and then learn to deal with it."[24]

Adaptive equipment such as braces and wheelchairs were visible symbols of crippling to both the polio survivor and to the rest of the world, symbols reinforced in the 1940s and 1950s by the massive publicity campaigns of the March of Dimes to raise funds for the NFIP. And the images stuck, especially in the minds of polio survivors who had struggled so hard to abandon these devices as quickly as they could. So, when the time came to use a wheelchair once again, all the old feelings about being disabled and crippled surged to the fore. In the case of Hugh Gallagher, these feelings were engendered by the necessity to switch from a manual chair to a powered one. He had relied on a manual chair following polio in 1952 and he had learned "to manipulate my old chair with a skill and precision borne of years of practice." His often-repaired manual chair had "been an integral part of my life, good days and bad, sickness and health, for more than a quarter century." With the onset of post-polio syndrome, Gallagher became less and less able to propel himself, more dependent on others for locomotion, and "less independent, more invalid." But he resisted the thought of a powered chair: "Electric wheelchairs are for *crippled* people, not for folks like me. I am one of those lean, mean athletic wheelies who compete in the marathon and get their pictures on the back of Wheaties boxes." When he finally acquired an electric chair, he had "a sense of failure, a sense that I have given up, given in, after all these years of struggle, to my polio paralysis." He kept the chair in the corner for a long time, but gradually discovered what he could do with it. He could easily visit an art museum, go Christmas shopping on his own, or go for hikes along a canal towpath. He admits that he "enjoyed all this greatly," and "it was a liberation" for him to be able to "go out into the world independent of the strength of my arm muscles." Still, he was acutely self-conscious in public. It took Gallagher some six months of using the chair to begin to accept its usefulness. As he finally admits, "I am not a failure, I have not given up, I am just sensible. I am *no* vegetable." Given the way the electric wheelchair opened the world to him once again, Gallagher even acknowledges that the transition from manual to electric chair was one he "should have made years ago."[25]

Leonard Kriegel has also had a complicated relationship with wheelchairs, beginning when he received his first chair in the New York State Reconstruction Home in 1945. He had waited for a chair for more than two months while enduring the hot baths that were "baking the stiffness" out of his polio-paralyzed body. Because wheelchairs were rationed during the war for use by wounded soldiers and sailors, Kriegel was able to get a chair only when his parents found one to buy. "The wheelchair," as he wrote in his 1964 memoir, "was the way home." Kriegel recalls that he "loved that wheelchair with a passion that embarrasses" him now. However, at the time, the wheelchair provided a "newly won mobility" that brought with it "a gift of overwhelming freedom." After he returned home, however, Kriegel was determined to get out of the wheelchair and become a "crutchwalker." He pushed himself through the city streets, built up his upper body strength and his arms on a local jungle gym, and abandoned the wheelchair. He "swore, aloud, as solemnly as only adolescent boys can swear, that I would never again use a wheelchair." Kriegel remembers that as he rebuilt his life after polio, he "refused to think about a wheelchair as an alternative to walking on braces and crutches." Along with his compatriots in the rehabilitation hospital, Kriegel had adopted the belief "that using a wheelchair signified some sort of spiritual surrender," that a real man wouldn't use the device. However, in his fifties, as age and post-polio took their toll, Kriegel found himself returning to the wheelchair, and again began "to embrace the image of the wheelchair rider" he once was. While he thinks that he "might still have had a few years of walking on braces and crutches left—no matter how difficult," he also learns "that getting back into the wheelchair was not the spiritual death" he had feared.[26] What had seemed unimaginable to a young man testing his masculinity against his paralyzed body, had become, some forty years later, inevitable.

As these accounts suggest, the symptoms of post-polio confronted survivors with difficult emotional and psychological issues. Several studies of polio survivors have pointed to the challenges of dealing with a "second disability." Because American society still "devalues those with disabling conditions," polio survivors experiencing the new disabilities of post-polio syndrome "often devalue themselves as the rest of society does." As a result of this internalized devaluation, polio survivors with post-polio can be "psychologically traumatized by the devaluing attitudes usually associated with becoming disabled."[27] Polio survivors exhibit a range of emotional and psychological responses to the symptoms of post-polio syndrome, but the "emotional responses to experiencing new medical problems related to polio can be as traumatic and disabling as the physical problems." Individuals can "experience any combination of denial, anger, frustration and hopelessness," but one study identified "three distinct categories of psychological responses: (1) those who do not regard themselves as handicapped, regardless of the extent of involvement and presence of obvious deformities; (2) those who feel disabled now, but who never did in the past, even during the acute illness; and (3) those who feel that, because they are experiencing polio for the second time, they are 'twice cursed.'"[28] As polio survivor Edmund Sass observed, "polio is a particularly cruel disease. It steals your childhood, gives you 20 to 30 years to adjust to the disabilities with which you were left, and then threatens to return to complicate your life once again." Surveys of polio survivors indicate that self-reported symptoms of depression among polio survivors ranged from a low of 16 percent to a high of 51 percent. In addition, survivors often report other psychological effects such as anxiety and low mood.[29] Although these surveys are an imprecise measure of the emotional and psychological toll taken by post-polio, they do indicate that considerable distress has accompanied the physical problems of post-polio for many survivors.

The new disabilities reopened often-painful recollections, but the perspective gained in the intervening decades encouraged some survivors to write polio narratives. In part, it was an act of recovery for themselves. It was an effort to understand what polio had taken from them and what they had achieved in spite of their losses. But it was also an act of historical recovery. Some memoirists realized they were part of a slowly vanishing generation. The success of the Salk and Sabin vaccines in the 1950s and 1960s meant, in the United States at least, no new polio generations. If they did not write the story of polio from the inside, soon no one would be left to tell the tale.

Writing a polio narrative decades after the disease struck affords the writer an opportunity to assess the impact of the disease and its aftermath on his or her life. The memoirists who are also professional writers are, not surprisingly, the most self-conscious about their reasons for exploring their polio experience in print. As Hugh Gallagher puts it in the beginning of his narrative, "This book reflects the maturation of my thought on aspects—personal and public—of being disabled in an able-bodied society." In living more than forty years as a quadriplegic, Gallagher discovered that "disability is far more complex, more profound than mere physical impairment." The disabled, he asserts, gain a knowledge usually reserved for the "old and dying." The question for the disabled is whether "a life—with its share of joy and reward—[can] be wrested from this encompassing, ever-present knowledge." *Black Bird Fly Away: Disabled in an Able-Bodied World* is Gallagher's effort to reveal how he did it. For Leonard Kriegel, the essays he has written exploring the meaning of polio and disability in his life are "a way of meeting myself." Kriegel is not particularly interested in achieving "the philosophical detachment that comes with age." He wants instead to record the "absence and rage" he felt and still feels over the paralysis of his legs. Although he is still angry about his loss, Kriegel also wants to "speak of my pride in my performance. All things considered, I have done well." He had "made the only bargain with fate a cripple and a writer could make," he had "survived" and he "would preserve that survival in the language of record." Whether they regard their polio experience with the knowledge that comes with experience or whether they are still animated by rage over their losses, the writers of polio narratives have used these memoirs to try to understand how and why polio shaped their lives in the decades since their awful diagnosis.[30]

One of the most extensive accounts of dealing with the emotional and psychological consequences of polio and of post-polio is Dorothea Nudelman's *Healing the Blues,* written with her psychotherapist, David Willingham. Although her depression seems to have been triggered by the onset of post-polio syndrome, Nudelman discovers during a year of psychotherapy that the root of her depression lay in her experiences as a child with polio, in her responses to hospitalization, rehabilitation, and the expectations of parents, doctors, and therapists, and in her repression of powerful emotions during the many years she successfully functioned with a disability in an able-bodied world. Writing alternating chapters, Nudelman and Willingham describe the hard work of therapy, of calling up powerful fears, emotions, and anger, and of learning how to deal with the psychological consequences of her illness and disability. Willingham's diagnosis was that Nudelman was "experiencing a form of depression which is caused by a severe delayed grief reaction, a condition which is similar to post-traumatic stress syndrome. The childhood polio had caused terrible pain and paralysis and traumatic separation from the family." Willingham concluded that "this traumatization had been buried deep in Dorothea's psyche. Now, reactivated by new losses from post-polio syndrome, the old grief resurfaced and plunged her into depression." It took a year of frequent therapy sessions, disturbing dreams, emotional highs and lows, and the support of her husband for Nudelman to confront and deal with the emotional and psychological problems enmeshed in her experience of polio and post-polio syndrome. When she wrote her book some six years after finishing therapy, Nudelman acknowledged that "therapy did not change the negative realities—pain, fatigue, loss of strength, and decreased mobility." She admits that "therapy doesn't cure crippling although it helps to heal the 'wounds' so mind and body and emotions can coexist."[31] What helped Nudelman deal with her depression was the realization that living with polio and post-polio, living with a disability, was a lifelong process. You couldn't simply put polio behind you or out of your mind. Your "recovery" was never completely finished.

Another lengthy account of the depression that is sometimes associated with the late effects of polio is Hugh Gregory Gallagher's chronicle in his book *Black Bird Fly Away*. For some twenty years following his polio in 1952 Hugh Gallagher seemed to have made an excellent recovery. He finished his education at Claremont McKenna College and at Oxford University in England. When he returned to the United States he went to work in Washington, D.C. He also began to work on issues associated with accessability and rights for the disabled. His body was his "obedient servant; it did what I forced it to." Throwing himself into his work, he recalls that all of his "energy and effort were invested in maintaining the shaky façade I presented to the world. There was nothing behind it." In July 1974 Gallagher "collapsed both mentally and physically." He slipped into "a deep situational depression" and "spent the rest of the decade getting out of it."[32]

Gallagher's problems had begun in the spring of 1972 around the time of his fortieth birthday. After a year of struggling alone with his depression, he sought aid from a psychiatrist. Seeking psychiatric help was humiliating for Gallagher. As he put it, "Throughout my life, I had handled my emotional problems without help. I had handled polio and the resultant severe paralysis with my own resources. I had constructed a life of notable success. The fact that I was there in his office that rainy morning was a major admission that something beyond my control had gone wrong." During a year of therapy with the psychiatrist, Gallagher writes, he "came to accept that, for whatever reason, I was emotionally crippled." He concluded that he was "a sensitive, intelligent person of strong passion severely repressed." In the process of therapy Gallagher learned that he "had never accepted my physical handicap." He "despised" his "body and all its works." He had lived his "life on a surface that was without flaw. There could be no sign to others of what lay underneath." And he concluded, "I was trapped within my performance." It took Gallagher a long time to accept the psychiatrist's diagnosis. But this was only the first step for, as he notes, "a diagnosis is not a cure." Ultimately, Gallagher began to reconstruct his life and to achieve "emotional maturity."[33]

In the last two decades polio survivors have developed a number of strategies to deal with the physical changes they are experiencing and with the emotional and psychological problems that often accompany their increasing disability. For those most severely affected, like Nudelman and Gallagher, these strategies may include psychoanalysis and psychotherapy. But many polio survivors have found other sources of assistance. These sources include physiatrists and other physicians increasingly knowledgeable about post-polio syndrome and how to treat it, GINI and its meetings and publications, local support groups, and the Internet.

Scientific and clinical knowledge about post-polio syndrome has grown significantly since the early 1980s when large numbers of polio survivors began manifesting new symptoms. One measure of this growing interest in post-polio is the number of medical articles published. From 1967 to 1989, there were over 200 articles dealing with the syndrome and its neuromuscular and respiratory complications, its psychological and sociological aspects, and difficulty swallowing. Since then, more than 200 additional articles have appeared in the medical and scientific literature. In addition to these medical articles, several handbooks for survivors and for physicians dealing with post-polio patients have been published in order to provide accurate and up-to-date information on the syndrome. For example, GINI published the *Handbook on the Late Effects of Poliomyelitis for Physicians and Survivors* in 1984 and more recently a revised edition in 1999. The most recent edition contains 90 brief articles on a wide range of topics of interest both to physicians and survivors. More recently, the March of Dimes published two guidelines for dealing with post-polio. Both of these pamphlets were designed to disseminate widely the conclusions reached at a May 2000 conference on post-polio syndrome sponsored by the March of Dimes and the Roosevelt Warm Springs Institute for Rehabilitation (the successor to the Georgia Warm Springs Foundation). As the March of Dimes pamphlet notes, in spite of the "increasing numbers of post-polio patients" showing up in doctors offices, "few physicians and relevant allied health professionals have adequate knowledge of the syndrome or of best clinical practices for diagnosis and treatment."[34]

Information about post-polio syndrome and the new problems that polio survivors are experiencing has also appeared frequently in the mass media over the past two decades. Newspapers and news magazines with both local and national readerships have published articles on post-polio detailing personal accounts of survivors and the state of current medical knowledge. These articles were important both in making the public aware of the new problems of polio survivors and in informing polio survivors puzzled by what was happening to them that there was an explanation for their disturbing symptoms.[35] The newspapers almost always provided local sources of reliable information and medical assistance for those survivors still struggling on their own with post-polio.

More recent sources of information and advice regarding post-polio syndrome are three detailed guides for polio survivors. In 1998 Dr. Lauro Halstead, director of the Post-Polio Program at the National Rehabilitation Hospital in Washington, D.C., and a polio survivor, edited *Managing Post-Polio: A Guide to Living Well with Post-Polio Syndrome*. In thirteen chapters, the authors described the typical problems of post-polio and provided advice on finding expert medical care, conserving energy, changing one's lifestyle, applying for disability, and using the Internet. In addition, there were seven accounts by polio survivors describing how they personally were coping with the late effects of polio. Three years later, Dr. Julie Silver, who had contributed to Halstead's volume, published *Post-Polio Syndrome: A Guide for Polio Survivors and Their Families*. Dr. Silver, who directs the International Center for Polio Rehabilitation in Framingham, Massachusetts, and whose grandfather, mother, and uncle had polio, provides brief descriptions of polio and of post-polio syndrome before offering advice on a wide variety of topics. Her goal was "to write a comprehensive volume that would help prevent further disability in polio survivors as they age" and to provide "health-care professionals who are interested in medical issues germane to aging with polio" with accurate and up-to-date information. Finally, in 2002, Richard Bruno published *The Polio Paradox: What You Need to Know*. Bruno is a clinical psychophysiologist and directs the Post-Polio Institute at New Jersey's Englewood Hospital and Medical Center. Although a polio survivor can glean useful advice from Bruno, particularly with regard to managing pain and fatigue, his book focuses on his theories regarding the causes of the symptoms of post-polio and of such related conditions as chronic fatigue syndrome and fibromyalgia. Bruno argues that many of the contemporary cases of chronic fatigue syndrome and fibromyalgia may in fact be cases of post-polio syndrome in individuals who had very mild or inapparent cases of polio in the 1940s and 1950s.[36] In addition to directing their institutes and clinics and writing their books, all three authors are frequent speakers at post-polio conferences. These commercially published guides, along with the GINI and March of Dimes guides mentioned earlier, have made available to both polio survivors and their physicians the kind of information that was so sorely lacking in the late 1970s and early 1980s.

Since its establishment, GINI (the Gazette International Networking Institute) has served as a clearinghouse for information on post-polio syndrome. It has also fostered research into the causes and treatment of post-polio syndrome. GINI grew out of Gini Laurie's commitment to helping polio survivors lead productive and useful lives. Her family was devastated by polio in 1912, one year before she was born. Her "12-year-old sister was mildly disabled, a 6-year-old brother very severely disabled, and two sisters, aged 3 and 9, died" at St. John's Hospital in St. Louis where their father was a surgeon on the staff. During the epidemics of the 1950s Gini Laurie became a Red Cross volunteer at the respiratory center in Cleveland. In 1958, Laurie and her husband began publishing a newsletter for alumni of the respiratory center that featured "news of how polio survivors managed at home." In 1970 the newsletter was renamed *Rehabilitation Gazette,* and Laurie continued to publish it after she and her husband moved to St. Louis.[37]

In 1979 the *Rehabilitation Gazette* published Larry Schneider's letter describing both the new problems being experienced by polio survivors and the dearth of physicians who knew anything about polio or about these new symptoms. The response to that letter led to additional articles on the problem and ultimately to a conference in Chicago in 1981 on "Whatever Happened to the Polio Patient?" that brought together both physicians and polio survivors. This was the first of eight post-polio and independent living conferences sponsored by GINI, as the volunteer organization that Laurie headed became known as in 1981. These conferences, the last of which was in 2000, along with other conferences such as those sponsored by the March of Dimes or the Roosevelt Warm Springs Rehabilitation Center, mix presentations of the latest scientific discoveries from medical laboratories and studies with sessions led by polio survivors discussing ways of dealing with the many problems associated with post-polio syndrome. The conferences bring together in one place to talk to one another both polio survivors and the health professionals who treat them.[38] When Gini Lauri died of cancer in 1989, Joan Headley succeeded her as director. In 1995 GINI created a research fund to raise money for grants to support research into the causes and treatment of post-polio syndrome. By 2002 the GINI Research Fund had raised over $250,000 and had made its first grants.[39] In June 2003 GINI changed its name to Post-Polio Health International. The efforts of Gini Laurie, Joan Headley, and the volunteers who work with them have created networks of shared information that have helped many polio survivors realize the problems they are experiencing are not unique and that there are things that can be done to alleviate the symptoms of post-polio. Over the years, GINI became, in effect, a support group writ large.

If GINI functions as a kind of national support group for polio survivors, numerous local support groups of polio survivors have been established around the country. While some of these have been established in cooperation with rehabilitation hospitals that once treated polio patients or by Easter Seals, polio survivors themselves have organized many independently. By the late 1990s approximately 300 support groups were functioning, although the number changes constantly as new groups are formed and others disband. Post-polio support groups perform several functions for their members. First, they are sources of reliable information on the problems being experienced by polio survivors. Support groups also provide emotional support for members as they experience the new or intensified symptoms of post-polio. Many support groups arrange for speakers on a wide variety of topics related to post-polio and to living with a disability. Most of these support groups are run by polio survivors and run on very little money, although occasionally Easter Seals or other organizations contribute meeting spaces or funding. In addition to regular meetings, many of the support groups publish newsletters for members containing information derived from GINI publications and other disability-related sources. Part of the impetus for establishing support groups came from the example of other diseases and chronic conditions that had flourishing support groups by the early 1980s. But part of the impetus, as well, came from a desire to recapture the spirit of community and camaraderie that many polio survivors had experienced during their rehabilitation in the 1940s and 1950s. As Linda Priest, who helped establish the Atlanta Post-Polio Association, put it, at the end of rehabilitation "we had consciously separated ourselves from our peers because we did not think of ourselves as disabled." However, as she developed new problems and read about post-polio, Priest "remembered how much strength I received from being around other people like myself when I went to Warm Springs during my childhood. I began to think more and more about how good it would be to have that association again."[40]

Rebuilding a meaningful polio community has proven a challenge that post-polio support groups have only partly met. When symptoms of the late effects of polio began to appear and post-polio support groups began to form, it was sometimes difficult for polio survivors to make the decision to go to a meeting or to join a group. To go to a support group meeting was to admit, on some level at least, that you could no longer handle polio on your own and that, yes, you had disability. Many, however, have found in post-polio support groups the sense of the community that had sustained them in rehabilitation. Survivors discovered they were not alone in experiencing the distressing symptoms, and that the support and encouragement of men and women experiencing similar problems was reassuring. Although support groups have to some extent replicated the polio community of the rehabilitation wards, they are also significantly different. Unlike in the ward communities, polio survivors can choose whether to attend, and may participate at varying levels. Second, in the support group setting, simply sharing problems does not necessarily result in close communal ties. And finally, even for groups that meet monthly, the sense of community is necessarily more tenuous than that of the ward, where you shared one another's lives twenty-four hours a day, seven days a week, often for months. The challenge for post-polio support groups will be to sustain the programming and assistance that has been so helpful for so many survivors. As polio survivors age and as post-polio takes its toll, finding individuals to coordinate the activities and make arrangements for meetings is likely to become increasingly difficult.[41]

The Internet has become a major source of information for polio survivors experiencing the late effects of polio. Typing "polio" or "post-polio" into any Web browser brings up hundreds, if not thousands, of Web pages and sites devoted to polio and post-polio syndrome. These sites, of course, vary considerably in quality. Some sites are maintained by medical schools, rehabilitation facilities, polio clinics, and Post-Polio Health International, while others are simply the home pages of Internet-savvy polio survivors. In addition to the sites providing information on post-polio and its treatment, there are a number of discussion lists and chat rooms for polio survivors. These discussion lists function as a kind of online support group, especially for polio survivors who find it difficult to get out to support group meetings. The discussions on these lists can cover a wide variety of topics from advice on where to get help, to reminiscences of one's polio experience and discussions of the pains and occasional joys of living with post-polio. These discussion groups tend to have a fairly regular group of individuals who post regularly and individuals who post only occasionally or ask questions. For some, these discussion groups become a kind of "electronic backyard," or perhaps "rehabilitation ward" where the residents share each other's travails and triumphs on an almost daily basis. While the information on the Internet regarding polio and post-polio grows continually, the challenge for polio survivors, as for any user of the Internet, is to separate the accurate and valuable information from the vast quantity of material available electronically.[42]

While the polio epidemics are, I hope, a thing of the past, the history of post-polio syndrome is still being lived. It is hard to know how many Americans will experience some form of the late effects of polio. In the late nineties, Dr. Lauro Halstead estimated that there were perhaps 600,000 individuals who had had paralytic polio living in the United States. He estimated that between 20 and 40 percent of these survivors were experiencing post-polio syndrome, which would suggest that between 120,000 and 240,000 had developed symptoms. Dr. Julie Silver, however, suggests that "as polio survivors age, it is expected that the majority will experience symptoms related to PPS."[43] The experience of these new sufferers will be different from the experience of many of those discussed in this chapter. In the first place, physicians and health professionals now generally recognize the late effects of polio as having a physiological basis, even though not all the mechanisms behind the many symptoms are fully understood. It is much rarer for a polio survivor seeking medical assistance to be told that her symptoms are "all in her head." The growing body of research on the problems of polio survivors has not only unraveled some of the mysteries of the phenomena, it has also led to a growing consensus on the best treatment. New sufferers will much more easily find reliable information about post-polio syndrome and how to cope with it. The publications of GINI and the March of Dimes, the handbooks of Halstead, Silver, and Bruno, the frequent attention given to the problems by the popular media, the establishment of local support groups, and the explosive growth of Internet resources have all made this information much more accessible than it was ten to fifteen years ago. If indeed most polio survivors will experience at least some of the symptoms of post-polio syndrome, now at least they will be better informed about the difficulties facing them and better able to secure reliable and helpful medical assistance.

The real challenge for polio survivors is not the physical deterioration, as difficult as that can be, but the emotional and psychological costs of coping with a "second disability." But polio survivors have once again proven resilient, recreating networks of support like those that sustained them in rehabilitation, pushing the medical profession to recognize their condition and to begin to understand it and treat it effectively, and finding ways of dealing with these physical and psychological changes late in life. Living with post-polio syndrome is not easy, but then living with polio, living with a permanent disability, has never been easy. While living with post-polio requires polio survivors to unlearn many of the lessons of polio rehabilitation, many are finding themselves slowly and often painfully adjusting to this new phase in their evolving relationship with polio.

| 10 |

Epilogue

EPIDEMIC POLIOMYELITIS in the United States was a disease of the twentieth century. Although the first recorded epidemic occurred in Vermont in 1894, it was in the twentieth century that polio became the feared crippler of children and adolescents. From the first large outbreaks in New York in 1907 and 1916 to the success of the Salk and Sabin vaccines in the 1950s and 1960s, polio epidemics occurred somewhere in the United States virtually every year.

The lifelong experience of the boys and girls, men and women, who had polio has been obscured by the moving story of Franklin D. Roosevelt's rise from polio victim to president of the United States, by the many activities of the National Foundation for Infantile Paralysis and the March of Dimes on behalf of polio research and care of victims, and by the dramatic accounts of Jonas Salk and Albert Sabin developing their successful vaccines. When the polio epidemics were at their height in the late forties and early fifties the published accounts of an encounter with polio emphasized the acute disease and the subsequent rehabilitation. These triumphant overcoming narratives celebrated the resilience of the human spirit in surmounting the challenge of a crippling disease.[1] Most polio survivors fought their way into the mainstream of American life burdened by a permanent disability, and the narratives that emerged toward the end of the century told a more complicated tale of a continuing struggle against the impairments of the body and the disabilities imposed by teachers, employers, and sometimes parents and spouses. The sense of triumph in regaining function as a result of the hard work of rehabilitation was real, but these later narratives have enabled us to explore what it has been like to live with the lasting impairments of paralytic polio.

The polio experience in the mid-twentieth century was deeply embedded in American culture and society. Paralytic polio struck hard at the American Dream of post–World War II America, which envisioned healthy happy children growing up to be successful adults through hard work and individual achievement. Because improved sanitation and living standards ironically fostered epidemic polio and deferred exposure to the virus until a later age when it was more likely to cause paralysis, polio seemed particularly cruel to those families poised to embrace the peace and prosperity of the postwar world. Parents often felt that their child's polio had killed the American Dream. In fact, those virtues of self-help, individual achievement, and hard work embodied in the Protestant work ethic were the very values that sustained many polio survivors through the long, arduous process of rebuilding muscle strength and function in rehabilitation.

Refocusing our attention on the lived experience of polio draws our attention to the limitations of the commonplace view in popular culture and indeed within much of the polio community that hard work, determination and persistence enabled one to overcome polio and its attendant paralysis. One didn't so much overcome polio as learn to live with its legacies and compensate for its losses. Polio survivors have endured and have succeeded in many things at many levels, but no one who had paralytic polio truly overcame the disease.

Polio is quickly becoming a forgotten disease. Americans under the age of fifty have few memories of fearful summers when one couldn't go swimming or to the movies, of classmates and friends encased in steel and leather braces or reliant on a wheelchair, or of the relief a nation felt when Dr. Thomas Francis announced on April 12, 1955, that the polio vaccine developed by Dr. Jonas Salk successfully protected children against the disease. Many physicians in the United States have never seen an active acute case of poliomyelitis. If polio is recalled at all, it is Franklin D. Roosevelt, the March of Dimes, Jonas Salk and, perhaps, Albert Sabin who are most likely to come to mind. For most Americans polio is a thing of the past, an example of triumph over adversity in the case of FDR and of the triumph of American science in the development of the Salk and Sabin vaccines. But for the many polio survivors, their families and friends, polio has never been a thing of the past. They have lived with its consequences since the day they were diagnosed and they will continue to have lives shaped and shadowed by a disease acquired fifty and more years ago. Although the day-to-day struggle against the impairments of polio may lack the drama of Roosevelt's rise to power or the Salk vaccine trial of 1954–55, the story of how polio survivors dealt with the disease and with permanent paralysis and disability deserves to be remembered as well. It is not a story of overcoming the disease, but of learning how to live well with a permanent disability. And that, as we have seen, was no small achievement.

Notes

1. The disease caused by the poliovirus has, as John R. Paul pointed out, been given several different names since the late eighteenth century. In the twentieth century, three names have predominated, *infantile paralysis, poliomyelitis,* and *polio.* "Poliomyelitis," which is the term preferred by scientists and physicians, refers to an inflammation of the gray marrow of the spinal cord as a result of the actions of the poliovirus. "Infantile paralysis" was first used by French authors to describe the visible effect on very young children who were the typical victims in the nineteenth century. It was, as Paul observed, "a name with a descriptive appeal that few others had," and was widely used in the first part of the twentieth century. However, as the epidemics continued and the age of patients increased, "infantile paralysis" seemed more and more inappropriate. It remained in use, however, to the end of the epidemics. For example, the National Foundation for Infantile Paralysis did not change its name until it refocused its energies on birth defects. "Polio" became in the twentieth century "a common term for parents and science writers." I will generally refer to the disease as "polio," except when dealing with the scientific and medical literature when I will use "poliomyelitis." "Infantile paralysis" will be used when the historical context seems appropriate. John R. Paul, *A History of Poliomyelitis* (New Haven: Yale University Press, 1971), 4–9.

2. Paul, *A History of Poliomyelitis,* 3–4; Dorothy M. Horstmann, "The Clinical Epidemiology of Poliomyelitis," *Annals of Internal Medicine* 43 (1955): 526–28.

3. Horstmann, "Clinical Epidemiology of Poliomyelitis," 528; Paul, *A History of Poliomyelitis,* traces the disease from ancient Egyptian and other very early records through the development of the vaccines.

4. John R. Paul, "Epidemiology of Poliomyelitis," in *Poliomyelitis* (Geneva, Switzerland: World Health Organization, 1955), 27; Paul, *A History of Poliomyelitis,* 364–65.

5. Paul, *A History of Poliomyelitis,* 365; Neal Nathanson and John R. Martin, "The Epidemiology of Poliomyelitis: Enigmas Surrounding Its Appearance, Epidemicity, and Disappearance," *American Journal of Epidemiology* 110 (1979): 676; Carl C. Dauer, "The Changing Age Distribution of Paralytic Poliomyelitis," *Annals of the New York Academy of Science* 61 (1955): 943–55; U.S. Department of Commerce, Bureau of the Census, *Historical Statis-*

tics of the United States: Colonial Times to 1970, Bicentennial Edition (Washington, DC: Government Printing Office, 1975), 1:77.

6. Reported cases from *Morbidity and Mortality Weekly Report* cited in "Incidence Rates of Poliomyelitis in the USA," *Polio Network News* 15 (Fall 1999): 3. Note that these figures probably understate the actual number of polio cases. In this period states did not have uniform reporting requirements and it is likely that not all cases were reported to the proper authorities.

7. The best source on the epidemics in the early twentieth century is Naomi Rogers, *Dirt and Disease: Polio before FDR* (New Brunswick, NJ: Rutgers University Press, 1990). See also Paul, *A History of Poliomyelitis,* especially chapters 9, 15, and 21.

8. On Roosevelt's polio see, Hugh Gregory Gallagher, *FDR's Splendid Deception,* rev. ed. (Arlington, VA: Vandamere Press, 1994); Richard Thayer Goldberg, *The Making of Franklin D. Roosevelt: Triumph over Disability* (Cambridge, MA: Abt Books, 1981); and Geoffrey C. Ward, *A First-Class Temperament: The Emergence of Franklin Roosevelt* (New York: Harper and Row, 1989). On Roosevelt as a model for other polio patients and survivors see, John Duffy, "Franklin Roosevelt: Ambiguous Symbol for Disabled Americans," *Midwest Quarterly* 29 (1987): 113–35; Daniel J. Wilson, "A Crippling Fear: Experiencing Polio in the Era of FDR," *Bulletin of the History of Medicine* 72 (1998): 464–95; and Amy L. Fairchild, "The Polio Narratives: Dialogues with FDR," *Bulletin of the History of Medicine* 75 (2001): 488–534.

9. On Roosevelt and Warm Springs see, Turnley Walker, *Roosevelt and the Warm Springs Story* (New York: A. A. Wyn, 1953); Theo Lippman, Jr., *The Squire of Warm Springs: FDR in Georgia, 1924–1945* (Chicago: Playboy Press, 1977); Tony Gould, *A Summer Plague: Polio and Its Survivors* (New Haven: Yale University Press, 1995), 41–84; Goldberg, *The Making of Franklin D. Roosevelt,* 73–104; Ward, *A First-Class Temperament,* 704–54; and Gallagher, *FDR's Splendid Deception,* 34–58.

10. On the March of Dimes and the National Foundation for Infantile Paralysis see Paul, *A History of Poliomyelitis,* chapters 29–30; Jane S. Smith, *Patenting the Sun: Polio and the Salk Vaccine* (New York: William Morrow and Co., 1990), part 1; David L. Sills, *The Volunteers: Means and Ends in a National Organization* (Glencoe, IL: Free Press, 1957); and Richard Carter, *The Gentle Legions* (Garden City, NY: Doubleday, 1961), chapter 4.

11. I will generally use "polio patient" when writing about individuals under the care of a physician, or in an acute or rehabilitation hospital. In nonhospital settings I will generally refer to individuals who had polio as "polio survivors." Some individuals who had polio refer to themselves and others as "polios." Although I don't use the term, it will appear in quotations.

12. I have used 81 male narratives and 73 female narratives. (Several individuals wrote more than one account.) Most of the book-length narratives are autobiographies, although there are several "as told to" books and biographies in the collection.

13. Fairchild, "The Polio Narratives," 492–93, 516–17.

14. Anne Hunsaker Hawkins, *Reconstructing Illness: Studies in Pathography* (West Lafayette, IN: Purdue University Press, 1993), 2, 3, 12; Arthur W. Frank, *The Wounded Sto-*

ryteller: Body, Illness, and Ethics (Chicago: University of Chicago Press, 1995), xi, 53; G. Thomas Couser, *Recovering Bodies: Illness, Disability, and Life Writing* (Madison: University of Wisconsin Press, 1997), 293.

15. Hawkins, *Reconstructing Illness,* 159; Couser, *Recovering Bodies,* 4; Harlan Hahn, "'The Good Parts': Interpersonal Relationships in the Autobiographies of Physically Disabled Persons," Wenner-Gren Foundation Working Papers in Anthropology (New York: Wenner-Gren Foundation, 1983), 10–11.

16. Ibid.

17. Frank, *The Wounded Storyteller,* 21–22; Fairchild, "The Polio Narratives," 492–93. Anne Hawkins argues that illness narratives generally adopted a new "tone and intent" by the end of the 1970s in which anger played a more prominent role, a change visible in some of the more recent polio narratives. Hawkins, *Reconstructing Illness,* 5–6.

18. Hawkins, *Reconstructing Illness,* 14–15; Frank, *Wounded Storyteller,* 22.

19. See the sources cited in note 8.

20. See the sources cited in note 9.

21. See the sources cited in note 10.

22. Paul, *A History of Poliomyelitis;* Richard Carter, *Breakthrough: The Saga of Jonas Salk* (New York: Trident Press, 1966); Smith, *Patenting the Sun;* and Gould, *A Summer Plague,* 111–58.

CHAPTER TWO

1. Neal Nathanson and John R. Martin, "The Epidemiology of Poliomyelitis: Enigmas Surrounding Its Appearance, Epidemicity, and Disappearance," *American Journal of Epidemiology,* 110 (1979): 681.

2. John R. Paul, *A History of Poliomyelitis* (New Haven: Yale University Press, 1971), 159, 165, 283.

3. Paul, *A History of Poliomyelitis,* 320; Maxine Davis, "*Good Housekeeping's* Home Chart for Infantile Paralysis," *Good Housekeeping* 113 (August 1941): 40–41.

4. U.S. Department of Commerce, Bureau of the Census, *Historical Statistics of the United States: Colonial Times to 1970,* Bicentennial Edition (Washington, DC: Government Printing Office, 1975), 1:77; "Incidence Rates of Poliomyelitis in the USA," *Polio Network News* 15 (Fall 1999): 3. Because reporting was inconsistent in these years, these figures probably understate the full number of polio cases.

5. Nathanson and Martin, "The Epidemiology of Poliomyelitis," 681; C. C. Dauer, "Prevalence of Poliomyelitis in 1948," *Public Health Reports* 64 (1949): 733. The aggregate cases were cited in "Incidence Rates of Poliomyelitis in the USA," *Polio Network News* 15 (Fall 1999): 3.

6. Nathanson and Martin, "Epidemiology of Poliomyelitis," 676; Paul, *A History of Poliomyelitis,* 365.

7. Nathanson and Martin, "Epidemiology of Poliomyelitis," 678–79; Dauer, "Prevalence of Poliomyelitis in 1948," 735; see also Selwyn D. Collins, "The Incidence of Po-

liomyelitis and Its Crippling Effects, As Recorded in Family Surveys," *Public Health Reports* 61 (1946): 328–32.

8. David L. Sills, *The Volunteers: Means and Ends in a National Organization* (Glencoe, IL: Free Press, 1957), 123–24.

9. Sills, *Volunteers,* 127–28.

10. Paul, *A History of Poliomyelitis,* 309; Sills, *Volunteers,* 118–21; Fred Davis, *Passage through Crisis: Polio Victims and Their Families* (1963; reprint, with a new introduction by the author, New Brunswick: Transaction Publishers, 1991), 24.

11. Jane S. Smith, *Patenting the Sun: Polio and the Salk Vaccine* (New York: William Morrow and Co., 1990), 158–60; Elaine Tyler May, *Homeward Bound: American Families in the Cold War Era* (New York: Basic Books, 1988), 160; Steven Mintz and Susan Kellogg, *Domestic Revolutions: A Social History of American Family Life* (New York: Free Press, 1988), 188.

12. Davis, *Passage,* xv, 41; see also Sills, *Volunteers,* 126–30.

13. Hart E. Van Riper, "What Parents Should Know about Polio This Summer," *Look* 17 (June 2, 1953): 52; Annie Dillard, *An American Childhood* (New York: Perennial Library, 1988), 168; Gerald A. Shepherd, "Years of Fear: The Time When Polio Was Everywhere," *City Paper* (Baltimore), 8 (August 14, 1984), 15; Noreen Linduska, *My Polio Past* (Chicago: Pellegrini & Cudahy, 1947), 23.

14. Janice Johnson Gradin in *Polio's Legacy: An Oral History,* ed. Edmund J. Sass with George Gottfried and Anthony Sorem (Lanham, MD: University Press of America, 1996), 256; Kathryn Black, *In the Shadow of Polio: A Personal and Social History* (Reading, MA: Addison Wesley, 1996), 45–46; Luther Robinson, *We Made Peace with Polio* (Nashville: Broadman Press, 1960), 11; Smith, *Patenting the Sun,* 156–57; Elaine Lodermeier in Sass, *Polio's Legacy,* 196; Charlene Pugleasa in *A Paralyzing Fear: The Triumph over Polio in America,* ed. Nina Gilden Seavey, Jane S. Smith, and Paul Wagner (New York: TV Books, 1998), 119.

15. Harold M. Visotsky, David A. Hamburg, Mary E. Goss, and Binyamin Z. Lebovits, "Coping Behavior under Extreme Stress: Observations of Patients with Severe Poliomyelitis," *Archives of General Psychiatry* 5 (1961): 30.

16. John Earl Lindell and Ethel Brooks Lindell, *Oh God, Help Me! For I Cannot Help Myself: A True Story of Faith in the Life of a Polio Survivor* (Tempe, AZ: John Earl Lindell, 1988), 7.

17. Lindell and Lindell, *Oh God,* 7–8; Mark Sauer in Seavey, Smith, and Wagner, *Paralyzing Fear,* 245.

18. Regina Woods, *Tales from Inside the Iron Lung (And How I Got Out of It)* (Philadelphia: University of Pennsylvania Press, 1994), 2–3; Hugh Gregory Gallagher, *Black Bird Fly Away: Disabled in an Able-Bodied World* (Arlington, VA: Vandamere Press, 1998), 18–19.

19. Kay Brutger in Sass, *Polio's Legacy,* 71.

20. Sarah Hunt in *The Grit behind the Miracle: A True Story of the Determination and Hard Work behind an Emergency Infantile Paralysis Hospital, 1944–1945, Hickory, North Carolina,* ed. Alice E. Sink (Lanham, MD: University Press of America, 1998), 125–27; Pugleasa in Seavey, Smith, and Wagner, *Paralyzing Fear,* 120; Arvid Schwartz in Seavey, Smith, and Wagner, *Paralyzing Fear,* 253.

21. Linda Atkins, *Jamaica and Me: The Story of an Unusual Friendship* (New York: Random House, 1998), xiii; Carol Meyer, e-mail to SJU Polio and Post Polio Syndrome List, June 18, 1998.

22. Richard Owen in Seavey, Smith, and Wagner, *Paralyzing Fear,* 235; Richard Owen in Sass, *Polio's Legacy,* 30; Paul Longmore, "Role Models: Paul Longmore," *Exceptional Parent* 26 (October 1996): 24.

23. Woods, *Tales,* 3–4; Gallagher, *Black Bird,* 18–24.

24. Schwartz in Seavey, Smith, and Wagner, *Paralyzing Fear,* 253; Schwartz in Sass, *Polio's Legacy,* 143–44; Lindell and Lindell, *Oh God,* 8–9.

25. Pat Morgan, e-mail to SJU Polio and Post Polio Syndrome List, January 5, 1998; Grace Audet in Sass, *Polio's Legacy,* 249; Carol Meyer, e-mail to SJU Polio and Post Polio Syndrome List, June 18, 1998; Carol Lewis, e-mail to SJU Polio and Post Polio Syndrome List, June 18, 1998; Mary Ann Hoffman in Sass, *Polio's Legacy,* 134; Denise Mealy, e-mail to SJU Polio and Post Polio Syndrome List, January 21, 1997; Schwartz in Sass, *Polio's Legacy,* 143; Robert F. Hall, *Through the Storm: A Polio Story* (St. Cloud, MN: North Star Press, 1990), 3; Jennifer Williams in Sass, *Polio's Legacy,* 240; Woods, *Tales,* 4; Pugleasa in Seavey, Smith, and Wagner, *Paralyzing Fear,* 120; Gerry, e-mail to SJU Polio and Post Polio Syndrome List, January 2, 1998; Elaine Lodermeier in Sass, *Polio's Legacy,* 196; John Swett, "Florida's Fourth of July '53," *APPA News* 12 (October–December 1997): n.p.; Millie Teders in Sass, *Polio's Legacy,* 194.

26. Teders in Sass, *Polio's Legacy,* 194.

27. "Clinical Diagnosis of Poliomyelitis," *Therapeutic Notes* 62 (July–August 1955), 181; Dr. Dorothy M. Horstmann, interview by author, tape recording, New Haven, CT, April 26, 1990.

28. Robert Britt, Amos Christie, and Randolph Batson, "Pitfalls in the Diagnosis of Poliomyelitis," *JAMA* 154 (April 24, 1954): 1401; Russell J. Blattner, "Recent Advances in Clinical Aspects of Poliomyelitis," *JAMA* 156 (September 4, 1954): 9.

29. Draper's original drawings describing the two phases are reproduced in George Draper, *Infantile Paralysis* (New York: D. Appleton-Century Co., 1935), 117–18; Britt, Christie, and Batson estimate that about half of polio patients experience the two phases, "Pitfalls," 1403.

30. Britt, Christie, and Batson, "Pitfalls," 1403; Alex J. Steigman, "Diagnosis and General Care of Acute Poliomyelitis," *Pediatric Clinics of North America* 1 (1953): 12–16; Clifford G. Grulee, Jr., "Differential Diagnosis of Poliomyelitis," *JAMA* 152 (August 22, 1953): 1588–89.

31. Philip Lewin, *Infantile Paralysis: Anterior Poliomyelitis* (Philadelphia: W. B. Saunders Co., 1941), 74–77 (quotation, 74); Grulee, "Differential Diagnosis," 1587.

32. Steigman, "Diagnosis," 16–17; National Foundation for Infantile Paralysis, *Definitive and Differential Diagnosis of Poliomyelitis* (New York: National Foundation for Infantile Paralysis, 1954), 3–6.

33. Blattner, "Recent Advances," 9–10; Britt, Christie, and Batson, "Pitfalls," 1401–2.

34. Blattner, "Recent Advances," 9; Richard Aldrich in Seavey, Smith, and Wagner, *Paralyzing Fear*, 115; Davis, *Passage*, 30.

35. Davis, *Passage*, 24.

36. Hall, *Through the Storm*, 4; Dorothea Nudelman and David Willingham, *Healing the Blues: Drug-Free Psychotherapy for Depression* (Pacific Grove, CA: Boxwood Press, 1994), 36.

37. June Radosovich in Sass, *Polio's Legacy*, 158.

38. Davis, *Passage*, 25–29; Bias in Sass, *Polio's Legacy*, 78; Lindell and Lindell, *Oh God*, 7; Sarah Hunt in Sink, *Grit behind the Miracle*, 125.

39. Mary-Lou Whitaker, e-mail to SJU Polio and Post Polio Syndrome List, September 16, 1996; Ray K. Gullickson in Sass, *Polio's Legacy*, 41–42; see also Marilyn Rogers in Sass, *Polio's Legacy*, 54; Richard Owen in Seavey, Smith, and Wagner, *Paralyzing Fear*, 235; and Marlene Krumrie in Sass, *Polio's Legacy*, 199.

40. L. McCarty Fairchild, "Some Psychological Factors Observed in Poliomyelitis Patients," *American Journal of Physical Medicine* 31 (1952): 276.

41. Louise Lake, *Each Day a Bonus: Twenty-five Courageous Years in a Wheelchair* (Salt Lake City: Deseret Book Co., 1971), 5–6; Lindell and Lindell, *Oh God*, 9; Eleanor Chappell, *On the Shoulders of Giants: The Bea Wright Story* (Philadelphia: Chilton Co., 1960), 20–22; Luther Robinson, *We Made Peace with Polio*, 27; Pugleasa in Seavey, Smith, and Wagner, *Paralyzing Fear*, 122; Owen in Sass, *Polio's Legacy*, 30–31; Owen in Seavey, Smith, and Wagner, *Paralyzing Fear*, 235–36; Leonard Kriegel, *The Long Walk Home* (New York: Appleton-Century, 1964), 14.

42. Gallagher, *Black Bird*, 27; and Nudelman and Willingham, *Healing the Blues*, 41

43. Nudelman and Willingham, *Healing the Blues*, 36, 41; Kriegel, *Long Walk Home*, 14; Louis Sternburg and Dorothy Sternburg, with Monica Dickens, *View from the Seesaw* (New York: Dodd, Mead & Co., 1986). Fred Davis noted that the first reliable estimates of the extent of permanent disability could not be made until six weeks to three months after the acute attack: Davis, *Passage*, 49.

44. Sauer in Seavey, Smith, and Wagner, *Paralyzing Fear*, 246; Audet in Sass, *Polio's Legacy*, 249.

45. Franklin G. Ebaugh and Clarence S. Hoekstra, "Psychosomatic Relationships in Acute Anterior Poliomyelitis," *American Journal of the Medical Sciences* 213 (January 1947): 117 (quotation); William S. Langford, "Physical Illness and Convalescence: Their Meaning to the Child," *Journal of Pediatrics* 33 (1948): 242; Richard H. Young, "The Patient's Attitude toward Poliomyelitis," *Mental Hygiene* 33 (1949): 263–64; and Davis, *Passage*, 32.

46. Nudelman and Willingham, *Healing the Blues*, 36; Kriegel, *Long Walk Home*, 13–14; and Charles H. Andrews, *No Time for Tears* (Garden City, NY: Doubleday & Co., 1951), 24.

47. Langford, "Physical Illness," 243–44; Davis, *Passage*, 22, 36; see also H. A. Robinson, J. E. Finesinger, and J. S. Bierman, "Psychiatric Considerations in the Adjustment of Patients with Poliomyelitis," *New England Journal of Medicine* 254 (1956): 978. Mary T. Westbrook, in a recent study of polio survivors, found that those who were young children when they had polio were more likely to have experienced guilt: "Early Survivors Mem-

ories of Having Polio: Survivors' Memories versus the Official Myths," Presented at the First Australian International Post-Polio Conference, Sydney, November 1996, http://www.zynet.co.uk/ott/polio/lincolnshire.

48. Tobin Siebers, "My Withered Limb," *Michigan Quarterly Review* 37 (1998): 197.

49. Dorothy M. Horstmann, "The Clinical Epidemiology of Poliomyelitis," *Annals of Internal Medicine* 43 (1955): 532; see also Morris Siegel and Morris Greenberg, "Risk of Paralytic and Nonparalytic Forms of Poliomyelitis to Household Contacts," *JAMA* 155 (May 29, 1954): 429–31.

50. Lindell and Lindell, *Oh God*, 8–9; Robinson, *Peace with Polio*, 27, 29, 74–76; Josephine Howard in Seavey, Smith, and Wagner, *Paralyzing Fear*, 39.

51. Because it was recognized by the midforties that the poliovirus circulated widely during any epidemic, official quarantines of affected families were ordered less frequently than earlier in the century.

52. Alice and Agnes Dalton in Sink, *Grit behind the Miracle*, 116–17; Schwartz in Sass, *Polio's Legacy*, 144; Andrews, *No Time for Tears*, 42–43; Sternburg and Sternburg, *View from the Seesaw*, 10–11.

53. Davis, *Passage*, 38–39.

CHAPTER THREE

1. "How Hospitals Fought Chicago's Polio Threat," *Hospitals* 30 (November 1956): 43; Robert S. Marshall, "Polio Epidemic Hits Massachusetts," *Hospitals* 29 (October 1955): 148; Herbert J. Kaufmann, "The Impact of the 1955 Poliomyelitis Outbreak on the Boston City Hospital," *Boston Medical Quarterly* 7 (March 1956): 4, 9.

2. Max Seham, "Discrimination against Negroes in Hospitals," *New England Journal of Medicine* 271 (October 29, 1964): 940–43; John Hume in *A Paralyzing Fear: The Triumph over Polio in America*, ed. Nina Gilden Seavey, Jane S. Smith, and Paul Wagner (New York: TV Books, 1998), 157; and W. Montague Cobb, "Medical Care for Minority Groups," *Annals of the American Academy of Political and Social Science* 273 (January 1951): 169–75; Alice E. Sink, ed., *The Grit behind the Miracle: A True Story of the Determination and Hard Work behind an Emergency Infantile Paralysis Hospital, 1944–1945, Hickory, North Carolina* (Lanham, MD: University Press of America, 1998), 73–74.

3. Philip Lewin, *Infantile Paralysis: Anterior Poliomyelitis* (Philadelphia: W. B. Saunders Co., 1941), 117–18; Shirley Paul, e-mail to SJU Polio and Post Polio Syndrome List, October 23, 1996; Charlene Pugleasa in *A Paralyzing Fear: The Triumph over Polio in America*, ed. Nina Gilden Seavey, Jane S. Smith, and Paul Wagner (New York: TV Books, 1998), 122.

4. Guenter B. Risse, "Revolt against Quarantine: Community Responses to the 1916 Polio Epidemic, Oyster Bay, New York," *Transactions and Studies of the College of Physicians of Philadelphia*, ser. 5, vol. 14, no. 1 (1992): 37, 40, 42; Naomi Rogers, *Dirt and Disease: Polio before FDR* (New Brunswick, NJ: Rutgers University Press, 1992), 41; Robert Gurney in *Polio's Legacy: An Oral History*, ed. Edmund J. Sass with George Gottfried and Anthony Sorem

(Lanham, MD: University Press of America, 1996), 22; Sheila Tohn, e-mail to SJU Polio and Post Polio Syndrome List, April 14, 1995.

5. Jane Boyle Needham, as told to Rosemary Taylor, *Looking Up* (New York: G. P. Putnam's Sons, 1959), 52–53; Charles L. Mee, *A Nearly Normal Life: A Memoir* (Boston: Little, Brown and Co., 1999), 14–15.

6. David Kangas in Seavey, Smith, and Wagner, *A Paralyzing Fear*, 268; David Kangas in Sass, *Polio's Legacy*, 62; Hugh Gregory Gallagher, *Black Bird Fly Away: Disabled in an Able-Bodied World* (Arlington, VA: Vandamere Press, 1998), 22.

7. Lewin, *Infantile Paralysis*, 74–76; Alex J. Steigman, "Diagnosis and General Care of Acute Poliomyelitis," *Pediatric Clinics of North America* 1 (1953): 17.

8. Marilyn Rogers in Seavey, Smith, and Wagner, *A Paralyzing Fear*, 25; Stanley L. Lipshultz, "Tough Love in the 50s, Mainstreaming and Support Groups," in *Managing Post-Polio: A Guide to Living Well with Post-Polio Syndrome*, ed. Lauro S. Halstead and Naomi Naierman (Washington, DC: NRH Press, 1998), 211; Robert Hudson in Sink, *The Grit behind the Miracle*, 143; Dorothea Nudelman and David Willingham, *Healing the Blues: Drug-Free Psychotherapy for Depression* (Pacific Grove, CA: Boxwood Press, 1994), 13.

9. Pugleasa in Seavey, Smith, and Wagner, *Paralyzing Fear*, 124; Mary E. Cook, "The Boy Who Never Came in Last," *Redbook* 120 (January 1963): 8.

10. Kenneth Kingery, *As I Live and Breathe* (New York: Grosset & Dunlap, 1966), 21; Mee, *A Nearly Normal Life*, 16.

11. Herbert J. Kaufmann, "The Impact of the 1955 Poliomyelitis Outbreak on the Boston City Hospital," *Boston Medical Quarterly* 7 (March 1956): 7; Grace Audet in Sass, *Polio's Legacy*, 249; Mary P. Wilson, interview by author, tape recording, Allentown, PA, October 10, 1989; Martha Mason, *Breath: Life in the Rhythm of an Iron Lung* (Asheboro, NC: Down Home Press, 2003), 172, 175–76.

12. Irving Kenneth Zola, "The Continuing Odyssey of a Medical Sociologist," in *Socio-Medical Inquiries: Recollections, Reflections, and Reconsiderations* (Philadelphia: Temple University Press, 1983), 9; Pugleasa in Seavey, Smith, and Wagner, *A Paralyzing Fear*, 125; Shirley A. Whisman, e-mail to SJU Polio and Post Polio Syndrome List, October 22, 1998; Mary P. Wilson interview; Kathryn Black, *In the Shadow of Polio: A Personal and Social History* (Reading, MA: Addison-Wesley Publishing Co., 1996), 68–69; Mee, *A Nearly Normal Life*, 26; Josephine Howard in Seavey, Smith, and Wagner, *A Paralyzing Fear*, 39.

13. Morris Siegel and Morris Greenberg, "Risk of Paralytic and Nonparalytic Forms of Poliomyelitis to Household Contacts," *JAMA* 155 (May 29, 1954): 430; Dorothy M. Horstmann, "Clinical Epidemiology of Poliomyelitis," *Annals of Internal Medicine* 43 (1955): 532; Richard Aldrich, M.D., in Seavey, Smith, and Wagner, *A Paralyzing Fear*, 115; Black, *In the Shadow of Polio*, 28–29; William S. Langford, "Physical Illness and Convalescence: Their Meaning to the Child," *Journal of Pediatrics* 33 (1948): 242–43; L. McCarty Fairchild, "Some Psychological Factors Observed in Poliomyelitis Patients," *American Journal of Physical Medicine* 31 (1952): 277; Richard H. Young, "The Patient's Attitude toward Po-

liomyelitis," *Mental Hygiene* 33 (1949): 265; Steigman, "Diagnosis and General Care of Poliomyelitis," 18.

14. Nudelman and Willingham, *Healing the Blues,* 40; Mee, *A Nearly Normal Life,* 17–18; Zola, "Continuing Odyssey," 9.

15. Larry Alexander, as told to Adam Barnett, *The Iron Cradle* (New York: Thomas Y. Crowell Co., 1954), 17, 19.

16. Gallagher, *Black Bird Fly Away,* 29–32; for another account of a tracheotomy without anesthesia, see Roger Winter, with Kenneth F. Hall, *Point after Touchdown* (Anderson, IN: Warner Press, 1944), 44.

17. David J. Rothman, *Beginnings Count: The Technological Imperative in American Health Care,* A Twentieth Century Fund Book (New York: Oxford University Press, 1997), 42–66; Robert M. Eiben, "The Polio Experience and the Twilight of the Contagious Disease Hospital," in *Polio,* ed. Thomas M. Daniel and Frederick C. Robbins (Rochester, NY: University of Rochester Press, 1997), 104.

18. John R. Paul, *A History of Poliomyelitis* (New Haven: Yale University Press, 1971), 331; Rothman, *Beginnings Count,* 45; Louise Lake, *Each Day a Bonus: Twenty-five Courageous Years in a Wheelchair* (Salt Lake City: Deseret Book Co., 1971), 10.

19. Paralytic cases typically made up less than 3 percent of infections and typically there was one death for every 11–13 paralytic cases. Neal Nathanson and John R. Martin, "The Epidemiology of Poliomyelitis: Enigmas Surrounding Its Appearance, Epidemicity, and Disappearance," *American Journal of Epidemiology* 110 (1979): 681; Josephine Howard in Seavey, Smith, and Wagner, *A Paralyzing Fear,* 39; Luther Robinson, *We Made Peace with Polio* (Nashville, TN: Broadman Press, 1960), 51–52, 76.

20. Lynne Dunphy, "'Constant and Relentless': The Nursing Care of Patients in Iron Lungs, 1928–1955," in *Nursing Research: A Qualitative Perspective,* 3rd ed., ed. Patricia L. Munhall (Sudbury, MA: Jones and Bartlett Publishers, 2001), 422.

21. Black, *In the Shadow of Polio* 54 (quotation), 64.

22. Dunphy, "'Constant and Relentless,'" 417–38; *Nursing for the Poliomyelitis Patient* (New York: The Joint Orthopedic Nursing Advisory Service of the National Organization for Public Health Nursing and the League of Nursing Education, 1948); Gallagher, *Black Bird Fly Away,* 26, 34; and Anne Walters and Jim Marugg, *Beyond Endurance* (New York: Harper & Brothers Publishers, 1954), 54.

23. Louis Sternburg and Dorothy Sternburg, with Monica Dickens, *View from the Seesaw* (New York: Dodd, Mead & Co., 1986), 14, 23; Gallagher, *Black Bird Fly Away,* 42–43; see also, Alexander, *Iron Cradle,* 48–49; Winter, *Point after Touchdown,* 45–46.

24. Walters and Marugg, *Beyond Endurance,* 54, 57; Gallagher, *Black Bird Fly Away,* 37, 46.

25. Walters and Marugg, *Beyond Endurance,* 55–56; Arnold Beisser, *Flying without Wings: Personal Reflections on Being Disabled* (New York: Doubleday, 1989), 18–19, 38; Howard Brody, *Stories of Sickness* (New Haven: Yale University Press, 1987), 133–34; Gallagher, *Black Bird Fly Away,* 44.

26. Beisser, *Flying*, 34; Regina Woods, *Tales from Inside the Iron Lung* (Philadelphia: University of Pennsylvania Press), 6; Rogers in Seavey, Smith, and Wagner, *A Paralyzing Fear*, 27–28.

27. Sternburg and Sternburg, *View from the Seesaw*, 19, 26; Woods, *Tales from Inside the Iron Lung*, 7, see also Mason, *Breath*, 175–76.

28. The following two paragraphs were originally published in Daniel J. Wilson, "Crippled Manhood: Infantile Paralysis and the Construction of Masculinity," *Medical Humanities Review* 12 (Fall 1998): 14–15.

29. Kingery, *As I Live and Breathe*, 46–47, 50–51; Beisser, *Flying*, 21–22.

30. Beisser, *Flying*, 22; Kingery, *As I Live and Breathe*, 79; Lorenzo Milam, *Cripple Liberation Front Marching Band Blues* (San Diego: Mho & Mho Works, 1984), 24.

31. John Affeldt in Seavey, Smith, and Wagner, *A Paralyzing Fear*, 143.

32. Woods, *Tales from Inside the Iron Lung*, 6–7; Kingery, *As I Live and Breathe*, 49, 51; Gallagher, *Black Bird Fly Away*, 47; see also, Alexander, *The Iron Cradle*, 49.

33. Polio often affected the lower leg. Many polio patients were unable to keep their feet at a 90-degree angle to their legs, a deformity called foot drop. If a patient couldn't keep her feet flat against the footboard (fig. 4), her feet were tied to the board. The theory was that keeping them in the natural position would lessen the deformity. Lewin, *Infantile Paralysis*, 138 (quotation), 136–55; Paul, *A History of Poliomyelitis*, 338.

34. Paul, *A History of Poliomyelitis*, 339.

35. Gallagher, *Black Bird Fly Away*, 37–38; Robert F. Hall, *Through the Storm: A Polio Story* (St. Cloud, MN: North Star Press, 1990), 7; Richard Owen in Sass, *Polio's Legacy*, 32; Gurney in Sass, *Polio's Legacy*, 25; and Paul, *A History of Poliomyelitis*, 339–340.

36. Elizabeth Kenny, *The Treatment of Infantile Paralysis in the Acute Stage* (Minneapolis: Bruce Publishing Co., 1941), 21–22.

37. Kenny, *Treatment of Infantile Paralysis in the Acute Stage*, 91; and John F. Pohl, in collaboration with Sister Elizabeth Kenny, *The Kenny Concept of Infantile Paralysis and Its Treatment* (Minneapolis: Bruce Publishing Co., 1943), 46–51.

38. Roland H. Berg, *The Challenge of Polio: The Crusade against Infantile Paralysis* (New York: Dial Press, 1946), 164; Paul, *A History of Poliomyelitis*, 344.

39. Kenny, *Treatment of Infantile Paralysis in the Acute Stage*, 97–118; Pohl, *The Kenny Concept of Infantile Paralysis and Its Treatment*, 64–73.

40. Margaret Benbow in Sink, *The Grit behind the Miracle*, 149–50; Mee, *A Nearly Normal Life*, 64–65; Nudelman and Willingham, *Healing the Blues*, 55–57; Kimball in Sass, *Polio's Legacy*, 113; see also, Gallagher, *Black Bird Fly Away*, 43.

41. Nudelman and Willingham, *Healing the Blues*, 59–60, 56.

42. Hall, *Through the Storm*, 7–8; Joyce Ann Tepley, "Polio Memories from the Class of 1952 and Maturing with Polio," in Halstead and Naierman, *Managing Post-Polio*, 193.

43. Grile, 203; Audet, 251; Kimball, 113; Gurney, 23; and Edmund J. Sass, 94; all in Sass, *Polio's Legacy*; Victor Raisman, "Orthopedic Treatment of Acute and Subacute Poliomyelitis with Curare and Stretching," *New York State Journal of Medicine* 52 (May 1, 1952): 1147–49.

44. Mee, *A Nearly Normal Life,* 64, 70.

45. Hall, *Through the Storm,* 12, 14, 7; Milam, *Cripple Liberation Front Marching Band Blues,* 23–25.

46. Hall, *Through the Storm,* 13; Milam, *Cripple Liberation Front Marching Band Blues,* 11, 24; Beisser, *Flying,* 33.

47. Charles L. Mee, Jr., *A Visit to Haldeman and Other States of Mind* (New York: M. Evans and Co., 1977), 146; Mee, *A Nearly Normal Life,* 31–32; Irving Kenneth Zola, *Missing Pieces: A Chronicle of Living with a Disability* (Philadelphia: Temple University Press, 1982), 218–19, see also 210.

48. Hall, *Through the Storm,* 20, 22.

49. Kingery, *As I Live and Breathe,* 56; Sternburg and Sternburg, *View from the Seesaw,* 26; Mee, *A Nearly Normal Life,* 26; for Linda Atkins it was the sound of her father's footsteps: *Jamaica and Me: The Story of an Unusual Friendship* (New York: Random House, 1998), xii.

50. Fred Davis, *Passage through Crisis: Polio Victims and Their Families* (1963; reprint, with a new introduction, New Brunswick, NJ: Transaction Publishers, 1991), 68–69; see also, Joseph Greenblum, "The Control of Sick-Care Functions in the Hospitalization of a Child: Family versus the Hospital," *Journal of Health and Human Behavior* 11 (Spring 1961): 34–35.

51. Alex Steigman recommended home care "when clinical and domestic circumstances permit": "Diagnosis and General Care of Acute Poliomyelitis," 18. Philip Lewin provides guidelines for home care of poliomyelitis in *Infantile Paralysis,* 118.

52. Dick Weir, "Memories from Dick Weir," in *Memories: A Tribute to Polio Survivors* (Atlanta, GA: Atlanta Post-Polio Association, 1997), 18–19.

53. Gallagher, *Black Bird Fly Away,* 38; Audet in Sass, *Polio's Legacy,* 250; Sternburg and Sternburg, *View from the Seesaw,* 26.

54. John R. Paul, "Epidemiology of Poliomyelitis," *Poliomyelitis* (Geneva: World Health Organization, 1955), 18–19; Siegel and Greenberg, "Risk of Paralytic and Nonparalytic Forms of Poliomyelitis to Household Contacts," 430; Ann L. McLaughlin, "One Couple's Journey from Paralysis to Post-Polio," in *Polio,* ed. Thomas M. Daniel and Frederick C. Robbins (Rochester, NY: Rochester University Press, 1997), 46–65, quotation on 46; Black, *In the Shadow of Polio,* 20–22.

55. John Earl Lindell and Ethel Brooks Lindell, *Oh God, Help Me!* (Tempe, AZ: John Earl Lindell, 1988), 10; Sternburg and Sternburg, *View from the Seesaw,* 27–28.

56. James Carroll, *An American Requiem: God, My Father, and the War That Came Between Us* (Boston: Houghton Mifflin Co., 1996), 44, 46; Kathryn Vastyshak interview, by author, Allentown, PA, June 25, 2002.

57. Mary P. Wilson interview; Pugleasa in Seavey, Smith, and Wagner, *A Paralyzing Fear,* 128; Davis, *Passage through Crisis,* 38.

58. Kingery, *As I Live and Breathe,* 62; Alexander, *Iron Cradle,* 42; Schwartz in Seavey, Smith, and Wagner, *A Paralyzing Fear,* 257; David L. Sills, *The Volunteers: Means and Ends in a National Organization* (Glencoe, IL: Free Press, 1957), 131.

59. Sills, *The Volunteers,* 133–35, quotations on 134, 135; Rosemary Marx in Sass, *Polio's Legacy,* 233; Sass in Sass, *Polio's Legacy,* 95.

60. Horstmann, "Clinical Epidemiology of Poliomyelitis," 528.

CHAPTER FOUR

1. Steven E. Koop, *We Hold This Treasure: The Story of Gillette Children's Hospital* (Afton, MN: Afton Historical Society Press, 1998); Colleen Adair Fliedner, *Rancho: Rancho Los Amigos Medical Center Centennial, 1888–1988* (Downey, CA: Rancho Los Amigos Medical Center, 1990); George J. Boines, "The Kenny Treatment of Anterior Poliomyelitis," typescript, Elizabeth Kenny Papers, box 4, Minnesota Historical Society; Turnley Walker, *Roosevelt and the Warm Springs Story* (New York: A. A. Wyn, 1953). The narratives describe the types of facilities mentioned in the text and the varying treatment they provided.

2. Fred Davis, "Definitions of Time and Recovery in Paralytic Polio Convalescence" in *An Introduction to Deviance: Readings in the Process of Making Deviants,* ed. William J. Filstead (Chicago: Markham Publishing Co., 1972), 115–16. Parts of this paragraph have been adapted from my "Covenants of Work and Grace: Themes of Recovery and Redemption in Polio Narratives," *Literature and Medicine* 13 (1994): 22–41. Multiple sclerosis patients in the 1950s were also told that hard work and determination would help them conquer their illness: Colin Talley, "The Treatment of Multiple Sclerosis in Los Angeles and the United States, 1947–1960," *Bulletin of the History of Medicine* 77 (Winter 2003): 896–97.

3. Ruth O'Brien, *Crippled Justice: The History of Modern Disability Policy in the Workplace* (Chicago: University of Chicago Press, 2001), 5–8; Elaine Tyler May, *Homeward Bound: American Families in the Cold War Era* (New York: Basic Books, 1988), 3–11.

4. John E. Affeldt, "Recent Advances in the Treatment of Poliomyelitis," *JAMA* 156 (September 4, 1954): 13; Philip Lewin, *Infantile Paralysis: Anterior Poliomyelitis* (Philadelphia: W. B. Saunders Co., 1941), 136, 138; Miland E. Knapp, "Rehabilitation in Severe Poliomyelitis," reprint from *Journal of the Iowa State Medical Society* (September 1953): n.p. Sister Kenny Papers, box 6, Minnesota Historical Society. See also, John F. Pohl, in collaboration with Elizabeth Kenny, *The Kenny Concept of Infantile Paralysis and Its Treatment* (Minneapolis: Bruce Publishing Co., 1943), 153; and Elizabeth Kenny, *The Treatment of Infantile Paralysis in the Acute Stage* (Minneapolis: Bruce Publishing Co., 1941), 45–79.

5. "Infantile Paralysis: Pioneers in Treatment," *Physical Therapy* 56 (January 1976): 42, 44; Glenn Gritzer and Arnold Arluke, *The Making of Rehabilitation: A Political Economy of Medical Specialization, 1890–1980* (Berkeley: University of California Press, 1985), 38–39.

6. Jay Schleichkorn, "Physical Therapist, 98, Recalls Rehabilitating Franklin Roosevelt," *PT Bulletin* (March 16, 1988): 24–26.

7. John R. Paul, *A History of Poliomyelitis* (New Haven: Yale University Press, 1971), 344; Gritzer and Arluke, *The Making of Rehabilitation,* 90; Roland H. Berg, *The Challenge of Polio: The Crusade against Infantile Paralysis* (New York: Dial Press, 1946), 166; O'Brien, *Crippled Justice,* 6–8.

8. Lewin, *Infantile Paralysis*, 190; William T. Green, "Orthopedic Management of Poliomyelitis," *Pediatric Clinics of North America* 1 (1953): 36.

9. Lewin, *Infantile Paralysis*, 156, 157, 166.

10. Green, "Orthopedic Management," 37.

11. See, for example, Harold A. Littledale, "Hope and Courage . . . That Is Warm Springs," reprinted from the *New York Times Magazine,* January 23, 1944, Georgia Warm Springs File, Franklin D. Roosevelt Library; "The Georgia Warm Springs Foundation at Warm Springs, Georgia" (Warm Springs, GA: The Foundation, 1932), Georgia Warm Springs File, Franklin D. Roosevelt Library; Turnley Walker, *Roosevelt and the Warm Springs Story* (New York: A. A. Wyn, 1953); Theo Lippman, Jr., *The Squire of Warm Springs: FDR in Georgia, 1924–1945* (Chicago: Playboy Press Paperbacks, 1977); Hugh Gregory Gallagher, *FDR's Splendid Deception,* revised (Arlington, VA: Vandamere Press, 1994), 34–67; Tony Gould, *A Summer Plague: Polio and Its Survivors* (New Haven: Yale University Press, 1995), 29–84; and Geoffrey C. Ward, *A First-Class Temperament: The Emergence of Franklin Roosevelt* (New York: Harper & Row, Publishers, 1989), 704–99.

12. Gallagher, *Splendid Deception,* 55, 56–57.

13. Letter, H. N. Hooper to Basil O'Connor, May 8, 1937, President's Personal File 76, Franklin D. Roosevelt Library; Letter, Basil O'Connor to Franklin D. Roosevelt, May 11, 1937, President's Personal File 76, Franklin D. Roosevelt Library.

14. John Hume in *A Paralyzing Fear: The Triumph over Polio in America,* ed. Nina Gilden Seavey, Jane S. Smith, and Paul Wagner (New York: TV Books, 1998), 157–61; Clara Yelder in Seavey, Smith, and Wagner, *A Paralyzing Fear,* 155.

15. "The Kenny Concept and Technique of Poliomyelitis," 1, 3, 5–6, 11, typescript, Sister Kenny Papers, box 2, Minnesota Historical Society; Pohl and Kenny, *The Kenny Concept,* 153. For detailed instructions on applying foments, see Kenny, *Treatment of Infantile Paralysis,* 64–69; and Pohl, *The Kenny Concept,* 97–118.

16. Knapp, "Rehabilitation in Severe Poliomyelitis."

17. James E. Dyson, "The Kenny Treatment of Infantile Paralysis," reprinted from the *Journal of the Iowa State Medical Society* (July 1942 and August 1943), n.p., Sister Kenny Papers, box 4; George J. Boines, "The Kenny Treatment of Anterior Poliomyelitis: Report of Cases and a Preliminary Report on the Use of Prostigmin," typescript, 14, 19, Sister Kenny Papers, box 4; Milton J. Wilder and John J. Untereker, "Evaluation of Results of Sister Kenny Treatment of Infantile Paralysis of 1942 Epidemic at the Kosair Crippled Children's Hospital [Louisville, KY]," typescript, n.p., Sister Kenny Papers, box 4; all in the Minnesota Historical Society.

18. Jesse Wright, "Physical and Occupational Therapy in Poliomyelitis," *Pediatric Clinics of North America* (1953), 27–28, 31, 32–34.

19. Lewin, *Infantile Paralysis,* 191; Green, "Orthopedic Management of Poliomyelitis," 38.

20. Lewin, *Infantile Paralysis,* 209; Green, "Orthopedic Management of Poliomyelitis," 39.

21. Green, "Orthopedic Management of Poliomyelitis," 39–41. Philip Lewin describes a wide variety of soft- and hard-tissue surgeries; Lewin, *Infantile Paralysis*, 209–322.

22. Davis, "Definitions of Time and Recovery in Paralytic Polio Convalescence," 110, 111–12.

23. Ibid., 112.

24. Ibid., 112–13.

25. Ibid., 113–14.

26. Green, "Orthopedic Management of Poliomyelitis," 35.

27. Arnold Beisser, *Flying without Wings: Personal Reflections on Loss, Disability, and Healing* (New York: Bantam Books, 1990), 53–54; Bell Gale Chevigny also uses the image of the medieval rack: Bell Gale Chevigny, "Eclipse: A Theater Workshop on Disability or, Reflections on Ahab's Tribe," *Michigan Quarterly Review* 37 (Spring 1998): 272.

28. Lorenzo Milam, *The Cripple Liberation Front Marching Band Blues* (San Diego: Mho & Mho Works, 1984), 16, 17; Hugh Gregory Gallagher, *Black Bird Fly Away: Disabled in an Able-Bodied World* (Arlington, VA: Vandamere Press, 1998), 44, 53.

29. Ed Keohan, e-mail to SJU Polio and Post Polio Syndrome List, June 17, 1999; David G. Henson, e-mail to SJU Polio and Post Polio Syndrome List, June 21, 1999.

30. Irving Kenneth Zola, "The Continuing Odyssey of a Medical Sociologist," in *Socio-Medical Inquiries: Recollections, Reflections, and Reconsiderations* (Philadelphia: Temple University Press, 1983), 9; Charles L. Mee, *A Nearly Normal Life: A Memoir* (Boston: Little, Brown and Co., 1999), 69–70; Wilfred Sheed, *In Love with Daylight: A Memoir of Recovery* (New York: Simon & Schuster, 1995), 29.

31. Robert F. Hall, *Through the Storm: A Polio Story* (St. Cloud, MN: North Star Press), 84; Edward Le Comte, *The Long Road Back: The Story of My Encounter with Polio* (Boston: Beacon Press, 1957), 96–97.

32. Fred Davis, *Passage through Crisis: Polio Victims and Their Families* (Indianapolis: Bobbs-Merrill Co., 1963; reprint, with a new forward by Fred Davis, New Brunswick, NJ: Transaction Publishers, 1991), 71.

33. Sheed, *In Love with Daylight*, 29; Zola, "Continuing Odyssey," 9; Kenneth Kingery, *As I Live and Breathe* (New York: Grosset & Dunlap, 1966), 87; Charles L. Mee, Jr., *A Visit to Haldeman and Other States of Mind* (New York: M. Evans and Co., 1977), 152–53.

34. See especially Gallagher, *FDR's Splendid Deception*, xiii–xiv, 91–105, and Ward, *A First-Class Temperament*, 781–83.

35. Jan Little, *If It Weren't for the Honor—I'd Rather Have Walked: Previously Untold Tales of the Journey to the ADA* (Cambridge, MA: Brookline Books, 1996), 10–12; Mee, *A Nearly Normal Life*, 95.

36. Mee, *A Nearly Normal Life*, 97; Leonard Kriegel, *The Long Walk Home* (New York: Appleton-Century, 1964), 75; Leonard Kriegel, *Falling into Life: Essays* (San Francisco: North Point Press, 1991), 9; and Ray K. Gullickson in *Polio's Legacy: An Oral History*, ed. Edmund J. Sass, with George Gottfried and Anthony Sorem (Lanham, MD: University Press of America, 1996), 46.

37. Le Comte, *The Long Road Back,* 88; Mee, *A Nearly Normal Life,* 98–100.

38. Le Comte, *The Long Road Back,* 96; Hall, *Through the Storm,* 79–80; Robert Gurney in Sass, *Polio's Legacy,* 26–27.

39. Mee, *A Nearly Normal Life,* 102; Hall, *Through the Storm,* 97; Kriegel, *Falling into Life,* 9–14.

40. Richard Field, "Cases from the Medical Grand Rounds, Massachusetts General Hospital: Case 243, Respiratory and Other Problems in the Adult with Poliomyelitis," *American Practitioner and Digest of Treatment* (April 4, 1953): 272; see also John E. Affeldt, "Recent Advances in the Treatment of Poliomyelitis," *JAMA* 156 (September 4, 1954): 12–15.

41. John Affeldt in Seavey, Smith, and Wagner, *A Paralyzing Fear,* 142–43; Fliedner, *Rancho,* 227; Robert M. Eiben, "The Polio Experience and the Twilight of the Contagious Disease Hospital," in *Polio,* ed. Thomas M. Daniel and Frederick C. Robbins (Rochester, NY: University of Rochester Press, 1997), 114–16.

42. Kathryn Black, *In the Shadow of Polio: A Personal and Social History* (Reading, MA: Addison-Wesley Publishing Co., 1996), 117–21; see also Thomas M. Daniel, "Polio and the Making of a Doctor," in Daniel and Robbins, *Polio,* 93–94; and Anne Walters and Jim Marugg, *Beyond Endurance* (New York: Harper and Brothers, 2001), 100–101.

43. Helen M. Wallace and Leona Baumgartner, "New York City Plan for Care of Poliomyelitis Patients in Respirators," *JAMA* 152 (August 15, 1953): 1506; Black, *In the Shadow of Polio,* 123–24; Eiben, "The Polio Experience and the Twilight of the Contagious Disease Hospital," 108–12; Affeldt in Seavey, Smith, and Wagner, *A Paralyzing Fear,* 139–44; Affeldt, "Recent Advances in the Treatment of Poliomyelitis," 12–15; John F. Marchand, "Care of Respiratory Paralysis from Poliomyelitis," *JAMA* 155 (August 7, 1954): 1297–1302; David J. Rothman, *Beginnings Count: The Technological Imperative in American Health Care,* A Twentieth Century Fund Book (New York: Oxford University Press, 1997), 63–64.

44. Louis Sternburg and Dorothy Sternburg, with Monica Dickens, *View from the Seesaw* (New York: Dodd, Mead & Co., 1986), 36, 46; Regina Woods, *Tales from Inside the Iron Lung (And How I Got Out of It)* (Philadelphia: University of Pennsylvania Press, 1994), 8–9.

45. Affeldt in Seavey, Smith, and Wagner, *A Paralyzing Fear,* 143; Larry Alexander, as told to Adam Barnett, *The Iron Cradle* (New York: Thomas Y. Crowell Co., 1954), 33; Sternburg and Sternburg, *View from the Seesaw,* 38.

46. Gallagher, *Black Bird Fly Away,* 51–53.

47. Sternburg and Sternburg, *View from the Seesaw,* 38–39, 63–65.

48. Sternburg and Sternburg, *View from the Seesaw,* 59, 62; Alexander, *The Iron Cradle,* 99–101.

49. Gallagher, *Black Bird Fly Away,* 54–57.

50. Mee, *A Nearly Normal Life,* 65.

51. Louise Lake, *Each Day a Bonus: Twenty-five Courageous Years in a Wheelchair* (Salt Lake City: Deseret Book Co., 1971), 31; Joan Hardee in Edith Henrich and Leonard Kriegel, eds. *Experiments in Survival* (New York: Association for the Aid of Crippled Children, 1961), 169.

52. O'Brien, *Crippled Justice*, 29–30, 52, 59.

53. Howard A. Rusk, "Rehabilitation in Poliomyelitis," *Pediatric Clinics of North America* 1 (1953): 42–43.

54. Harold M. Visotsky, David A. Hamburg, Mary E. Goss, and Binyamin Z. Lebovits, "Coping Behavior under Extreme Stress: Observations of Patients with Severe Poliomyelitis," *Archives of General Psychiatry* 5 (1961): 29, 48–49.

55. Ibid., 49–51.

56. Gallagher, *Black Bird Fly Away*, 54–57, 88–89; Sternburg and Sternburg, *View from the Seesaw*, 37, 125–27; Black, *In the Shadow of Polio*, 139.

57. Gallagher, *Black Bird Fly Away*, 44; Alexander, *The Iron Cradle*, 103–4.

58. Sternburg and Sternburg, *View from the Seesaw*, 52, 60; Alexander, *The Iron Cradle*, 239; Black, *In the Shadow of Polio*, 136–40, 196–97.

59. There were, of course, exceptions to this generalization. Dottie Sternburg spent most days with her husband: Sternburg and Sternburg, *View from the Seesaw*, 56. Anne and Charles McLaughlin had polio at the same time and stayed in the same hospital, and once Anne was mobile she spent most of the time in Charles's room: Anne L. McLaughlin, "One Couple's Journey from Paralysis to Post-Polio," in Daniel and Robbins, *Polio*, 47.

60. Sternburg and Sternburg, *View from the Seesaw*, 46, 42; Hall, *Through the Storm*, 84.

61. Dorothea Nudelman and David Willingham, *Healing the Blues: Drug-Free Psychotherapy for Depression* (Pacific Grove, CA: Boxwood Press, 1994), 22, 64–65; Mee, *A Nearly Normal Life*, 93.

CHAPTER FIVE

1. Harold A. Littledale made this point in "Hope and Courage . . . That Is Warm Springs," a pamphlet reprint from the *New York Times Magazine*, January 23, 1944, unpaginated, Georgia Warm Springs File, Franklin D. Roosevelt Library.

2. Larry Alexander, as told to Adam Barnett, *The Iron Cradle* (New York: Thomas Y. Crowell Co., 1954), 84–85; Hugh Gregory Gallagher, *Black Bird Fly Away: Disabled in an Able-Bodied World* (Arlington, VA: Vandamere Press, 1998), 71, 74. On Warm Springs, see also Bentz Plagemann, *My Place to Stand* (New York: Farrar, Straus, and Co., 1949), 150–51, 176, and Lorenzo Milam, *Cripple Liberation Front Marching Band Blues* (San Diego: Mho & Mho Works, 1984), 53.

3. Mary Phraner Warren and Don Kirkendall, *Bottom High to the Crowd* (New York: Walker and Co., 1973), 56–57; Milam, *Cripple Liberation Front*, 18–19, 53; John Swett, "Florida's Fourth of July '53," *APPA News* 12 (October–December 1997): n.p.

4. Steven E. Koop, *We Hold This Treasure: The Story of Gillette Children's Hospital* (Afton, MN: Afton Historical Society, 1998), 100; Gail Bias in *Polio's Legacy: An Oral History*, ed. Edmund J. Sass with George Gottfried and Anthony Sorem (Lanham, MD: University Press of America, 1996), 78.

5. Arvid Schwartz in *A Paralyzing Fear: The Triumph over Polio in America,* ed. Nina Gilden Seavey, Jane S. Smith, and Paul Wagner (New York: TV Books, 1998), 256; Arvid Schwartz in Sass, *Polio's Legacy,* 145–47; Larry Fournier, *I Did It! So Can You!* (Gilberg, AZ: Pussywillow Publishing House, 1988), 8; Joyce Ann Tepley, "Polio Memories from the Class of 1952 and Maturing with Polio," in *Managing Post-Polio: A Guide to Living Well with Post-Polio Syndrome,* ed. Lauro S. Halstead and Naomi Naierman (Washington, DC: NRH Press, 1998), 193–94.

6. Irving Kenneth Zola, "The Continuing Odyssey of a Medical Sociologist," in *Socio-Medical Inquiries: Recollections, Reflections, and Reconsiderations* (Philadelphia: Temple University Press, 1983), 9; Norma Duchin in Edith Henrich and Leonard Kriegel, eds., *Experiments in Survival* (New York: Association for the Aid of Crippled Children, 1961), 15; Gallagher, *Black Bird Fly Away,* 88.

7. Louis Sternburg and Dorothy Sternburg, with Monica Dickens, *View From the Seesaw* (New York: Dodd, Mead & Co., 1986), 47; Robert F. Hall, *Through the Storm: A Polio Story* (St. Cloud, MN: North Star Press, 1990), 22.

8. Kathryn Black, *In the Shadow of Polio: A Personal and Social History* (Reading, MA: Addison-Wesley Publishing Co., 1996), 127–28; Arnold Beisser, *Flying without Wings: Personal Reflections on Loss, Disability, and Healing* (New York: Bantam Books, 1989), 53–54; Plagemann, *My Place to Stand,* 180.

9. Hall, *Through the Storm,* 35–36; Dorothea Nudelman and David Willingham, *Healing the Blues: Drug-Free Psychotherapy for Depression* (Pacific Grove, CA: Boxwood Press, 1994), 52–53; Black, *In The Shadow of Polio,* 56.

10. Charlene Pugleasa in Seavey, Smith, and Wagner, *A Paralyzing Fear,* 129–30; Ray K. Gullickson in Sass, *Polio's Legacy,* 47–48; Hugh Gallagher in Seavey, Smith, and Wagner, *A Paralyzing Fear,* 57.

11. Swett, "Florida's Fourth of July '53," n.p.; Richard Foley quoted in Koop, *We Hold This Treasure,* 108.

12. Zola, "Continuing Odyssey," 15.

13. Tepley, "Polio Memories," 195; Nudelman and Willingham, *Healing the Blues,* 64–65; Charles L. Mee, *A Nearly Normal Life: A Memoir* (Boston: Little, Brown and Co., 1999), 93.

14. Mee, *A Nearly Normal Life,* 93.

15. Bill Van Cleve in Sass, *Polio's Legacy,* 185; Beisser, *Flying without Wings,* 38.

16. David Oakley, e-mail to SJU Polio and Post Polio List, June 1, 1999; Fournier, *I Did It! So Can You!,* 10; Mark O'Brien, with Gillian Kendall, *How I Became a Human Being: A Disabled Man's Quest for Independence* (Madison: University of Wisconsin Press, 2003), 91; Kenneth Kingery, *As I Live and Breathe* (New York: Grosset & Dunlap, 1966), 79.

17. Nudelman and Willingham, *Healing the Blues,* 70–71; Alice E. Sink, *The Grit behind the Miracle: A True Story of the Determination and Hard Work behind an Emergency Infantile Paralysis Hospital, 1944–1945, Hickory, North Carolina* (Lanham, MD: University Press of America, 1998), 141.

18. Clara Yelder in Seavey, Smith, and Wagner, *A Paralyzing Fear,* 154; Fournier, *I Did It! So Can You!,* 10; Leonard Kriegel, *The Long Walk Home* (New York: Appleton-Century, 1964), 58; Hall, *Through the Storm,* 64; Sternburg and Sternburg, *View from the Seesaw,* 47.

19. Tepley, "Polio Memories," 194; Grace Audet in Sass, *Polio's Legacy,* 250; Arvid Schwartz in Sass, *Polio's Legacy,* 147; David Kangas in Sass, *Polio's Legacy,* 63; Zola, "Continuing Odyssey," 10–11.

20. Len Jordan in Sass, *Polio's Legacy,* 128–29; Fournier, *I Did It! So Can You!,* 9; Bias in Sass, *Polio's Legacy,* 80; Hall, *Through the Storm,* 85–86; Kriegel, *The Long Walk Home,* 75, 92.

21. David Graham e-mail to SJU Polio and Post Polio Syndrome List, April 23, 1995; Larry Kohout, e-mail to SJU Polio and Post Polio Syndrome List, April 23, 1995; Schwartz in Sass, *Polio's Legacy,* 147; Kangas in Sass, *Polio's Legacy,* 63.

22. Kriegel, *The Long Walk Home,* 45–47, 52–55, 62–72, 76–87, 98–106.

23. Erika, April 1, 1998; Ed Wood, April 18, 1995; and Joy Hillhouse, April 2, 1998, all e-mail to SJU Polio and Post Polio Syndrome List.

24. W. H. Henderson, November 5, 1996; David Olson, April 18, 1995; David Graham, April 18, 1995, all e-mail to SJU Polio and Post Polio Syndrome List; Hall, *Through the Storm,* 86.

25. Charles L. Mee, Jr., *A Visit to Haldeman and Other States of Mind* (New York: M. Evans and Co., 1977), 146; Mee, *A Nearly Normal Life,* 31–32; Irving Kenneth Zola, *Missing Pieces: A Chronicle of Living with a Disability* (Philadelphia: Temple University Press, 1982), 218; Sternburg and Sternburg, *View from the Seesaw,* 41; Michael W. R. Davis, "Personal Memoir from the 1944 Kentucky Polio Epidemic," in *Polio,* ed. Thomas M. Daniel and Frederick C. Robbins (Rochester, NY: University of Rochester Press, 1997), 35.

26. Zola, "Continuing Odyssey," 10; Warren and Kirkendall, *Bottom High to the Crowd,* 100; Beisser, *Flying without Wings,* 53–54.

27. Billie McCabe, April 22, 1995; Ed Keohan, October 12, 1998; both e-mail to SJU Polio and Post Polio Syndrome List; Warren and Kirkendall, *Bottom High to the Crowd,* 80.

28. Zola, *Missing Pieces,* 206; Milam, *Cripple Liberation Front,* 61; Gallagher, *Black Bird Fly Away,* 81.

29. Gallagher, *Black Bird Fly Away,* 71.

30. Gallagher, *Black Bird Fly Away,* 81; Milam, *Cripple Liberation Front,* 82–83.

31. Milam, *Cripple Liberation Front,* 83; Gallagher, *Black Bird Fly Away,* 81; Milam, *Cripple Liberation Front,* 82; Gallagher, *Black Bird Fly Away,* 88–89.

32. Beisser, *Flying without Wings,* 53; Teders in Sass, *Polio's Legacy,* 195; Omega, e-mail to SJU Polio and Post Polio Syndrome List, December 7, 1995; Fournier, *I Did It! So Can You!,* 9–10; Nudelman and Willingham, *Healing the Blues,* 73.

33. W. Weatherbee, e-mail to SJU Polio and Post Polio Syndrome List, June 22, 1999; Tepley, "Polio Memories," 194; Schwartz in Seavey, Smith, and Wagner, *A Paralyzing Fear,* 257–58.

34. Bias in Sass, *Polio's Legacy*, 80–81.

35. Warren and Kirkendall, *Bottom High to the Crowd*, 57–58; RoxieLady, December 6, 1995; and David Graham, April 27, 1995; both e-mail to SJU Polio and Post Polio Syndrome List.

36. Edmund J. Sass in Sass, *Polio's Legacy*, 102; Roxann O'Brien, e-mail to SJU Polio and Post Polio Syndrome List, June 21, 1999.

37. Koop, *We Hold This Treasure*, 102.

38. Kingery, *As I Live and Breathe*, 56–57.

39. Yelder in Seavey, Smith, and Wagner, *A Paralyzing Fear*, 154; MGB, e-mail to SJU Polio and Post Polio Syndrome List, June 22, 1999; Schwartz in Sass, *Polio's Legacy*, 147–48.

40. Jana Weston, September 25, 1996; and RoxieLady, November 9, 1995; both e-mail to SJU Polio and Post Polio Syndrome List; Kathryn Vastyshak, Interview by Daniel J. Wilson, June 25, 2002, Allentown, PA; Ed Keohan, June 16, 1999; and Iva Grover, April 13, 1995; both e-mail to SJU Polio and Post Polio Syndrome List.

41. Fournier, *I Did It! So Can You!*, 9; and Jana Weston, September 25, 1996; and RoxieLady, November 9, 1995; both e-mail to SJU Polio and Post Polio Syndrome List.

42. Davis, *Passage through Crisis*, 66; and "Progress Notes, May 16, 1954" for Janice Knight from State Hospital for Crippled Children, Elizabethtown, PA, used by permission of Janice (Knight) Hartman.

43. Zola, "Continuing Odyssey," 9–10; and Gus Petitt, e-mail to SJU Polio and Post Polio Syndrome List, April 12, 1995.

44. Fournier, *I Did It! So Can You!*, 11; Swett, "Florida's Fourth of July '53," n.p.; Larry Alexander, as told to Adam Barnett, *The Iron Cradle* (New York: Thomas Y. Crowell Co., 1954), 77.

45. Schwartz in Seavey, Smith, and Wagner, *A Paralyzing Fear*, 259–60; Anne Walters and Jim Marugg, *Beyond Endurance* (New York: Harper & Brothers, Publishers, 1954), 105, 119.

46. Sternburg and Sternburg, *View from the Seesaw*, 66, 71; Walters and Marugg, *Beyond Endurance*, 121; John Affeldt in Seavey, Smith, and Wagner, *A Paralyzing Fear*, 141–42.

CHAPTER SIX

1. Philip Lewin, *Infantile Paralysis: Anterior Poliomyelitis* (Philadelphia: W. B. Saunders Co., 1941), 166, 190; John F. Pohl, in collaboration with Sister Elizabeth Kenny, *The Kenny Concept of Infantile Paralysis and Its Treatment* (Minneapolis: Bruce Publishing Co., 1943), 333.

2. William T. Green, "The Management of Poliomyelitis: The Convalescent Stage," in *Poliomyelitis: Papers and Discussions Presented at the First International Poliomyelitis Conference* (Philadelphia: J. B. Lippincott Co., 1949), 165, 181–82.

3. Fred Davis, *Passage through Crisis: Polio Victims and Their Families* (Indianapolis: Bobbs-

Merrill Co., 1963; reprint, with a new forward by Fred Davis, New Brunswick, NJ: Transaction Publishers, 1991), 49, 64, 51.

4. Ibid., 73–74.

5. John Earl Lindell and Ethel Brooks Lindell, *Oh God, Help Me! For I Cannot Help Myself: A True Story of Faith in the Life of a Polio Survivor* (Tempe, AZ: John Earl Lindell, 1988), 40; Turnley Walker, *Rise Up and Walk* (New York: E. P. Dutton, 1950), 92–93; Louise Lake, *Each Day a Bonus: Twenty-five Courageous Years in a Wheelchair* (Salt Lake City: Deseret Book Co., 1971), 43; Leonard Kriegel, *The Long Walk Home* (New York: Appleton-Century, 1964), 116–17.

6. Kathryn Black, *In the Shadow of Polio: A Personal and Social History* (Reading, MA: Addison-Wesley, 1996), 149; Louis Sternburg and Dorothy Sternburg, with Monica Dickens, *View from the Seesaw* (New York: Dodd, Mead & Co., 1986), 64–65, 70–71, 75; Marilyn Rogers in Sass, *Polio's Legacy,* 57; and Roger Winter with Kenneth F. Hall, *Point after Touchdown* (Anderson, IN: Warner Press, 1964), 58.

7. David Kangas in Sass, *Polio's Legacy,* 64; Ray K. Gullickson in Sass, *Polio's Legacy,* 48.

8. Charles H. Andrews, *No Time for Tears* (Garden City, NY: Doubleday & Co., 1951), 136–37.

9. Sternburg and Sternburg, *View from the Seesaw,* 72–73; Regina Woods, *Tales from Inside the Iron Lung (And How I Got Out of It)* (Philadelphia: University of Pennsylvania Press, 1994), 9; Kriegel, *Long Walk Home,* 117–18; Ken W. Purdy, " . . . The Rest of Me Is Alive," *McCall's* 81 (October 1953): 71.

10. Woods, *Tales from Inside the Iron Lung,* 8; Hugh Gregory Gallagher, *Black Bird Fly Away: Disabled in an Able-Bodied World* (Arlington, VA: Vandamere Press, 1998), 88–89; Lorenzo W. Milam, *The Cripple Liberation Front Marching Band Blues* (San Diego: Mho & Mho Works, 1984), 88.

11. Joyce Ann Tepley, "Polio Memories from the Class of 1952 and Maturing with Polio" in *Managing Post-Polio: A Guide to Living Well with Post-Polio Syndrome,* ed. Lauro S. Halstead and Naomi Naierman (Washington, DC: NRH Press, 1998), 196; Leonard Kriegel, "Uncle Tom and Tiny Tim: Some Reflections on the Cripple as Negro," *American Scholar* 38 (Summer 1969): 417–18.

12. Arvid Schwartz in *A Paralyzing Fear: The Triumph over Polio in America,* ed. Nina Gilden Seavey, Jane S. Smith, and Paul Wagner (New York: TV Books, 1998), 261–62; Charles L. Mee, *A Nearly Normal Life: A Memoir* (Boston: Little, Brown and Co., 1998), 121.

13. Richard Owen in Seavey, Smith, and Wagner, *A Paralyzing Fear,* 238–39; Mary Grimley Mason, *Life Prints: A Memoir of Healing and Discovery* (New York: Feminist Press at City University of New York, 1999), 7; Clara Yelder in Seavey, Smith, and Wagner, *A Paralyzing Fear,* 155–56; Paul Reitmeir, interview by Daniel J. Wilson, Bethlehem, PA, August 2, 2002.

14. Lynne Dunphy, "'Constant and Relentless': The Nursing Care of Patients in Iron Lungs, 1928–1955," in *Nursing Research: A Qualitative Perspective,* 3rd ed., ed. Patricia L. Munhall (Sudbury, MA: Jones and Bartlett Publishers, 2001), 433; Sternburg and Stern-

burg, *View from the Seesaw*, 75; Marilyn Rogers in Seavey, Smith, and Wagner, *A Paralyzing Fear*, 30; Winter, *Point after Touchdown*, 59–62.

15. Dick Weir, "Illinois Memories," in *Memories: A Tribute to Polio Survivors* (Atlanta: Atlanta Post-Polio Association, 1997), 18–19; Worth Younts in *The Grit behind the Miracle: A True Story of the Determination and Hard Work behind an Emergency Infantile Paralysis Hospital, 1944–1945, Hickory, North Carolina*, ed. Alice E. Sink (Lanham, MD: University Press of America, 1998), 122; Grace Audet in Sass, *Polio's Legacy*, 251; Charlene Pugleasa in Seavey, Smith, and Wagner, *A Paralyzing Fear*, 131; Anita Bjorling, e-mail to SJU Polio and Post Polio Syndrome List, March 17, 1999; Franklin D. Roosevelt to Edward H. Barker, December 19, 1934, and attached newspaper clipping "Victim Has Own 'Warm Springs,'" President's Personal File 50, Franklin D. Roosevelt Library.

16. Kathryn Vastyshak, interview by Daniel J. Wilson, Allentown, PA, June 25, 2002; Paul Reitmeir interview; James Berry in Sass, *Polio's Legacy*, 226; Weir, "Illinois Memories," 18–19; Alexandra York, "My Father Gave Me Life—Twice," *Reader's Digest* 133 (August 1988): 55; Purdy, " . . . The Rest of Me Is Alive," 71; Mary E. Cook, "The Boy Who Never Came in Last," *Redbook* 120 (January 1963): 8.

17. Bill Van Cleve in Sass, *Polio's Legacy*, 184; Jack Schwartz, June 17, 1998; and Loreen Wells, May 29, 1995; both e-mail to SJU Polio and Post Polio Syndrome xList.

18. Edmund J. Sass in Sass, *Polio's Legacy*, 96; Stuart Goldschen in Sass, *Polio's Legacy*, 201; Wanda Peterson, May 24, 1997; and Marsha in Texas, May 25, 1997; both e-mail to SJU Polio and Post Polio List; Bonnie Bonham, "Memories," in *Memories: A Tribute to Polio Survivors* (Atlanta: Atlanta Post-Polio Association, 1997), 11; Mary Phraner Warren and Don Kirkendall, *Bottom High to the Crowd* (New York: Walker and Co., 1973), 44; Sharon Kimball in Sass, *Polio's Legacy*, 116.

19. James Carroll, *An American Requiem: God, My Father, and the War That Came Between Us* (Boston: A Mariner Book, Houghton Mifflin, 1996), 44–46.

20. Paul Reitmeir interview; Nancy Brotzman, February 19, 1999, Dick Giddings, January 29, 1999, and Linda Donahue, February 2, 1999, all e-mail to SJU Polio and Post Polio Syndrome List; Mee, *A Nearly Normal Life*, 165–66.

21. John Swett, "Florida's Fourth of July '53," *APPA News* 12 (October–December 1997): n.p.; Hugh Gallagher in Seavey, Smith, and Wagner, *A Paralyzing Fear*, 59.

22. Carroll, *An American Requiem*, 45; Kriegel, "Uncle Tom and Tiny Tim," 420.

23. Lindell and Lindell, *Oh God, Help Me!*, 45; Larry Alexander, as told to Adam Barnett, *The Iron Cradle* (New York: Thomas Y. Crowell Co., 1954), 234; Sternburg and Sternburg, *View from the Seesaw*, 77, 130.

24. Lake, *Each Day a Bonus*, 63; Black, *In the Shadow of Polio*, 137, 196, 249–51.

25. Robert C. Kammerer, "An Exploratory Psychological Study of Crippled Children," *Psychological Record* 4 (July 1940): 98; Mary Frances Gates, "A Comparative Study of Some Problems of Social and Emotional Adjustment of Crippled and Non-Crippled Girls and Boys," *Journal of Genetic Psychology* 68 (1946): 236–37; H. A. Robinson, J. E. Finesinger, and J. S. Bierman, "Psychiatric Considerations in the Adjustment of Patients with Polio-

myelitis," *New England Journal of Medicine* 254 (1956): 978; Harold M. Visotsky, David A. Hamburg, Mary E. Goss, and Binyamin Z. Lebovits, "Coping Behavior under Extreme Stress: Observations of Patients with Severe Poliomyelitis," *Archives of General Psychiatry* 5 (1961): 45.

26. Sass in Sass, *Polio's Legacy,* 96; Diane Baggett, "We Both Had Polio," in *Memories,* 10; Mary Grimley Mason, *Life Prints: A Memoir of Healing and Discovery* (New York: Feminist Press at City University of New York, 2000), 12, 32.

27. Wilma Rudolph, *Wilma* (New York: Signet, 1977), 30–35.

28. Mary P. Wilson, interviewed by Daniel J. Wilson, Allentown, PA, October 10, 1989; Kathryn Vastyshak, interviewed by Daniel J. Wilson, Allentown, PA, June 25, 2002; Gail Bias in Sass, *Polio's Legacy,* 81; Rosemary Marx in Sass, *Polio's Legacy,* 233.

29. Gradin in Sass, *Polio's Legacy,* 259–60.

30. Paul Reitmeir, interview; Warner and Kirkendall, *Bottom High to the Crowd,* 48–50.

31. Elinor Young, June 29, 1995; Judy Garrison, August 12, 1997; Tom in Cal, June 26, 1995, all e-mail to SJU Polio and Post Polio Syndrome List.

32. Dennis Lang, June 27, 1995, e-mail to SJU Polio and Post Polio Syndrome List; Leonard C. Hawkins with Milton Lomask, *The Man in the Iron Lung: The Frederick B. Snite, Jr., Story* (Garden City, NY: Doubleday & Co., 1956). On Catholic beliefs about suffering and healing, see Robert A. Orsi, " 'Mildred, Is It Fun to Be a Cripple?': The Culture of Suffering in Mid-Twentieth-Century American Catholicism," *South Atlantic Quarterly* 93 (Summer 1994): 547–90.

33. Jan Little, *If It Weren't for the Honor—I'd Rather Have Walked: Previously Untold Tales of the Journey to the ADA* (Cambridge, MA: Brookline Books, 1996), 3–5.

34. Leonard Kriegel, *The Long Walk Home* (New York: Appleton-Century, 1964), 154; Leonard Kriegel, *Falling into Life: Essays* (San Francisco: North Point Press, 1991), 57. For a discussion of masculinity and polio see, Daniel J. Wilson, "Crippled Manhood: Infantile Paralysis and the Construction of Masculinity," *Medical Humanities Review* 12 (Fall 1998): 11–28.

35. Edward Le Comte, *The Long Road Back: The Story of My Encounter with Polio* (Boston: Beacon Press, 1957), 105.

36. Irving Kenneth Zola, "The Continuing Odyssey of a Medical Sociologist," in *Socio-Medical Inquiries: Recollections, Reflections, and Reconsiderations* (Philadelphia: Temple University Press, 1983), 11.

37. Larry Fournier, *I Did It, So Can You!* (Gilbert, AZ: Pussywillow Publishing House, 1988), 5–7; Kay Brutger in Sass, *Polio's Legacy,* 73. For a discussion of eligibility criteria for NFIP aid, see David L. Sills, *The Volunteers: Means and Ends in a National Organization* (Glencoe, IL: Free Press, 1957), 132–34.

38. Le Comte, *The Long Road Back,* 106–7.

39. Tepley, "Polio Memories," 197; Richard Owen in Sass, *Polio's Legacy,* 36.

40. Mary Ann Hoffman in Sass, *Polio's Legacy,* 138; Diane Keyser in Sass, *Polio's Legacy,* 154; Mee, *A Nearly Normal Life,* 124.

41. Jim O'Meara in Sass, *Polio's Legacy*, 215; Jeraldine, e-mail to SJU Polio and Post Polio Syndrome List, April 12, 1995.

42. Lewin, *Infantile Paralysis*, 181; Joseph S. Barr, "The Management of Poliomyelitis: The Late Stage," in *Poliomyelitis: Papers and Discussion Presented at the First International Poliomyelitis Conference*, compiled and edited for the International Poliomyelitis Conference (Philadelphia: J. B. Lippincott Co., 1949), 210; Elizabeth Kenny with Martha Ostenso, *And They Shall Walk: The Life Story of Sister Elizabeth Kenny* (New York: Dodd, Mead & Co., 1943).

43. Davis, *Passage through Crisis*, 89; Leonard Kriegel, "Wheelchairs," in *Flying Solo: Reimagining Manhood, Courage, and Loss* (Boston: Beacon Press, 1998), 40.

44. Reitmeir interview; Little, *If It Weren't for the Honor*, 10–12; Robert Lovering, *Out of the Darkness: Coping with Disability* (Phoenix, AZ: Associated Rehabilitation Counseling Specialists, 1993), 65.

45. Barr, "Management of Poliomyelitis," 204; Lewin, *Infantile Paralysis*, 209; Dorothea Nudelman and David Willingham, *Healing the Blues: Drug-Free Psychotherapy for Depression* (Pacific Grove, CA: Boxwood Press, 1994), 204.

46. Barr, "Management of Poliomyelitis," 204–5, 216; Lewin, *Infantile Paralysis*, 209–322.

47. Nudelman and Willingham, *Healing the Blues*, 135.

48. Kay Brutger in Sass, *Polio's Legacy*, 72–75; Barb Johnson in Sass, *Polio's Legacy*, 87.

49. Nudelman and Willingham, *Healing the Blues*, 135–38; LGM, June 21, 1999; and David G. Henson, June 21, 1999; both e-mail to SJU Polio and Post Polio Syndrome List.

50. Barr, "Management of Poliomyelitis," 210.

51. Edmund J. Sass in Sass, *Polio's Legacy*, 97–98, 100–101; Chava Willig Levy, e-mail to SJU Polio and Post Polio Syndrome List, August 20, 1997.

52. David G. Oakley, October 19, 1998; Elinor Young, September 20, 1995; Erika Inkster, October 15, 1998; and Chava Willig Levy, August 20, 1997; all e-mail to SJU Polio and Post Polio Syndrome List; and personal reminiscence.

53. Franklin D. Roosevelt to Ruth Weinberg, December 21, 1934; Walter Weinberg to Franklin D. Roosevelt, December 19, 1934; and five undated letters from Ruth Weinberg to her parents, all in President's Personal File 50, Franklin D. Roosevelt Library.

54. Lewin, *Infantile Paralysis*, 246–51; Sass in Sass, *Polio's Legacy*, 101–2; Carole Sauer in Sass, *Polio's Legacy*, 108–9; Sharon Kimball in Sass, *Polio's Legacy*, 118.

55. Sauer in Sass, *Polio's Legacy*, 109–10.

56. Sass in Sass, *Polio's Legacy*, 102; Kimball in Sass, *Polio's Legacy*, 118–19.

57. Mee, *A Nearly Normal Life*, 174–75.

58. Warner and Kirkendall, *Bottom High to the Crowd*, 99–100; Mee, *A Nearly Normal Life*, 175–76.

59. Kenneth Kingery, *As I Live and Breathe* (New York: Grosset & Dunlop, 1966), 104.

60. Kingery, *As I Live and Breathe*, 87; Sternburg and Sternburg, *View from the Seesaw*, 64–65; Black, *In the Shadow of Polio*, 149.

61. Roger Winter, with Kenneth F. Hall, *Point after Touchdown* (Anderson, IN: Warner Press, 1964), 58–59; Arnold R. Beisser, *Flying without Wings: Personal Reflections on Being Disabled* (New York: Doubleday, 1989), 60–61; Sternburg and Sternburg, *View from the Seesaw,* 75; Larry Alexander, as told to Adam Barnett, *The Iron Cradle* (New York: Thomas Y. Crowell, 1954), 185; Kingery, *As I Live and Breathe,* 102–5; Mark O'Brien, with Gillian Kendall, *How I Became a Human Being: A Disabled Man's Quest for Independence* (Madison: University of Wisconsin Press, 2003), 30, 31–65; Regina Woods, *Tales from Inside the Iron Lung (And How I Got Out of It)* (Philadelphia: University of Pennsylvania Press, 1994), 9–10, 42–43; Luther Robinson, *We Made Peace with Polio* (Nashville, TN: Broadman Press, 1960), 154–55, 159; Marilyn Rogers in Sass, *Polio's Legacy,* 57; Martha Mason, *Breath, Life in the Rhythm of an Iron Lung: A Memoir* (Asheboro, NC: Down Home Press, 2003), 183–85; and Black, *In the Shadow of Polio,* 191–210, 238.

62. O'Brien, *How I Became a Human Being,* 30–32, 109–78; Black, *In the Shadow of Polio,* 191–210, 238.

63. Sternburg and Sternburg, *View from the Seesaw,* 120–21, 130; Alexander, *The Iron Cradle,* 239; Black, *In the Shadow of Polio,* 205–6.

64. Black, *In the Shadow of Polio,* 179, 184.

65. Harold M. Visotsky, David A. Hamburg, Mary E. Goss, and Binyamin Z. Lebovits, "Coping Behavior under Extreme Stress: Observations of Patients with Severe Poliomyelitis," *Archives of General Psychiatry* 5 (November 1961): 49, 51.

66. Woods, *Tales from Inside the Iron Lung,* 59–63.

67. Sternburg and Sternburg, *View from the Seesaw,* 117–20, 125–30.

68. Daniel J. Wilson, "Covenants of Work and Grace: Themes of Recovery and Redemption in Polio Narratives," *Literature and Medicine* 13 (Spring 1994): 24; Woods, *Tales from Inside the Iron Lung,* 98; Sternburg and Sternburg, *View from the Seesaw,* 182–83, 210.

69. Beisser, *Flying without Wings,* 119, 126, 131, 169.

70. Woods, *Tales from Inside the Iron Lung,* 67; Black, *In the Shadow of Polio,* 184–85, 245–46.

CHAPTER SEVEN

1. Fred Davis, *Passage through Crisis: Polio Victims and Their Families* (Indianapolis: Bobbs-Merrill Co., 1963; reprint, with a new forward by Fred Davis, New Brunswick, NJ: Transaction Publishers, 1991), 132–33; Ellen Whelan Coughlin, "Some Parental Attitudes toward Handicapped Children," *Child* 6 (1941): 45; Fay S. Copellman, "Follow-up of One Hundred Children with Poliomyelitis," *Family* 25 (1944): 293; and Robert C. Kammerer, "An Exploratory Psychological Study of Crippled Children," *Psychological Record* 4 (1940): 93.

2. Kammerer, "An Exploratory Psychological Study," 93; Davis, *Passage through Crisis,* 163; Coughlin, "Some Parental Attitudes," 41–42; and Roger G. Barker, in collaboration

with Beatrice A. Wright, Lee Meyerson, and Mollie R. Gonick, *Adjustment to Physical Handicap and Illness: A Survey of the Social Psychology of Physique and Disability* (New York: Social Science Research Council, 1953), 67.

3. Ken W. Purdy, " . . . The Rest of Me Is Alive," *McCall's* 81 (October 1953): 71; Dorothea Nudelman and David Willingham, *Healing the Blues: Drug-Free Psychotherapy for Depression* (Pacific Grove, CA: Boxwood Press, 1994), 209–10; Stanley L. Lipshultz, "Tough Love in the 50s, Mainstreaming and Support Groups," in Lauro S. Halstead and Naomi Naierman, *Managing Post-Polio: A Guide to Living Well with Post-Polio Syndrome* (Washington, DC: NRH Press, 1998), 212; and Gail Bias in *Polio's Legacy: An Oral History*, ed. Edmund J. Sass, with George Gottfried and Anthony Sorem (Lanham, MD: University Press of America, 1996), 82–83.

4. Charles L. Mee, *A Nearly Normal Life: A Memoir* (Boston: Little, Brown and Co., 1999), 122; Richard L. Bruno and Nancy M. Frick, "The Psychology of Polio as Prelude to Post-Polio Sequelae: Behavior Modification and Psychotherapy," *Orthopedics* 14 (November 1991): 1187–88.

5. Don Kirkendall and Mary Phraner Warren, *Bottom High to the Crowd* (New York: Walker and Co., 1973), 15, 68; Kay Brutger in Sass, *Polio's Legacy*, 73.

6. Marilyn Rogers in *A Paralyzing Fear: The Triumph over Polio in America*, ed. Nina Gilden Seavey, Jane S. Smith, and Paul Wagner (New York: TV Books, 1998), 31; Mark O'Brien with Gillian Kendall, *How I Became a Human Being* (Madison: University of Wisconsin Press, 2003), 33; Regina Woods, *Tales from Inside the Iron Lung (And How I got Out of It)* (Philadelphia: University of Pennsylvania Press, 1994), 10.

7. Harold M. Visotsky, David A. Hamburg, Mary E. Goss, and Binyamin Z. Lebovits, "Coping Behavior under Extreme Stress: Observations of Patients with Severe Poliomyelitis," *Archives of General Psychiatry* 5 (1961): 45–48.

8. Kenneth Kingery, *As I Live and Breathe* (New York: Grosset & Dunlap, 1966), 104, 110, 192.

9. Roger Winter, with Kenneth F. Hall, *Point after Touchdown* (Anderson, IN: Warner Press, 1964), 61, 64.

10. Louis and Dorothy Sternburg, with Monica Dickens, *View from the Seesaw* (New York: Dodd, Mead, and Co., 1986), 75–77, 92.

11. Kathryn Black, *In the Shadow of Polio: A Personal and Social History* (Reading, MA: Addison-Wesley, 1996), 192, 249–50.

12. Sternburg and Sternburg, *View from the Seesaw*, 84, 102–4, 162, 107–8, 167–69.

13. Black, *In the Shadow of Polio*, 205–6, 246.

14. Fred Davis, "Deviance Disavowal: The Management of Strained Interaction by the Visibly Handicapped," *Social Problems* 9 (Fall 1961): 121–22, 125–31.

15. Tobin Siebers, "My Withered Limb," in "Disability, Art, and Culture (Part One)," ed. Susan Crutchfield and Marcy Epstein, special issue, *Michigan Quarterly Review* 37 (Spring 1998): 199–200.

16. Jan Little, *If It Weren't for the Honor—I'd Rather Have Walked* (Cambridge, MA: Brookline Books, 1996), 10; Arnold R. Beisser, *Flying without Wings: Personal Reflections on Loss, Disability, and Healing* (New York: Bantam Books, 1988), 52; Hugh Gregory Gallagher, *Black Bird Fly Away: Disabled in an Able-Bodied World* (Arlington, VA: Vandamere Press, 1998), 65; Sternburg and Sternburg, *View from the Seesaw*, 67, 79, 98, 115, 117.

17. Nudelman and Willingham, *Healing the Blues*, 159; Irving Kenneth Zola, "The Continuing Odyssey of a Medical Sociologist," in *Socio-Medical Inquiries: Recollections, Reflections, and Reconsiderations* (Philadelphia: Temple University Press, 1983), 10; Irving Kenneth Zola, *Missing Pieces: A Chronicle of Living with a Disability* (Philadelphia: Temple University Press, 1982), 234.

18. Rogers in Seavey, Smith, and Wagner, *A Paralyzing Fear*, 31–32; Mark O'Brien in Seavey, Smith, and Wagner, *A Paralyzing Fear*, 110; O'Brien, *How I Became a Human Being*, 37, 41.

19. Little, *If It Weren't for the Honor*, 12–14.

20. Clara Yelder in Seavey, Smith, and Wagner, *A Paralyzing Fear*, 156.

21. Kathryn Vastyshak, interview with Daniel J. Wilson, June 25, 2002, Allentown, PA; Paul Reitmeir, interview with Daniel J. Wilson, August 2, 2002, Bethlehem, PA.

22. Brutger in Sass, *Polio's Legacy*, 75; Ray K. Gullickson in Sass, *Polio's Legacy*, 49; Zola, *Missing Pieces*, 234; David Kangas in Sass, *Polio's Legacy*, 65.

23. Richard Owen in Seavey, Smith, and Wagner, *A Paralyzing Fear*, 241; Bias in Sass, *Polio's Legacy*, 81; Nudelman and Willingham, *Healing the Blues*, 11; Edmund Sass in Sass, *Polio's Legacy*, 97–98.

24. Jennifer Williams in Sass, *Polio's Legacy*, 242; Bias in Sass, *Polio's Legacy*, 81–82; Siebers, "My Withered Limb," 197.

25. Williams in Sass, *Polio's Legacy*, 242; Vivian Johnson Reagin, "Before the War," in *Memories: A Tribute to Polio Survivors* (Atlanta, GA: Atlanta Post-Polio Association, 1997), 21; Sass in Sass, *Polio's Legacy*, 98.

26. Joyce Ann Tepley, "Polio Memories from the Class of 1952 and Maturing with Polio," in Halstead and Naierman, *Managing Post-Polio*, 196–97.

27. Grace Audet in Sass, *Polio's Legacy*, 252; Williams in Sass, *Polio's Legacy*, 243; Sass in Sass, *Polio's Legacy*, 103; Siebers, "My Withered Limb," 201.

28. Millie Malone, October 19, 1998; and Bob Sellars, March 19, 1999; both e-mail to SJU Polio and Post Polio Syndrome List.

29. Little, *If It Weren't for the Honor*, 10, 14; Arvid Schwartz in Sass, *Polio's Legacy*, 150; Arvid Schwartz in Seavey, Smith, and Wagner, *A Paralyzing Fear*, 264; Mary Ann Hoffman in Sass, *Polio's Legacy*, 140.

30. Jim Doherty, "Chicago Changes," in *Memories*, 39–40.

31. Little, *If It Weren't for the Honor*, 14; Williams in Sass, *Polio's Legacy*, 242; Wanda Peterson, e-mail to SJU Polio and Post Polio Syndrome List, October 5, 1996.

32. Schwartz in Sass, *Polio's Legacy*, 150; Bias in Sass, *Polio's Legacy*, 82; James Frederick Berry in Sass, *Polio's Legacy*, 228.

33. Hoffman in Sass, *Polio's Legacy,* 140; Zola, *Missing Pieces,* 234; Mee, *A Nearly Normal Life,* 168–69.

34. Doherty, "Chicago Changes," 40; Bill Van Cleve in Sass, *Polio's Legacy,* 188.

35. Little, *If It Weren't for the Honor,* 16–17, 20.

36. Joseph P. Shapiro, *No Pity: People with Disabilities Forging a New Civil Rights Movement* (New York: Times Books, 1993), 44–45; Paul K. Longmore and Lauri Umansky, "Introduction: Disability History: From the Margins to the Mainstream," in *The New Disability History: American Perspectives,* ed. Paul K. Longmore and Lauri Umansky (New York: New York University Press, 2001), 7.

37. Richard Owen in Sass, *Polio's Legacy,* 35; David Kangas in Sass, *Polio's Legacy,* 66–67.

38. Little, *If It Weren't for the Honor,* 20–22, 31, 34.

39. Shapiro, *No Pity,* 45–51.

40. Shapiro, *No Pity,* 51–54; see also, Doris Zames Fleischer and Frieda Zames, *The Disability Rights Movement: From Charity to Confrontation* (Philadelphia: Temple University Press, 2001), 37–43.

41. Brenda Bell, "The Man in the Iron Lung," *Los Angeles Times Magazine* (July 31, 1994): 14, 35; see also, O'Brien, *How I Became a Human Being,* chapters 8–11.

42. Charles LeRoy Lowman and Morton A. Seidenfeld, "A Preliminary Report of the Psychosocial Effects of Poliomyelitis," *Journal of Consulting Psychology* 11 (1947): 32–33; and Margaret L. Campbell, " 'Aging with Polio—101': Risk Factors and Protective Influences?" (paper presented at the Seventh International Post-Polio and Independent Living Conference, May 29, 1997), 3.

43. Ann Walters and Jim Marugg, *Beyond Endurance* (New York: Harper & Brothers Publishers, 1954), 159–60, 165–66; Eleanor Chappell, *On the Shoulders of Giants: The Bea Wright Story* (Philadelphia: Chilton Co., 1960), 26, 45, 49; Edward Le Comte, *The Long Road Back: The Story of My Encounter with Polio* (Boston: Beacon Press, 1957), 5–6, 143; William Foote Whyte, *Participant Observer: An Autobiography* (Ithaca, NY: ILR Press, 1994), 131, 141.

44. John Earl Lindell and Ethel Brooks Lindell, *Oh God, Help Me! For I Cannot Help Myself: A True Story of Faith in the Life of a Polio Survivor* (Tempe, AZ: John Earl Lindell, 1988), 38–39, 48–49.

45. Kirkendall and Warren, *Bottom High to the Crowd,* 135, 208–10; Doherty, "Chicago Changes," 40–41.

46. Schwartz in Sass, *Polio's Legacy,* 151–52.

47. Ibid.; Kangas in Sass, *Polio's Legacy,* 67–69.

48. Beisser, *Flying without Wings,* 51, 57–59, 61, 68–69.

49. Daniel J. Wilson, "Crippled Manhood: Infantile Paralysis and the Construction of Masculinity," *Medical Humanities Review* 12 (Fall 1998): 21–22.

50. Winter, *Point after Touchdown,* 58, 61–63; Sternburg and Sternburg, *View from the Seesaw,* 92–93, 95, 191, 199–203.

51. Sylvia Gray, "Mississippi Memories," *Memories,* 24; Harriet Ford Griswold, "I Had Polio," *Collier's* 123 (January 29, 1949): 56.

52. Louise Lake, *Each Day a Bonus: Twenty-five Courageous Years in a Wheelchair* (Salt Lake City: Deseret Book Co., 1971), 43–44, 55, 63–64.

53. Jane Boyle Needham, as told to Rosemary Taylor, *Looking Up* (New York: G. P. Putnam's Sons, 1959), 12–13, 68–69, 76–77, 189.

CHAPTER EIGHT

1. Not all polio survivors were kept out of the military. In 1943, Charles Stone talked his way into the army air corps in spite of having one leg that was smaller than the other. He retired from the air force as a lieutenant colonel in 1968. Charles A. Stone in *Polio's Legacy: An Oral History*, ed. Edmund J. Sass with George Gottfried and Anthony Sorem (Lanham, MD: University Press of America, 1996), 176–83; Jack Dominik in Sass, *Polio's Legacy,* 174–75; Bill Van Cleve in Sass, *Polio's Legacy,* 186–87; Arnold Beisser, *Flying without Wings: Personal Reflections on Loss, Disability, and Healing* (New York: Bantam Books, 1989), 4. Polio also kept Ray Gullickson out of the Korean Conflict; Ray K. Gullickson in Sass, *Polio's Legacy,* 49.

2. Richard Owen in Sass, *Polio's Legacy,* 33–34; Dale Jacobson in Sass, *Polio's Legacy,* 211–12; Mary Ann Hoffman in Sass, *Polio's Legacy,* 140–42.

3. Jim Doherty, "Chicago Changes," in *Memories: A Tribute to Polio Survivors* (Atlanta, GA: Atlanta Post-Polio Association, 1997), 40; Van Cleve in Sass, *Polio's Legacy,* 187–88; Joseph P. Shapiro, *No Pity: People with Disabilities Forging a New Civil Rights Movement* (New York: Times Books, 1993), 44–45, 47, 53–54. I should note that the Wisconsin Division of Vocational Rehabilitation paid my undergraduate tuition.

4. Shapiro, *No Pity,* 27–29.

5. Shapiro, *No Pity,* 56–57; Cass Irvin, *Home Bound: Growing Up with a Disability in America* (Philadelphia: Temple University Press, 2004), 81, 99; Robert Gurney in Sass, *Polio's Legacy,* 28–29.

6. Naomi Wernick, "Role Models: Paul Longmore," *Exceptional Parent* 26 (October 1996): 25–26; Paul Longmore, *Why I Burned My Book and Other Essays* (Philadelphia: Temple University Press, 2003), 232–37; Shapiro, *No Pity,* 29.

7. Kay Brutger in Sass, *Polio's Legacy,* 77; Edmund Sass in Sass, *Polio's Legacy,* 105; Len Jordan in Sass, *Polio's Legacy,* 131; Mary Ann Hoffman in Sass, *Polio's Legacy,* 142; Pat Zahler in Sass, *Polio's Legacy,* 224.

8. Amy Fairchild, "The Polio Narratives: Dialogues with FDR," *Bulletin of the History of Medicine* 75 (2001): 493; Dorothea Nudelman and David Willingham, *Healing the Blues: Drug-Free Psychotherapy for Depression* (Pacific Grove, CA: Boxwood Press, 1994), 210; Leonard Kriegel, *The Long Walk Home* (New York: Appleton-Century, 1964), 56–58; Daniel J. Wilson, "A Crippling Fear: Experiencing Polio in the Era of FDR," *Bulletin of the History of Medicine* 72 (1998): 487–94; Hugh Gregory Gallagher, *FDR's Splendid Deception,* rev. ed. (Arlington, VA: Vandamere Press, 1994), xiv.

9. Fairchild, "The Polio Narratives," 515; Hugh Gregory Gallagher, *Black Bird Fly Away: Disabled in an Able-Bodied World* (Arlington, VA: Vandamere Press, 1998), 207–9; Irving Kenneth Zola, *Missing Pieces: A Chronicle of Living with a Disability* (Philadelphia: Temple University Press, 1982), 204–5.

10. Steven Mintz and Susan Kellogg, *Domestic Revolutions: A Social History of American Family Life* (New York: Free Press, 1988), 180; Elaine Tyler May, *Homeward Bound: American Families in the Cold War Era* (New York: Basic Books, 1988), 18, 160. Margaret Campbell's survey of 120 polio survivors reported that only 11 percent had never married. ("Aging with Polio—101" [paper presented at the Seventh International Post-Polio and Independent Living Conference, St. Louis, MO, May 29, 1997], 3). Sandra S. French and G. Sam Sloss's survey of 295 polio survivors showed that only 13 percent were single ("Health and Demographic Characteristics of Polio Survivors" [A Lincolnshire Post-Polio Library Publication, April 1999], 2). And respondents to the 1990 National Post-Polio Survey reported that 11 percent were single (Richard L. Bruno and Nancy M. Frick, "The Psychology of Polio as Prelude to Post-Polio Sequelae: Behavior Modification and Psychotherapy," *Orthopedics* 14 [November 1991]: 1188).

11. Lorenzo Milam, *The Cripple Liberation Front Marching Band Blues* (San Diego: Mho & Mho Works, 1984), 116–17, 123–25, 141, 147–53, 171–86.

12. Hoffman in Sass, *Polio's Legacy*, 142; Sass in Sass, *Polio's Legacy*, 105; Jordan in Sass, *Polio's Legacy*, 131; June Radosovich in Sass, *Polio's Legacy*, 163; Millie Teders in Sass, *Polio's Legacy*, 195.

13. Arvid Schwartz in Sass, *Polio's Legacy*, 150–51.

14. Roger Winter, with Kenneth F. Hall. *Point after Touchdown* (Anderson, IN: Warner Press, 1964), 51, 56–59, 61–63; Roger Winter, *I'll Walk Tomorrow* (Anderson, IN: Warner Press, 1971), 16, 24–25.

15. Beisser, *Flying without Wings*, 54–55, 57–61; Arnold R. Beisser, *A Graceful Passage: Notes on the Freedom to Live or Die* (New York: Bantam Books, 1990), 208.

16. Louis and Dorothy Sternburg with Monica Dickens, *View from the Seesaw* (New York: Dodd, Mead and Co., 1986).

17. Ibid., 19, 23, 25–26, 82–84.

18. Ibid., 95.

19. Ibid., 130, 140, 186–87.

20. Kenneth Kingery, *As I Live and Breathe* (New York: Grosset & Dunlap, 1966), 53.

21. Ibid., 85, 97–98.

22. Ibid., 104, 112–13.

23. Ibid., 126, 147.

24. Ann L. McLaughlin, "One Couple's Journey from Paralysis to Post-Polio," in *Polio*, ed. Thomas M. Daniel and Frederick C. Robbins (Rochester, NY: University of Rochester Press, 1997), 47, 51–52, 57–58, 63–64, 66.

25. Bonnie Bonham, "Memories," in *Memories: A Tribute to Polio Survivors*, 13. ·

26. Ibid., 13–14.

27. Louise Lake, *Each Day a Bonus: Twenty-five Courageous Years in a Wheelchair* (Salt Lake City: Deseret Book Co., 1971), 49, 63.

28. Jane Boyle Needham, as told to Rosemary Taylor, *Looking Up* (New York: G. P. Putnam's Sons, 1959), 13, 15, 19, 73–74, 76–77.

29. Ibid., 84, 100–101, 12–13, 102–3, 114–15, 14.

30. Don Kirkendall and Mary Phraner Warren, *Bottom High to the Crowd* (New York: Walker and Co., 1973), 152–53, 158, 174, 176, 178–79, 189.

31. Mary Grimley Mason, *Life Prints: A Memoir of Healing and Discovery* (New York: Feminist Press at City University of New York, 2000), 82, 90–91, 97.

32. Ibid., 98, 183, 186–87, 209.

33. Regina Woods, *Tales from Inside the Iron Lung (And How I Got Out of It)* (Philadelphia: University of Pennsylvania Press, 1994), 67, 69–70.

34. Mark O'Brien, "On Seeing a Sex Surrogate," *Sun* 174 (May 1990), available at http://www.pacificnews.org/marko/sex-surrogate.html, 1–2, 4–10. A slightly different version of the essay is chapter 13 in Mark O'Brien with Gillian Kendall, *How I Became a Human Being* (Madison: University of Wisconsin Press, 2003), 213–21. See also Mark O'Brien, "Tracy Would've Been a Pretty Girl," available at http://www.pacificnews.org/marko/tracy.html; and Jane Meredith Adams, "Not Just Alive . . . But Living," *Biography* (September 1997): 60–64.

35. O'Brien, "On Seeing a Sex Surrogate," 11.

36. Gurney in Sass, *Polio's Legacy,* 29; Owen in Sass, *Polio's Legacy,* 39–40.

37. Sternburg and Sternburg, *View from the Seesaw,* 102–3, 104–5, 107–8.

38. Ibid., 162–63, 165, 166.

39. Ibid., 167, 168–69.

40. Ibid., 104.

41. Black, *In the Shadow of Polio,* 18–19, 57–58, 65.

42. Ibid., 122–23, 136, 186–89, 190.

43. Ibid., 192, 196–97, 100, 205, 238–41, 249, 250–51.

44. Ibid., 254–55.

45. Martha Mason, *Breath: Life in the Rhythm of an Iron Lung* (Asheboro, NC: Down Home Press, 2003), 205–6, 246–50, 21, 275–88.

46. Jessica Scheer and Mark L. Luborsky, "The Cultural Context of Polio Biographies," *Orthopedics* 14 (November 1991): 1177–79.

47. Lauro S. Halstead, "Introduction," in *Managing Post-Polio: A Guide to Living Well with Post-Polio Syndrome,* ed. Lauro S. Halstead and Naomi Naierman (Washington, DC: NRH Press, 1998), xi–xii; Carol J. Gill, "Overcoming Overcoming," in *Managing Post-Polio,* 208, 209.

48. Lennard Davis, *Enforcing Normalcy: Disability, Deafness, and the Body* (New York: Verso, 1995), 23, 29.

CHAPTER NINE

1. David O. Wiechers, "Late Effects of Polio: Historical Perspectives," *Birth Defects Original Article Series* 23 (1987): 1, 2–4; Naomi Rogers, *Dirt and Disease: Polio before FDR* (New Brunswick, NJ: Rutgers University Press, 1990), 1–2.

2. Wiechers, "Late Effects of Polio," 5, 6, 8.

3. For example, on the possibility that Franklin Roosevelt was experiencing the symptoms of post-polio syndrome during his last years in the White House, see Hugh Gregory Gallagher, *FDR's Splendid Deception*, rev. ed. (Arlington, VA: Vandamere Press, 1994), 189–90; Richard Thayer Goldberg, *The Making of Franklin D. Roosevelt: Triumph over Disability* (Cambridge, MA: Abt Books, 1981), 183; and John F. Ditunno, Jr., and Gerald J. Herbison, "Franklin D. Roosevelt: Diagnosis, Clinical Course, and Rehabilitation from Poliomyelitis," *American Journal of Physical Medicine and Rehabilitation* 81 (August 2002): 565.

4. The most thorough account of the medical and scientific inquiry into understanding and preventing polio is still John R. Paul, *A History of Poliomyelitis* (New Haven: Yale University Press, 1971).

5. The *Morbidity and Mortality Weekly Report* cited in *Polio Network News* 15 (Fall 1999): 3.

6. Lauro S. Halstead, "Acute Polio and Post-Polio Syndrome," in *Managing Post-Polio: A Guide to Living Well with Post-Polio Syndrome*, ed. Lauro S. Halstead and Naomi Naierman (Washington, DC: NRH Press, 1998), 11–12. Dr. Julie K. Silver discusses the risk of post-polio syndrome for survivors who had nonparalytic polio in *Post-Polio Syndrome: A Guide for Polio Survivors and Their Families* (New Haven: Yale University Press, 2001), 19, 21–22.

7. Over four hundred scientific and medical articles have been devoted to the late effects of polio since 1967. Lori J. Klein, *Post-Polio Syndrome: January 1967 through September 1989*, Current Bibliographies in Medicine (Bethesda, MD: National Library of Medicine, 1989); and search of the National Library of Medicine's online bibliography, PubMed, April 2003.

8. Tony Gould, *A Summer Plague: Polio and Its Survivors* (New Haven: Yale University Press, 1995), 205–6, 214; Gertrud Weiss, "Gini and G.I.N.I. Conferences: Pioneering Independent Living," *Polio Network News* 9 (Fall 1993): 1–2; Joan Headley, "Independent Living: The Role of Gini Laurie," *Rehabilitation Gazette* 38 (Winter 1998): 1–3; Nora Groce, *The U.S. Role in International Disability Activities: A History and a Look towards the Future* (Oakland, CA: The World Institute on Disability, The World Rehabilitation Fund, and Rehabilitation International, 1992), 150–52. In June 2003, the Gazette International Networking Institute changed its name to Post-Polio Health International.

9. Silver, *Post-Polio*, 16–18; see also Lauro S. Halstead, "New Health Problems in Persons with Polio," in Halstead, *Managing Post-Polio*, 20–27.

10. Halstead, "New Health Problems," 29–33, 35–37; see also Silver, *Post-Polio*, 60–79, 103–21, 122–39.

11. Halstead, "New Health Problems," 53.

12. Tobin Siebers, "My Withered Limb," *Michigan Quarterly Review* 37 (Spring 1998):

202; William Foote Whyte, *Participant Observer: An Autobiography* (Ithaca, NY: ILR Press, 1994), 328.

13. Dorothea Nudelman and David Willingham, *Healing the Blues: Drug-Free Psychotherapy for Depression* (Pacific Grove, CA: Boxwood Press, 1994), 7–10.

14. Leonard Kriegel, *Falling into Life: Essays* (San Francisco: North Point Press, 1991), 12–15, 16, 17–18.

15. Linda Priest, "APPA: The Birth of an Organization," in *Memories: A Tribute to Polio Survivors* (Atlanta: Atlanta Post-Polio Association, 1997), 6–7.

16. Ibid., 7–8.

17. Nancy Baldwin Carter, "How I Learned to Make Peace with My Disability," in Halstead, *Managing Post-Polio,* 220–21.

18. Stanley L. Lipshultz, "Tough Love in the 50s, Mainstreaming and Support Groups," in Halstead, *Managing Post-Polio,* 213–14.

19. Wilfred Sheed, *In Love with Daylight: A Memoir of Recovery* (New York: Simon & Schuster, 1995), 50.

20. Carol J. Gill, "Overcoming Overcoming," in Halstead, *Managing Post-Polio,* 208; Carter, "How I Learned to Make Peace with My Disability," 222.

21. Janice Johnson Gradin in *Polio's Legacy: An Oral History,* ed. Edmund J. Sass with George Gottfried and Anthony Sorem (Lanham, MD: University Press of America, 1996), 261; Jennifer Williams in Sass, *Polio's Legacy,* 245; Carter, "How I Learned to Make Peace with My Disability," 221.

22. Silver, *Post-Polio,* 16.

23. Ray Gullickson in Sass, *Polio's Legacy,* 50; Sharon Kimball in Sass, *Polio's Legacy,* 122.

24. Kimball in Sass, *Polio's Legacy,* 122–23; Gradin in Sass, *Polio's Legacy,* 261.

25. Hugh Gregory Gallagher, *Black Bird Fly Away: Disabled in an Able-Bodied World* (Arlington, VA: Vandamere Press, 1998), 216–19.

26. Leonard Kriegel, "Wheelchairs," in *Flying Solo: Reimagining Manhood, Courage, and Loss* (Boston: Beacon Press, 1998), 30–34, 38–40, 42–45: see also, Leonard Kriegel, *The Long Walk Home* (New York: Appleton-Century, 1964), 52–55, 62.

27. Nancy M. Frick and Richard L. Bruno, "Post-Polio Sequelae: Physiological and Psychological Overview," *Rehabilitation Literature* 47 (May–June 1986): 109. See also, Denise Tate et al., "Coping with the Late Effects: Differences between Depressed and Nondepressed Polio Survivors," *American Journal of Physical Medicine and Rehabilitation* 73 (February 1994): 27; and Jessica Scheer and Mark Luborsky, "The Cultural Context of Polio Biographies," *Orthopedics* 14 (November 1991): 1179.

28. Anne Carrington Gawne and Lauro S. Halstead, "Post-Polio Syndrome: Pathophysiology and Clinical Management," *Critical Reviews in Physical and Rehabilitation Medicine* 7 (1995): 180.

29. Edmund J. Sass in Sass, *Polio's Legacy,* 105; Margaret L. Campbell, "Aging with Polio—101: Risk Factors and Protective Influences?" (paper presented at the Seventh International Post-Polio and Independent Living Conference, St. Louis, MO, May 29, 1997), 6;

Sandra S. French and G. Sam Sloss, "Health and Demographic Characteristics of Polio Survivors" (Lincolnshire Post-Polio Library Publication, April 1999), 5–7, available at http://www.ott.zynet.co.uk/polio/lincolnshire/library/usa/kentuckysurvey.htm; National Post-Polio Survey (1990) cited in Richard L. Bruno and Nancy M. Frick, "The Psychology of Polio as Prelude to Post-Polio Sequelae: Behavior Modification and Psychotherapy," *Orthopedics* 14 (November 1991): 1189.

30. Gallagher, *Black Bird Fly Away*, 5, 2–3; Kriegel, *Falling into Life*, xiv–xv.

31. Nudelman and Willingham, *Healing the Blues*, 27, 229.

32. Gallagher, *Black Bird*, 95, 100, 106–10.

33. Ibid., 166–69, 177–80.

34. Klein, *Post-Polio Syndrome*; Literature search on the National Library of Medicine's electronic database, PubMed, with keyword "post polio" from January 1989 to April 2003; Gini Laurie, et al., eds., *Handbook on the Late Effects of Poliomyelitis for Physicians and Survivors* (St. Louis: Gazette International Networking Institute, 1984); Frederick M. Maynard and Joan L. Headley, *Handbook on the Late Effects of Poliomyelitis for Physicians and Survivors*, rev. ed. (St. Louis: Gazette International Networking Institute, 1999); *Guidelines for People Who Have Had Polio* (White Plains, NY: March of Dimes Birth Defects Foundation, 2001); *March of Dimes International Conference on Post-Polio Syndrome: Identifying Best Practices in Diagnosis and Care* (White Plains, NY: March of Dimes Birth Defects Foundation, 2001), 5.

35. Rosa Salter, "Post-Polio Syndrome: Many Recovered Patients Hit by Effects Long After," *Morning Call*, December 19, 1989; Jacqueline Shaheen, "New Woes for Polio Survivors," *New York Times*, June 27, 1993, sec. 13; Laura Klepacki, "Lives in Full Circle," *Newark (NJ) Star-Ledger*, September 1, 1996, sec. 6; Karen D. Brown, "Symptoms of Polio Haunt Survivors," *Philadelphia Inquirer*, April 14, 1977, sec. B; Huntly Collins, "Decades Later, a Trauma Revived," *Philadelphia Inquirer*, February 24, 1999, sec. A; Philip Elmer-Dewitt, "Reliving Polio," *Time* (March 24, 1994): 54–55; Joyce Ann Tepley, "Polio Memories from the Class of 1952 and Maturing with Polio," in Halstead, *Managing Post-Polio*, 198; and Lipshultz, "Tough Love in the 50s," 214.

36. Halstead, *Managing Post-Polio*, xii–xiii; Silver, *Post-Polio*, xiv–xv; Richard L. Bruno, *The Polio Paradox: What You Need to Know* (New York: Warner Books, 2002), 285–98.

37. Gould, *A Summer Plague*, 206; Joan Headley, "Independent Living: The Role of Gini Laurie," *Rehabilitation Gazette* 38 (Winter 1998): 1–2; Joan Headley, "Forty Years of GINI," *Rehabilitation Gazette* 38 (Winter 1998): 6.

38. Gould, *A Summer Plague*, 206; Headley, "Independent Living," 1–3; and see, for example, "Program: Eighth International Post-Polio and Independent Living Conference," St. Louis, MO, June 8–10, 2000.

39. Headley, "Independent Living," 3; Headley, "Forty Years of GINI," 6; Headley and Maynard, *Handbook on the Late Effects*, 103; Gould, *A Summer Plague*, 223; "GINI Research Fund Awards Grant of $25,000," *Polio Network News* 18 (Fall 2002): 10; "The GINI Research Fund First Award Recipient Releases Final Report," *Polio Network News* 18 (Fall 2002): 11.

40. Nancy Baldwin Carter and Ruth Wilder Bell, "Journeying Together: Post-Polio Support Groups," in Halstead, *Managing Post-Polio,* 146. The Lehigh Valley Post-Polio Support Group, where I serve on the steering committee, receives $1,000 from the local Easter Seals as well as the assistance of a liaison to help organize meetings. The group has met at Easter Seals, a local hospital, and a retirement community. Priest, "APPA: The Birth of an Organization," 7; Gould, *A Summer Plague,* 214–16.

41. Personal experience; Carter and Bell, "Journeying Together," 153–54.

42. Personal experience; Anne C. Gawne and Tom Walter, "A Guide to the Internet for Polio Survivors," in Halstead, *Managing Post-Polio,* 184–90.

43. Halstead, "Acute Polio and Post-Polio Syndrome," 11–12; Silver, *Post-Polio,* 19.

CHAPTER TEN

1. Amy L. Fairchild, "The Polio Narratives: Dialogues with FDR," *Bulletin of the History of Medicine* 75 (2001): 491–93.

Index

accommodations: lack of, 136–37, 179, 181, 182–83, 190

Affeldt, John, 51, 72, 92, 129

African Americans: excluded from Warm Springs, 75–76; outpatient therapy for, 146–47; and segregation in polio hospitals, 37, 146–47

Aldrich, Richard, 26–27

Alexander, Larry: attitude toward iron lung, 44, 92; on Christmas in the hospital, 127; financial worries of, 64; placed in iron lung, 44; on polio community, 104; psychological problems of, 94, 98–99, 104, 144; relations with wife, 144, 164

Alexander, Norma, 98–99, 163, 164

Andrews, Charles (Chuck), 33, 135

Atkins, Linda, 21

Atlanta Post-Polio Association, 236, 248

Audet, Grace, 30, 42, 57, 62, 113, 140

Baggett, Diane, 146

Barker, Edward, 140

Barr, Joseph, 154, 155, 156, 158

Beisser, Arnold: on accepting disability, 167; dependency of, 50, 209; discriminated against, 196; emotions of in iron lung, 48, 49; and family, 163; feelings of shame, 59, 179, 209; on role of "good handicapped person," 48; on hospital food, 121; on humor, 107; on lack of privacy, 59; marriage of, 208–9; and masculinity, 50; and muscle stretching, 81–82; and nurses, 49, 50–51, 111, 119; and physical therapists, 81–82; and sexual desires, 118; and work, 196, 201

Beisser, Rita, 208–9

Benbow, Margaret, 56

Berry, James, 140, 188

Bias, Gail: on dancing, 188; family's treatment of, 171; loneliness of, 105–6; on outpatient clinics, 147; in school, 183, 184, 185; on smuggled food, 122–23; and wheelchair races, 114

Bjorling, Anita, 140

Black, Kathryn, 46, 107; on impact of polio on family, 144–45, 163–64, 168, 176, 177, 223–24; on mother's polio, 98, 99, 134, 163–64, 168, 177, 223–24

Black, Virginia, 134, 144, 163–64, 168, 176, 177, 223–24

Blaine, Howard, 98

bonesetters, 148

Bonham, Bonnie, 141, 214–15

Bonham, George, 214–15

bowels, 58–59

braces, 78; attitudes toward, 151–53, 158, 184, 240; care of, 152; cost of, 151–52; decision against, 151; decision for, 150–51; ending use of, 153; functionality of, 152–53; for scoliosis, 158, 184; and walking, 153; wearing, 152–53, 183, 184

Brody, Howard, 48

Brotzman, Nancy, 142–43

Brown, Jerry, 203